Encyclopedia of Neurodegenerative Diseases: Advanced Researches

Volume VI

Encyclopedia of Neurodegenerative Diseases: Advanced Researches Volume VI

Edited by **Natalie Theresa**

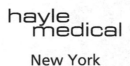

New York

Published by Hayle Medical,
30 West, 37th Street, Suite 612,
New York, NY 10018, USA
www.haylemedical.com

Encyclopedia of Neurodegenerative Diseases: Advanced Researches
Volume VI
Edited by Natalie Theresa

© 2015 Hayle Medical

International Standard Book Number: 978-1-63241-181-5 (Hardback)

Printed in the United States of America.

Contents

Preface

This book provides an extensive account of various diseases, such as Parkinson's disease, prion disease, motor neuron diseases like multiple sclerosis and spinal muscular atrophy. It also offers a profound explanation of various neurodegenerative diseases with novel theories of understanding the etiology, pathological mechanisms, drug screening methodology and new therapeutic interventions. It discusses how hormones and health food supplements influence disease progression of neurodegenerative diseases and it also deals with the collection of prion proteins in prion diseases along with discussing application of stem cells. This book is appropriate for various people: college students can utilize it as a textbook; researchers in academic institutions; pharmaceutical companies can use it as an up-to-date account of research information; health care professionals can take it as a reference book, and patients' families, relatives and friends can refer to it as a good means to understand neurodegenerative diseases.

This book is a result of research of several months to collate the most relevant data in the field.

When I was approached with the idea of this book and the proposal to edit it, I was overwhelmed. It gave me an opportunity to reach out to all those who share a common interest with me in this field. I had 3 main parameters for editing this text:

1. Accuracy – The data and information provided in this book should be up-to-date and valuable to the readers.

2. Structure – The data must be presented in a structured format for easy understanding and better grasping of the readers.

3. Universal Approach – This book not only targets students but also experts and innovators in the field, thus my aim was to present topics which are of use to all.

Thus, it took me a couple of months to finish the editing of this book.

I would like to make a special mention of my publisher who considered me worthy of this opportunity and also supported me throughout the editing process. I would also like to thank the editing team at the back-end who extended their help whenever required.

Editor

Part 1

Parkinson's Disease

Grape Secondary Metabolites – Benefits for Human Health

Teodora Dzhambazova, Violeta Kondakova,
Ivan Tsvetkov and Rossitza Batchvarova
AgroBioInstitute,
Bulgaria

1. Introduction

Grapevine is one of the ancient crops linked with human history during the evolutionary development of man. The fruits and wine have taken part in daily life and ancient ceremonies of our predecessors and currently grapevine is one of the most widely cultivated fruit crop in the world. It is consumed fresh, dry or as beverage but the most popular consumption form in the world is wine. Recent decades researchers found another reason to praise grape products: its beneficial effect on health. In the late Eighties grape and wine have been in the spotlight because of the finding of so called 'French Paradox' that linked moderate red wine consumption to a lower incidence of cardiovascular disease. As an addition, epidemiological studies demonstrated the beneficial effect of moderate wine intake on the neurodegenerative process (Marambaud et al., 2005). These findings gave boost to numerous studies of grape and wine effects on health, revealing evidences about the protective effect of grape compounds against cancer and age-related disorders, such as certain neurological diseases and metabolic disorders. Moreover, scientists proved that some compounds of grape are implicated in important biological functions in the body such as antioxidant defense system, immunological regulation and anti-inflammatory processes. The main question is what makes grape so useful and healthy?

The answer is found in the fruit and wine constituents, i.e. grape secondary metabolites. The secondary metabolites are exclusively produced by plants and represent more than 30 000 different substances that give individual properties of plant species and define them as healthy, healing or even poisonous. Grape is rich in secondary metabolites which makes this fruit crop so popular among the scientific society. Different research groups have undertaken the study of grape metabolomics and revealed the rich profile of grape and wine, including polyphenols such as resveratrol, caffeic acid, catechin, quercetin etc., all of which present highly bioactive substances. In recent years the analyses of grape composition and its effect on human health led to the conclusion that resveratrol is one of the key grape substances responsible for the preventive and therapeutic abilities of wine. Recent study of Iriti et al. (2006) discovered another key substance in grape - melatonin, which is considered for one of the most powerful antioxidants involved in various physiological functions in human body (Srinivasan et al., 2006). It is noteworthy that the health promoting effects of grape and wine are due to the secondary metabolites presented in them.

2. Resveratrol

Resveratrol is one of the polyphenol substances which are considered to have antioxidant activities and to extend life (Lagouge et al., 2006). Resveratrol is a stilbene which is produced naturally by more than 70 plant species as a defensive reaction against pathogens or under stress conditions (UV radiation). As far as resveratrol is a phytoalexin it is produced in plants during the process of a long-term resistance to a certain pathogens or abiotic stress and it is reported that in grapes resveratrol provides a resistance to fungal diseases (LeBlanc, 2006). Resveratrol is soluble in fats and exists in two isomeric forms: cis and trans. Both forms could be bound to a glucose molecule so that resveratrol also occurs naturally as glucoside in grapes which is known as piceid.

Resveratrol is naturally occurring in grapevines where it is almost exclusively synthesized in berry skins, but in muscadine grapes it is found also in seeds (LeBlanc, 2006). The content of this substance in red grapes is higher than in white ones. Total resveratrol content in 100 g red grapes varies between 0.15 mg and 0.78 mg. It is estimated that fresh grape skins contain between 50 and 100 µg resveratrol per gram wet weight (Baliga et al., 2005). The levels of resveratrol in grape are influenced by grape cultivar, its geographic origin and exposure to a fungal disease or other stress conditions. It is found that during the process of winemaking this substance could increase its content depending on fermentation time during which the wine spends in contact with the grape skins. Therefore, the content of resveratrol in white wines is considerably lower since this wine is made after removing the grape skins. In contrary red wine is fermented with the grape skins allowing the wine to absorb more quantity of resveratrol. Some reports suggest that during the winemaking process resveratrol glucosides (piceids) convert to resveratrol and thus the higher concentration of the substance in wine in comparison of that found in fresh grape juice is explained (LeBlanc, 2006).

Recently, scientists are interested in biological activity of phytoalexins and their effect on human health. According to data concerning incidences of coronary heart disease collected from World Health Organization (WHO) in the period of 80s-90s last century, it is reported that French people suffer less from this disease despite having a diet relatively rich in saturated fats and this fact is known as a French paradox (LeBlanc, 2006). Different research groups were investigating the reason for French paradox and why French people have less incidences of coronary heart disease in comparison with Americans although the fact that French consume daily in average more saturated fats (15,6% of total energy intake) than American people (11,3% of total energy intake) (Elmadfa & Kornsteiner, 2009). It has been suggested that the high consumption of red wine in France is a primary factor for the French paradox. The data suggest that wine consumption reduces coronary heart diseases much more than other alcohol beverages and therefore the presence of other wine components different from alcohol provide higher prevention of heart diseases. An increased interest in wine bioactive compounds gave a boost in research of resveratrol and its effect on human health.

2.1 Resveratrol and its cardioprotective effect

The occurrence of the French paradox boosted the researchers to analyze the effect of resveratrol on people with a known predisposition to cardiovascular heart disease. A recent study of Sacanella et al. (2007) reported that 2 glasses of 100 ml red wine per day for 4 weeks is resulting in a greater reduction of inflammatory biomarkers, cellular adhesion molecules and monocyte adhesion to endothelium, which is not found for the white wine. Resveratrol is a key constituent of red wine which has variety of activities associated with its cardioprotective effect. This assertion is well-founded with the results from Hung's research showing that synthesized and purified trans-resveratrol is effective to prevent reperfusion-induced arrhythmias and mortality in rats (Hung et al., 2000). It is considered that the protective mechanism of resveratrol is due to its activity as intracellular antioxidant, anti-inflammatory agent, and due to its ability to induce angiogenesis and expression of nitric oxide synthase (Bhat et al., 2001) as well to block low-density lipoprotein (LDL) peroxidation and increase the levels of high-density lipoprotein (HDL) (Petrovski et al., 2011). In the study conducted by Klinge et al. (2008) are analyzed the signaling pathways and molecular mechanisms by which resveratrol in concentrations compatible with oral consumption (nanomolar concentrations) is activating the protection against coronary heart diseases and is improving the function of endothelium of blood vessels. It is found that nanomolar concentration of this compound is enough to stimulate rapidly nitric oxide production in endothelial cells by increasing the interaction between estrogen receptor α-Src and calveolin-1, which is one of the components of signaling pathway of resveratrol's protective action. As far as inflammation plays a key role in atherosclerosis, resveratrol can attenuate the condition through its anti-inflammatory effect, which involves inhibition of the synthesis of pro-inflammatory compounds such as prostaglandin E_2 and interleukin-6 (Petrovski et al., 2011). Another cardioprotective mechanism of resveratrol is its ability to inhibit platelet aggregation, thus preventing formation of thrombi (Petrovski et al., 2011).

Another important side of resveratrol's heart protective effect is its participation in so called 'preconditioning' which is known to be one of the most powerful technique for promoting a cardioprotection (Das et al., 1993; Sato et al., 2000). The preconditioning includes several short cycles of reversible ischemia, each followed by another short duration of reperfusion. The process of preconditioning-mediated cardioprotection makes the heart resistant to subsequent lethal ischemic injury (Das & Maulik, 2006). Preconditioning induces the expression of some heat shock proteins and endogenous antioxidant enzymes such as superoxide dismutase and also enhances the signal transduction by activating the survival signals and inhibiting the death ones. Resent study of Das & Maulik (2006) reported that resveratrol may act as a phytopharmacological preconditioning agent by activation of signaling pathways of preconditioning. These pathways include activation of adenosine A_1 and A_3 receptors, multiple kinases, K_{ATP} mitochondrial ATP-sensitive potassium channel and nitric oxide production - all of them are important factors with crucial role in preconditioning-mediated cardioprotection (Das & Maulik, 2006; Petrovski et al., 2011). Resveratrol provides cardioprotection by improving postischemic recovery and reducing the size of myocardial infarct and cardiomyocyte apoptosis (Das & Maulik, 2006). However, the mechanisms of enhancing the heart endogenous defense are not completely clear and more studies are necessary for better understanding of these signaling pathways.

2.2 Resveratrol and its therapeutic potential in neurological disorders

In addition to the cardioprotective effect of resveratrol, recent data suggest that this phytoalexine has protective and therapeutic potential against certain neurological disorders. Neurodegenerative diseases are one of the significant challenges of medicine and involve malfunction or progressive loss of structure of neurons and even cell death. Although the profound research in this area, so far the mechanisms of diseases pathologies are poorly understood. Many of these diseases are heritable and caused by genetic mutations. Other causes of such disorders include toxins, chemicals and certain medical conditions such as alcoholism or stroke. With the research progress it has been hypothesized that the oxidative stress and damage caused by reactive oxygen species (ROS) play a major role in neurodegeneration (Pallàs et al., 2009). The oxidative stress is induced by imbalance between production and detoxification of ROS leading to damage of all cell components, including DNA, proteins, lipids and even neuronal messengers. This could lead to irreversible damage of neuron structure and function, thus contributing to the pathogenesis of neurodegeneration. Other toxic reactions that cause neurodegeneration involve inflammation and dysfunction of mitochondrial activity (Ramassamy, 2006). As far as resveratrol is reported to have a strong antioxidant and anti-inflammatory activity its beneficial properties could be used in the treatment and prevention of neurodegenerative diseases. Epidemiological studies have shown that the moderate red wine consumption is correlated with a significant reduction of Alzheimer's disease and dementia (Marambaud et al., 2005; Orgogozo et al., 1997). Furthermore, *in vivo* studies with animals demonstrate the protective effect of resveratrol in models of neurotoxicity (Virgili & Contestabile, 2000). These results gave boost of studying the molecular targets of resveratrol as a potential phytoceutical in neurological diseases. The most common neurodegenerative disorders include Alzheimer's, Parkinson's and Huntington's diseases.

2.2.1 Alzheimer's disease (AD)

AD is the most common form of dementia, which is associated with senile plaques caused by aggregation of β-amyloid peptide (βAP). It has been shown that intra- and extra-cellular βAP is responsible for the initiation of synaptic malfunctions and occurrence of AD-symptoms (Wirths et al., 2004). Yu and colleagues (2006) reported that βAPs can cause massive neuronal cell loss by inducing apoptosis. It is suggested that βAPs trigger the apoptosis by interaction with various neuronal receptors and free radical production that activate different cell-death-signalling pathways (Yuan & Yankner, 2000). Valerio et al. (2006) found that the activation of protein complex NF-kB in microglia plays a crucial role in βAP-induced neuronal cell death. This signaling pathway can be modulated and significantly reduced by inhibition of the degradation of cytoplasmatic protein IkB that acts as an inhibitor of NF-kB. That very pathway is reported to be a target of resveratrol, where the grape compound inhibits the degradation of IkB thus showing neuroprotective and therapeutic effect (Pallàs et al., 2009).

In a study Marambaud et al. (2005) investigated whether resveratrol is modulating the levels of βAPs in the neocortex and hippocampus of brains damaged from AD. The *in vitro* research reports that the βAP levels were significantly decreased in cells treated with resveratrol. Further *in vitro* experiments demonstrate that the polyphenol promotes intracellular degradation of βAPs without increasing the total protease activity (Marambaud et al., 2005).

Another possible therapeutic mechanism of resveratrol is its similarity with the effects of calorie restriction. In the survey of Pallàs et al. (2009) are discussed studies, which demonstrated that short-term calorie restriction is associated with reduction of βAP-plaques in transgenic mouse models of AD. It is suggested that the dietary regime promotes processing of the amyloid precursor protein via pathway that does not result in βAPs. This is possible when the processing is made by α-secretase cleavage instead of β- and γ-secretases. As far as resveratrol mimics the calorie restriction pathways, it can be hypothesized that it reduces the βAPs using the same pathway (Pallàs et al., 2009).

Moreover, βAPs induce apoptosis via production of reactive oxygen species, which can be scavenged by the strong anti-oxidation effect of resveratrol (Jang et al., 2007). These data prove that resveratrol stimulates the clearance of senile plaques and prevents from the neurotoxic effect of βAPs, thus having a neuroprotective effect.

Inflammation, being associated with the development of AD, is another target of resveratrol. The anti-inflammatory properties of resveratrol have a beneficial effect on prevention and treatment of neurodegenerative process.

2.2.2 Parkinson's disease (PD)

PD is another neurodegenerative disorder that is characterized by a selective death of dopamine-producing cells in the substantia nigra (Gao et al., 2002). As contributing factors to the disease, mitochondrial dysfunction, inflammation, oxidative stress and apoptosis appear to have a major role in the development and progression of PD. Recent studies showed that resveratrol has neuroprotective function against the deleterious effect of 6-hydroxydopamine (6-OHDA) in rat models of PD (Jin et al., 2008; Khan et al., 2010). The conducted trials revealed that resveratrol suppresses the expression of pro-inflammatory cytokines (TNF-α) and enzymes (COX-2), which play a key role in the inflammatory process that is related with the progression of neurodegenerative diseases. Jin et al. (2008) demonstrated that the overexpression of COX-2 and TNF-α mRNA is involved in the pathogenesis of PD and resveratrol can be used to reduce the levels of these proteins, resulting in improvement of pathological lesions in substantia nigra neurons in rat models of PD. These results confirm the beneficial effect of resveratrol in the treatment of PD.

2.2.3 Huntington's disease (HD)

HD is a neurodegenerative genetic disorder caused by a mutation of the gene coding Huntingtin protein. The mutation results in synthesis of a different form of the protein that forms aggregates with neurotoxic effect leading to degeneration of specific brain areas. The mutant protein damages mitochondria in the affected neurons, causing dysfunction and death of the cells. One of the experimental models of HD is the utilization of the neurotoxin 3-nitropropionic acid on rodents. One of the major mechanisms of toxin action is the induction of mitochondrial dysfunction via oxidative stress. Several studies reported the protection activity of resveratrol against this neurotoxin and suggested that it was its antioxidant properties that are responsible for the prevention of the functional effect of the toxin (Binienda et al., 2010; Kumar et al., 2006). Furthermore, some authors reported that the beneficial effect of resveratrol is through activation of SIRT1 (Howitz et al., 2003; Lagouge et al., 2006). However, Pallos et al. (2008), working with Drosophila model of HD, demonstrated that resveratrol has a neuroprotective effect in a dose-dependent manner but through mechanisms that are independent of Sir2 activation (the human ortholog is SIRT1).

Another research demonstrates that the phenolic constituents of red wine can inhibit the harmful effect of oxidative stress as a result of nitric oxide production (Bastianetto et al., 2000), which is neurodegenerative event with damages relevant to those occurring during chronic inflammation, cerebral ischemia or excitotoxicity. The in vitro study showed that resveratrol is capable of protecting and rescuing rat's hypothalamic cells against nitric oxide - induced toxicity (Bastianetto et al., 2000).

Hence, the results from the above mentioned studies lead to the conclusion that the red wine polyphenol constitute, resveratrol, possesses a therapeutic potential and has a beneficial effect for the prevention of age-related neurodegenerative disorders. The data about the antioxidant activities of resveratrol support the hypothesis of beneficial effects of moderate daily red wine consumption against the occurrence of neuropathological diseases of chronic or acute nature. Presented studies confirm the neuroprotective value of resveratrol and its ability to rescue neuron cells but yet the exact mechanisms and pathways of its action remain not fully revealed and further studies are needed.

2.3 Resveratrol and its longevity and anti-ageing properties

Ageing processes are determined by metabolic disorders which occur with the age increasing. Metabolic disorders are tightly linked to compromised mitochondrial functions (Petersen et al., 2003) as a result of reduced expression of genes controlling mitochondrial biogenesis in humans and animals (Lagouge et al., 2006). Numerous studies revealed that the gene PGC-1α (peroxisome proliferator-activated receptor γ co-activator) has a crucial role in mitochondrial activity (Wu et al., 1999), skeletal muscle fiber-type switching (Puigserver & Spiegelman, 2003), controlling of adaptive thermogenesis (Puigserver et al., 1998) and together with SIRT1 gene promotes the adaptation to caloric restriction (Rodgers et al., 2005). SIRT1 gene encodes a member of sirtuin family of proteins and interacts with PGC-1α, taking part in regulation of longevity, apoptosis and DNA repair (Sinclair, 2005). Recent studies showed that resveratrol significantly increases the SIRT1 activity through allosteric interaction (Howitz et al., 2003). In the *in vivo* animal studies conducted by Lagouge et al. (2006) is demonstrated that resveratrol impacts on the regulation of energy homeostasis by inducing mitochondrial activity through increasing SIRT1 activity and thus modulating PGC-1α functions. In series of experiments is demonstrated that the intake of resveratrol 200 or 400 mg/kg/day has a beneficial effect on body weight by inducing a resistance to weight gain and enhances the adaptive thermogenesis by increasing the cold tolerance (Lagouge et al., 2006). Resveratrol treatment induces mitochondrial morphological changes in muscles and brown adipose tissue such as enlarging of mitochondrial structures and increasing presence of cristae and thus the polyphenol has a beneficial influence on the energy homeostasis and reduces the weight gaining in conditions of high fat diet.

As far as resveratrol changes the morphological structure of mitochondria in muscles, this substance enhances the enzymatic activity of organelles and induces the muscle fiber-type switching resulting in increased resistance to muscle fatigue (Booth et al., 2002). All these data lead to the conclusion that resveratrol enhances mitochondrial activity resulting in suppression of ageing symptoms by increasing of fatty acid oxidation, amelioration of fat burning, maintaining of energy homeostasis and induction of muscle fatigue resistance.

Besides its anti-ageing properties, there are evidences that resveratrol works as a longevity agent. In year 2003 the team of David Sinclair reported that resveratrol increases cell survival by stimulating SIRT1-dependent deacetylation of p53 tumor suppressor (Howitz et al., 2003). Nevertheless, some studies with yeast (Kaeberlein et al., 2004) and nematode *Caenorhabditis elegans* (Guarente & Picard, 2005) questioned the involvement of sirtuin in lifespan extension leaving this assertion quite controversial (Markus & Morris, 2008). These results suggest that the wide effects of resveratrol are not always a result of sirtuin activation. In the recent review of Markus & Morris (2008) is revealed that resveratrol is also involved in sirtuin-independent pathway which is central to the control of lifespan. In this pathway the target of resveratrol is PI3K (phosphoinositide 3-kinase) which implicates the polyphenol in insulin-like signaling pathway for activating of mitochondrial biogenesis (Frojdo et al., 2007).

The reports that resveratrol has positive effect on lifespan extension in mice prompt to more extensive research of *in vivo* resveratrol's effects in mammals (Baur et al., 2006; Lagouge et al., 2006). The findings of the French (Lagouge et al., 2006) and American (Baur et al., 2006) research groups are promising for therapeutic properties of resveratrol in human metabolic disorders.

3. Melatonin

Melatonin (N-acetyl-5-methoxytryptamine) is an indoleamine, a naturally occurring compound found in animals, plants and microbes. In human body melatonin plays an important role for regulation of sleep-wake cycles, induction of immune system, sexual development and vascular tone (Iriti et al., 2006).

For a long time it was thought that melatonin is a neurohormone exclusively synthesized in vertebrates, but in recent years it was found that this substance is presented in plants, bacteria, algae, fungi and invertebrates (Iriti & Faoro 2006). Few years ago, Iriti et al. (2006) discovered melatonin in different grape cultivars, which gave a boost of series of studies concerning the presence and biosynthesis of this compound in grape and wine (Guerrero et al., 2008; Mercolini et al., 2008). Melatonin content in grape is reported to range from 5 to 96 pg/g, while in wine the content was found to vary from 50-80 pg/ml (Spanish wines) to 400-500 pg/ml (Italian wines) with higher content in red wines (Iriti et al., 2010). It was reported that the human serum concentration of melatonin significantly increases 1 hour after intake of 100 ml red wine (Guerrero et al., 2008), resulting in increased plasma antioxidant capacity. These results show that the effect of this neurohormone in humans could be modulated by moderate administration of wine. Recent studies are directed to melatonin treatment of cancer, immune disorders, cardiovascular diseases, depression, circadian rhythm sleep disorders and sexual dysfunction. Therefore, the reported presence of melatonin in grape and wine gives an additional support to the hypothesis about the beneficial health effects of moderate wine consumption.

3.1 Antioxidant properties of melatonin

Melatonin is a pervasive substance whose powerful antioxidant property is particularly directed to a protection of nuclear and mitochondrial DNA by scavenging OH, O_2^-, H_2O_2, NO and inhibition of lipid peroxidation. Reiter et al. (2003) reported melatonin to be an efficient scavenger of free radicals in mitochondria, which are a major source of reactive species in the cell. Moreover, the authors reported that melatonin suppresses the apoptotic signals originating in mitochondria, thus diminishing disorders that are related to mitochondrial dysfunction – brain damages, age-related disease, etc. It was found that melatonin is effective against brain damages caused by release of free radicals containing oxygen atom (Tütüncüler et al., 2005) and also can reduce the brain damages caused by some types of Parkinson's disease. The antioxidant effect of melatonin provides a protection from neurodegeneration as well as from the mutagenic and carcinogenic actions of free radicals and thus, melatonin contributes enhancing of longevity (Oaknin-Bendahan et al., 1995).

Other evidence concerning the strong antioxidative properties of melatonin is its positive effect for successful treatment for septic shock in newborns, which is discussed by Reiter et al. (2003). As far as the excessive free radical generation is considered to be one of the causes for sepsis the authors attributed the beneficial actions of melatonin to its antioxidant properties. Moreover, in this review the authors presented numerous evidences about the positive effect of melatonin in treatment of a variety of conditions associated with elevated oxidative stress in newborns, children and adults (Reiter et al., 2003).

So far, the obtained information from numerous studies, some of which are above mentioned, leads to the conclusion that melatonin acts on multiple ways for reduction of oxidative stress, i.e. direct scavenge of free radicals and reactive species, stimulation of antioxidative enzymes, stimulation of mitochondrial function, synergy with classic antioxidants, etc. The powerful direct and indirect antioxidant actions of melatonin, proved by *in vitro* and clinical tests, are promising for prevention and treatment of disease states that involve damage caused by free radicals.

3.2 Melatonin effects on nervous system

As far as melatonin in mammals plays a role of neurohormone, it is obviously that it is involved in various function associated with nervous system. It has a key role in regulation of circadian rhythm that coordinates sleep-wake cycle and takes part in modulation of mood and behavior. Since melatonin (exogenous and endogenous) possesses the ability to pass the blood-brain barrier it has a direct effect on brain. Moreover, it is reported that melatonin from edible plants binds to melatonin receptors in mammalian brain and exerts its biological activity (Iriti et al., 2010). Melatonin has a broad range of action, which is not limited only to the regulation of circadian rhythm. Findings from mice and rat trials have shown that melatonin receptors appear to play important role in mechanisms of learning and memory (Larson et al., 2006) as well as that melatonin facilitates short-term memory (Argyriou et al., 1998). The study conducted by Baydas and co-workers (2002) suggested that the beneficial effect of melatonin on memory and learning processes could be due to its involvement in structural remodeling of synaptic connections during these processes. In another study is demonstrated the powerful antioxidant effect of melatonin in ethanol-treated rats where melatonin prevents lipid peroxidation in brain resulting from chronic ethanol exposure (Gönenç et al., 2005).

The melatonin acts through three main mechanisms, namely receptor-mediated, protein-mediated and non-receptor-mediated. The receptor-mediated activity of melatonin involves membrane (MT_1 and MT_2) and nuclear receptors ($ROR\alpha$ and $RZR\beta$) and is responsible for the immune system and upregulation of antioxidant enzymes (Srinivasan et al., 2006). The non-receptor-madiated action of melatonin involves its antioxidant properties as a direct scavenger of reactive species.

Interestingly, melatonin secretion decreases with ageing, which was suggested to be associated with the manifestation of age-related neurodegenerative diseases (Srinivasan et al., 2006). Moreover, it is reported a significant reduction of melatonin secretion in people with dementia in comparison with nondemented controls (Papolla et al., 1997), thus, suggesting exogenous melatonin to be extensively explored as a therapeutic and preventive agent in neurodegenerative diseases.

3.2.1 Alzheimer's disease (AD)

It has been reported by many researchers that the melatonin levels are much lower in AD patients in comparison with the hormone levels detected in aged matched controls (Skene & Swaab, 2003). Another finding indicated one of the melatonin receptors (MT_2) to mediate the melatonin effects in human hippocampus – a mechanism that appear to be impaired in AD patients (Savaskan et al., 2005). The study of Savaskan et al. (2005) is the first immunohistochemical assay that identifies the exact cellular distribution of MT_2 in human hippocampus and proves the altered expression and cellular loss of this receptor in AD patients. All these data prove the importance of melatonin and its targets for the neurological processes and suggest its beneficial effect for treatment of AD.

As far as deposition of cerebral βAPs is a primary hallmark of AD, the effect of melatonin against the neurotoxic properties of βAPs is examined. It was found that melatonin prevents death of cultured neuronal cells caused by exposure to βAPs (Pappolla et al., 1997). As an addition, the oxidative stress, along with the neurotoxicity of βAPs, is proposed to play a significant role in the pathogenesis of AD lesions. Pappolla et al. (1992) first presented evidences that proof the role of oxidative damage in the development and progression of AD. These finding was confirmed by recent trial with transgenic mouse models of AD (Feng et al., 2006). Both, oxidative stress and deposition of βAPs, were found to be related with damage and severe modifications of brain lipids, proteins and DNA and to trigger apoptosis in AD brain (Feng et al., 2006). The authors summarize that these neuronal alterations in certain regions of AD brains are indicated by some pro-apoptotic markers such as increased levels of Par-4 (proapoptotic protein), elevated expression of Bax (apoptosis-effector gene) and upregulated caspases (enzymes, main executors of apoptosis). In this study the authors demonstrated that in transgenic mouse models of AD the early melatonin supplement prevents the abnormal upregulation of pro-apoptotic markers, thus inhibiting the consequential initiation of apoptotic cascade (Feng et al., 2006). However, melatonin fails in reducing βAPs-plaques and expressing antioxidant activity in old transgenic mouse models with already established AD (Quinn et al., 2005), thus limiting the therapeutic properties of exogenous melatonin only to the early stages of the disease. Nevertheless, the demonstrated neuroprotective effect of melatonin supplement in the early stage of AD (Feng et al., 2006) is promising for the prevention of AD development. Even though melatonin cannot inhibit the AD progression when it is in advanced stage, it shows to be useful in symptomatic treatment concerning sleep disturbance, sundowning etc. (Srinivasan et al., 2006).

3.2.2 Parkinson's disease (PD) and Huntington's disease (HD)

Several studies demonstrated the neuroprotective effect of melatonin in experimental models of PD. The protective effect is suggested to be complex due to the multiple targets involved in the melatonin action against oxidative stress, which is reviewed by Srinivasan (2002) and Srinivasan et al. (2005). However, some studies, summarized in the profound review of Srinivasan et al. (2006), reported about adverse effect of melatonin leading to aggravation of motor deficit in animal models of PD. The presence of such contradictory results concerning melatonin action in PD models calls for more profound studies in this area.

A large body of evidence supports the thesis that mitochondrial dysfunction and defects in brain energy metabolism trigger HD. Thus, the oxidative stress, excitotoxicity and apoptosis play crucial role in the pathogenesis of HD. Therefore, the powerful anti-oxidant property of melatonin is proposed to have beneficial effect in HD patients. The experimental animal models of the disease use neurotoxins, quinolinic acid or 3-nitropropionic acid, to mimic mitochondrial dysfunction. When the effect of melatonin is tested in both models, the results showed prevention of oxidative stress damage and cell death in the quinolinic acid-model (Southgate et al., 1998) and protection of brain structures after induced oxidative stress in 3-nitropropionic acid-models (Túnez et al., 2004). These results confirm the neuroprotective ability of melatonin against induced oxidative stress, but more experiments are needed to elucidate the melatonin effect on the other key factors of the disease - excitotoxicity and apoptosis.

Although various experimental models of AD, PD and HD prove the ability of exogenous melatonin to counteract diseases progression, the exact direct and indirect pleiotropic mechanisms of hormone actions are not completely revealed. Since central nervous system is highly susceptible to oxidative stress, it is suggested that the beneficial effect of melatonin is mostly due to its powerful antioxidant activity exerted at various levels. However, the research work in this area should be continued in order to elucidate the therapeutic potential of exogenous melatonin in neurodegenerative disorders.

All these data suggest that melatonin is an important substance associated with numerous health benefits. Recent results proved that melatonin presented in plant foods preserves its bioavailability and suggest that it may counteract numerous disease conditions, including age-related and neurological disorders, carcinogenesis, cardiovascular diseases and diabetes (Iriti et al., 2010). It is noteworthy that grape and wine appear to be a rich source of melatonin and interestingly, it is found that melatonin level in grape could be increased by agrochemical treatments, while its level in wine may be modulated during the indoleamine synthesis by yeasts during the fermentation process of winemaking (Iriti et al., 2006). The presence of melatonin in these products gives new evidence for the healthpromoting effect of grape and wine.

Grape and wine are rich in phytoceuticals but it is still little known about their beneficial effects on human health. Thus, metabolomics offers an opportunity for revealing the properties of a large number of plant secondary metabolites and for better understanding of their phytoceutical effects on humans.

4. Conclusions

So far, metabolite analyses of grape showed its rich content of secondary metabolites, which are highly beneficial for human health. This brief presenting of evidences about the beneficial effects of resveratrol and melatonin reveal only a little part of the effectiveness of grape secondary metabolites. The above reported data about very few grape secondary metabolites (resveratrol and melatonin) proved their biological potential as natural antioxidants, therapeutic agents for numerous pathological disorders and demonstrated the significance of grape and wine compounds. These natural substances showed an enormous promise for utilization as phytoceuticals for prevention and treatment of diseases (cancer, cardiovascular diseases, neurodegenerative disorders and others) which are so common for our society. However, it is still not completely clear which of the cellular mechanisms and signaling pathways are involved or activated by these phytoceuticals in the processes of disease prevention and therefore more detailed research in this area is necessary.

5. References

Argyriou, A.; Prast, H. & Philippu, A. (1998). Melatonin facilitates short-term memory. *European Journal of Pharmacology*, Vol.349, No2-3, pp. 159-162

Baliga, M.S.; Meleth, S. & Katiyar, S.K. (2005). Growth inhibitory and antimetastatic effect of green tea polyphenols on metastasis-specific mouse mammary carcinoma 4T1 cells in vitro and in vivo systems. *Clinical Cancer Research*, Vol.11, pp. 1918-1927

Bastianetto, S.; Zheng, W.-H. & Quirion, R. (2000). Neuroprotective abilities of resveratrol and other red wine constituents against oxide-related toxicity in cultured hippocampal neurons. *British Journal of Pharmacology*, Vol.131, No4, pp. 711-720

Baur, J.A.; Pearson, K.J.; Price, N.L.;Jamieson, H.A.; Lerin, C.; Karla, A.; Prabhu, V.V.; Allard, J.S.; Lopez-Lluch, G.; Lewis, K.; Pistell, P.J.; Poosala, S.; Becker, K.G.; Boss, O.; Gwinn, D.; Wang, M.; Ramaswamy, S.; Fishbein, K.W.; Spencer, R.G.; Lakatta, E.G.; Le Couteur, D.; Shaw, R.J.; Navas, P.; Puigserver, P.; Ingram, D.K.; de Cabo, R. & Sinclair, D.A. (2006). Resveratrol improves health and survival of mice on a high-calorie diet. *Nature*, Vol.444, (November 2006), pp. 337-342

Baydas, G.; Nedzvetsky, V.S.; Nerush, P.A.; Kirichenko, S.V.; Demechenko, H.M. & Reiter, R.J. (2002). A novel role for melatonin: regulation of the expression of cell adhesion molecules in the rat hippocampus and cortex. *Neuroscience Letters*, Vol.326, pp. 109-112

Bhat, K.P.; Kosmeder, J.W. & Pezzuto, J.M. (2001). Biological effects of resveratrol. *Antioxidants & Redox Signaling*, Vol.3, No6, (December 2001), pp. 1041-1064

Binienda, Z.K.; Beaudoin, M.A.; Gough, B.; Ali, S.F. & Virmani, A. (2010). Assessment of 3-nitropropionic acid-evoked peripheral neuropathy in rats: Neuroprotective effects of acetyl-L-carnitine and resveratrol. *Neuroscience Letters*, Vol.480, pp. 117-121

Booth, F.W.; Chakravarthy, M.V. & Spangenburg, E.E. (2002). Exercise and gene expression: physiological regulation of the human genome through physical activity. *The Journal of Physiology*, Vol.543, pp. 399-411

Das, D.K.; Engelman, R.M. & Kimura, Y. (1993). Molecular adaptation of cellular defenses following preconditioning of the heart by repeated ischemia. *Cardiovascular Research*, Vol.27, pp. 578-584

Das, D.K. & Maulik, N. (2006). Resveratrol in cardioprotection: A therapeutic promis of alternative medicine. *Molecular Interventions*, Vol.6, No1, pp. 36-47

Elmadfa, I. & Kornsteiner, M. (2009). Dietary Fat Intake – A Global Perspective. *Annals of Nutrition & Metabolism*, Vol. 54 (suppl 1), pp. 8-14

Feng, Z.; Qin, C.; Chang, Y. & Zhang, J.-T. (2006). Early melatonin supplementation alleviates oxidative stress in a transgenic mouse model of Alzheimer's disease. *Free Radical Biology & Medicine*, Vol. 40, pp. 101-109

Frojdo, S.; Cozzone, D.; Vidal, H. & Pirola, L. (2007). Resveratrol is a class IA phosphoinositide 3-kinase inhibitor. *Biochemical Journal*, Vol. 406, pp. 511-518

Gao, H.M.; Jiang, J.; Wilson, B.; Zhang, W.; Hong, J.S. & Liu, B. (2002). Microglial activation-mediated delayed and progressive degeneration of rat nigral dopaminergic neurons: relevance to Parkinson's disease. *Journal of Neurochemistry*, Vol. 81, No. 6, pp. 1285-1297

Gönenç, S.; Uysal, N.; Açikgöz, O.; Kayatekin, B.M.; Sönmez, A.; Kiray, M.; Aksu, İ.; Güleçer, B.; Topçu, A. & Şemin, İ. (2005). Effects of melatonin on oxydative stress and spatial memory impairment induced by acute ethanol treatment in rats. *Physiological Research*, Vol. 54, pp. 341-348

Guarente, L. & Picard, F. (2005). Calorie restriction – the SIR2 connection. *Cell*, Vol. 120, pp. 473-482

Guerrero, J.M.; Martínez-Cruz, F. & Elorza, F.L. (2008). Significant amount of melatonin in red wine: its consumption increases blood melatonin levels in humans. *Food Chemistry*, doi: 10.1016/j.foodchem.2008.02.007

Howitz, K.T.; Bitterman, K.J.; Cohen, H.Y.; Lamming, D.W.; Lavu, S.; Wood, J.G.; Zipkin, R.E.; Chung, P.; Kisielewski, A.; Zhang, L.L.; Scherer, B. & Sinclair, D.A. (2003). Small molecule activators of sirtuins extend Saccharomyces cerevisiae lifespan. *Nature*, Vol. 425, pp. 191-196

Hung, L.-M.; Chen, J.-K.; Huang, S.-S.; Lee, R.-S. & Su, M.-J. (2000). Cardioprotective effect of resveratrol, a natural antioxidant derived from grapes. *Cardiovascular Research*, Vol. 47, pp. 549-555

Iriti, M. & Faoro, F. (2006). Grape phytochemicals: a bouquet of old and new nutraceuticals for human health. *Medical Hypotheses,* Vol. 67, pp. 833-838

Iriti, M.; Rossoni, M. & Farao, F. (2006). Melatonin content in grape: myth or panacea? *Journal of the Science of Food & Agriculture,* Vol. 86, No. 10, pp. 1432-1438

Iriti, M.; Varoni, E.M. & Vitalini, S. (2010). Melatonin in traditional Mediterranean diets. Journal of Pineal Research, Vol. 49, No. 2, pp. 101-105

Jang, M.H.; Piao, X.L.; Kim, H.Y.; Cho, E.J.; Baek, S.H.; Kwon, S.W. & Park, J.H. (2007). Resveratrol oligomers from Vitis amurensis attenuate beta-amyloid-induced oxidative stress in PC12 cells. *Biological Pharmaceutical Bulletin,* Vol. 30, pp. 1130-1134

Jin, F.; Wu, Q.; Lu, Y.-F.; Gong, Q.-H. & Shi, J.-S. (2008). Neuroprotective effect of resveratrol on 6-OHDA-induced Parkinson's disease in rats. *European Journal of Pharmacology,* Vol. 600, No. 1-3, pp. 78-82

Kaeberlein, M.; Kirkland, K.T.; Fields, S. & Kennedy, B.K. (2004). Sir2-independent life span extension by calorie restriction in yeast. *PLoS Biology,* Vol. 2, No. 9, pp. 1381-1387

Khan, M.M.; Ahmad, A.; Ishrat, T.; Khan, M.B.; Hoda, M.N.; Khuwaja, G.; Raza, S.S.; Khan, A.; Javed, H.; Vaibhav, K. & Islam, F. (2010). Resveratrol attenuates 6-hydroxydopamine oxidative damage and dopamine depletion in rat model of Parkinson's disease. *Brain Research,* Vol. 1328, pp. 139-151

Klinge, C.M.; Wickramasinghe, N.S.; Ivanova, M.M. & Dougherty, S.M. (2008). Resveratrol stimulates nitric oxide production by increasing estrogen receptor and phosphorylation in human umbilical vein endothelial cells. *The FASEB Journal,* Vol. 22, pp. 2185-2197

Kumar, P.; Padi, S.S.W.; Naidu, P.S. & Kumar, A. (2006). Effect of resveratrol on 3-nitropropionic acid-induced biochemical and behavioural changes: possible neuroprotective mechanisms. *Behavioural Pharmacology,* Vol. 17, pp. 485-492

Lagouge, M.; Argmann, C.; Gerhart-Hines, Z.; Meziane, H.; Lerin, C.; Daussin, F.; Messadeg, N.; Milne, J.; Lambert, P.; Elliott, P.; Geny, B.; Laakso, M.; Puigserver, P. & Auwerx, J. (2006). Resveratrol Improves Mitochondrial Function and Protects against Metabolic Disease by Activating SIRT1 and PGC-1α. *Cell,* Vol. 127, No. 6, pp. 1109-1122

Larson, J.; Jessen, R.E.; Uz, T.; Arslan, A.D.; Kurtuncu, M.; Imbesi, M. & Manev, H. (2006). Impaired hippocampal long-term potentiation in melatonin MT$_2$ receptor-deficient mice. *Neuroscience Letters,* Vol. 393, No. 1, pp. 23-26

LeBlanc, M.R. (2006). Cultivar, Juice Extraction, Ultra Violet Irradiation and Storage Influence the Stilbene Content of Muscadine Grapes (Vitis Rotundifolia Michx.). Dissertation, Louisiana State University

Marambaud, P.; Zhao, H. & Davies, P. (2005). Resveratrol Promotes Clearance of Alzheimer's Disease Amyloid-β Peptides. *Journal of Biological Chemistry,* Vol. 280, No. 45, pp. 37377-37382

Mercolini, L.; Saracino, M.A.; Bugamelli, F.; Ferranti, A.; Malaguti, M.; Hrelia, S. & Raggi, M.A. (2008). HPLC-F analysis of melatonin and resveratrol isomers in wine using a SPE procedure. Journal of Separation Science, Vol. 31, No. 6-7, pp. 1007-1014

Markus, M. & Morris, B.J. (2008). Resveratrol in prevention and treatment of common clinical conditions of aging. *Clinical Interventions in Aging,* Vol. 3, No. 2, pp. 331-339

Oaknin-Bendahan, S.; Anis, Y.; Nir, I. & Zisapel, N. (1995). Effects of long-term administration of melatonin and a putative antagonist on the ageing rat. *NeuroReport,* Vol. 6, No. 5, pp. 785-788

Orgogozo, J.M.; Dartigues, J.F.; Lafont, S.; Letenneur, L.; Commenges, D.; Salamon, R.; Renaud, S. & Breteler, M.B. (1997). Wine consumption and dementia in the elderly:

a prospective community study in the Bordeaux area. *Revue Neurologique*, Vol. 153, No. 3, pp. 185-192

Pallàs, M.; Casadesús, G.; Smith, M.A.; Coto-Montes, A.; Pelegri, C.; Vilaplana, J. & Camins, A. (2009). Resveratrol and neurodegenerative diseases: Activation of SIRT1 as the potential pathway towards neuroprotection. *Current Neurovascular Research*, Vol. 6, pp. 70-81

Pallos, J.; Bodai, L.; Lukacsovich, T.; Purcell, J.M.; Steffan, J.S.; Thompson, L.M. & Marsh, J.L. (2008). Inhibition of specific HDACs and sirtuins suppresses pathogenesis in a Drosophila model of Huntington's disease. *Human Molecular Genetics*, Vol. 17, No. 23, pp. 3767-3775

Pappolla, M.A.; Omar, R.A.; Kim, R.S. & Robakis, N.K. (1992). Immunohistochemical evidence of oxidative stress in Alzheimer's disease. *The American Journal of Pathology*, Vol. 140, No. 3, pp. 621-628

Pappolla, M.A.; Sos, M.; Omar, R.A.; Bick, R.J.; Hickson-Bick, D.L.M.; Reiter, R.J.; Efthimiopoulos, S. & Robakis, N.K. (1997). Melatonin prevents death of neuroblastoma cells exposed to the Alzheimer amyloid peptide. The *Journal of Neuroscience*, Vol. 17, No. 5, pp. 1683-1690

Petersen, K.F.; Befroy, D.; Dufour, S.; Dziura, J.; Ariyan, C.; Rothman, D.L.; DiPietro, L.; Cline, G.W. & Shulman, G.I. (2003). Mitochondrial dysfunction in the elderly: possible role in insulin resistance. *Science*, Vol. 300, No. 5622, pp. 1140-1142

Petrovski, G.; Gurusamy, N. & Das, D.K. (2011). Resveratrol in cardiovascular health and disease. *Annals of the NY academy of sciences*, Vol. 1215, pp. 22-33

Puigserver, P. & Spiegelman, B.M. (2003). Peroxisome proliferator-activated receptor-gamma coactivator 1 alpha (PGC-1 alpha): transcriptional coactivator and metabolic regulator. *Endocrine Reviews*, Vol. 24, No. 1, pp. 78-90

Puigserver, P.; Wu, Z.; Park, C.W.; Graves, R.; Wright, M. & Spiegelman, B.M. (1998). A cold-inducible coactivator of nuclear receptors linked to adaptive thermogenesis. *Cell*, Vol. 92, No. 6, pp. 829-839

Quinn, J.; Kulhanek, D.; Nowlin, J.; Jones, R.; Pratico, D.; Rokach, J. & Stackman, R. (2005). Chronic melatonin therapy fails to alter amyloid burden or oxidative damage in old Tg2576 mice: implications for clinical trials. *Brain Research*, Vol. 1037, No. 1-2, pp. 209-213

Ramassamy, C. (2006). Emerging role of polyphenolic compounds in the treatment of neurodegenerative diseases: A review of their intracellular targets. *European Journal of Pharmacology*, Vol. 545, pp. 51-64

Reiter, R.J.; Tan, D.; Mayo, J.C.; Sainz, R.M., Leon, J. & Czarnocki, Z. (2003). Melatonin as an antioxidant: biochemical mechanisms and pathophysiological implications in humans. *Acta Biochimica Polonica*, Vol. 50, No. 4, pp. 1129-1146

Rodgers, J.T.; Lerin, C.; Haas, W.; Gygi, S.P.; Spiegelman, B.M. & Puigserver P. (2005). Nutrient control of glucose homeostasis through a complex of PGC-1alpha and SIRT1. *Nature*, Vol. 434, pp. 113-118

Sacanella, E.; Vazquez-Agell, M.; Mena, M.P.; Antúnez, E.; Fernández-Solá, J.; Nicolás, J.M.; Lamuela-Raventós, R.M.; Ros, E. & Estruch, R. (2007). Down-regulation of adhesion molecules and other inflammatory biomarkers after moderate wine consumption in healthy women: a randomized trial. *The American Journal of Clinical Nutrition*, Vol. 86, No. 5, pp. 1463-1469

Sato, M.; Cordis, G.A.; Maulik, N. & Das, D.K. (2000). SAPKs regulation of ischemic preconditioning. *American Journal of Physiology-Heart & Circulatory Physiology*, Vol. 279, No. 3, pp. H901-H907

Savaskan, E.; Ayoub, M.A.; Ravid, R.; Angeloni, D.; Fraschini, F.; Meier, F.; Eckert, A.; Müller-Spahn, F. & Jockers, R. (2005). Reduced hippocampal MT_2 melatonin receptor expression in Alzheimer's disease. *Journal of Pineal Research*, Vol. 38, pp. 10-16

Sinclair, D.A. (2005). Toward a unified theory of caloric restriction and longevity regulation. *Mechanisms of Ageing & Development*, Vol. 126, pp. 987-1002

Skene, D.J. & Swaab, D.F. (2003). Melatonin rhythmicity: effect of age and Alzheimer's disease. *Experimental Gerontology*, Vol. 38, pp. 199-206

Southgate, G.S., Daya, S. & Potgieter, B. (1998). Melatonin plays a protective role in quinolinic acid-induced neurotoxicity in the rat hippocampus. *Journal of Chemical Neuroanatomy*, Vol. 14, No. 3-4, pp. 151-156

Srinivasan, V. (2002). Melatonn oxidative stress and neurodegenerative diseases. *Indian Journal of Experimental Biology*, Vol. 40, pp. 668-679

Srinivasan, V.; Pandi-Perumal, S.R.; Cardinali, D.P.; Poeggeler, B. & Hardeland, R. (2006). Melatonin in Alzheimer's disease and other neurodegenerative disorders, In: *Behavioral and Brain Fnctions 2, doi: 10.1186/1744-9081-2-15*, 20.06.2011, Available from http://www.behavioralandbrainfunctions.com/content/2/1/15

Srinivasan, V.; Pandi-Perumal, S.R.; Maestroni, G.J.M.; Esquifino, A.I.; Hardeland, R. & Cardinali, D.P. (2005). Role of melatonin in neurodegenerative diseases. *Neurotoxicity Research*, Vol. 7, No. 4, pp. 293-318

Túnez, I.; Montilla, P.; Muñoz, M. del C. ; Feijóo, M. & Salcedo, M. (2004). Protective effect of melatonin on 3-nitropropionic acid-induced oxidative stress in synaptosomes in an animal model of Huntington's disease. *Journal of Pineal Research*, Vol. 37, No. 4, pp. 252-256

Tütüncüler, F.; Eskiocak, S.; Basaran, U.N.; Ekuklu, G.; Ayvaz, S. & Vatansever, U. (2005). The protective role of melatonin in experimental in experimental hypoxic brain damage. *Pediatrics International*, Vol. 47, No. 4, pp. 434-439

Valerio, A.; Boroni, F.; Benarese, M.; Sarnico, I.; Ghisi, V.; Bresciani, L.G.; Ferrario, M.; Borsani, G.; Spano, P. & Pizzi, M. (2006). NF-kappaB pathway: A target for preventing beta-amyloid (Abeta)-induced neuronal damage and Abeta42 production. *European Journal of Neuroscience*, Vol. 23, pp. 1711-1720

Virgili, M. & Contestabile, A. (2000). Partial neuroprotection of in vivo excitotoxic brain damage by chronic administration of the red wine antioxidant agent, trans-resveratrol in rats. *Neuroscience Letters*, Vol. 281, pp. 123-126

Wirths, O.; Multhaup, G. & Bayer, T.A. (2004). A modified beta-amyloid hypothesis: intraneuronal accumulation of the beta-amyloid peptide- the first step of a fatal cascade. *Journal of Neurochemistry*, Vol. 91, pp. 513-520

Wu, Z.; Puigserver, P.; Andersson, U.; Zhang, C.; Adelmant, G.; Mootha, V.; Troy, A.; Cinti, S.; Lowell, B.; Scarpulla, R. & Spiegelman, B.M. (1999). Mechanisms controlling mitochondrial biogenesis and respiration through the thermogenic coactivator PGC-1. *Cell*, Vol. 98, No. 1, pp. 115-124

Yu, M.-S.; Suen, K.-C.; Kwok, N.-S.; So, K.-F.; Hugon, J. & Chang R.C.-C. (2006). Beta-amyloid peptides induces neuronal apoptosis via a mechanism independent of unfolded protein responses. *Apoptosis*, Vol. 11, No. 5, pp. 687-700

Yuan, J. & Yankner, B.A. (2000). Apoptosis in the neuvous system. *Nature*, Vol. 407, pp. 802-809

2

Gut Hormones Restrict Neurodegeneration in Parkinson's Disease

Jacqueline Bayliss, Romana Stark,
Alex Reichenbach and Zane B. Andrews
Department of Physiology
Monash University
Australia

1. Introduction

Parkinson's disease is the most common neurodegenerative movement disorder and the second most common neurological disorder behind Alzheimer's disease in today's society. It is a progressive disorder that affects more than 1% of people older than 60. Cardinal features of Parkinson's disease include motor dysfunction such as rigidity, resting tremor, postural instability and bradykinesia. These debilitating symptoms manifest due to the massive loss of dopamine in the striatum, the nerve terminal region of dopamine neurons are located in the substantia nigra pars compacta (SNpc). This anatomical circuit is known as the nigrostriatal pathway and plays a critical role in fine tuning motor functions.

At present there are only a few known monogenic mutations accelerating the onset of Parkinson's disease, therefore most cases are considered sporadic and develop as a complex polygenic interaction with age and environment. Although the pathogenesis of Parkinson's disease is largely unknown, mitochondrial dysfunction, oxidative stress, intracellular protein accumulation (Lewy Bodies containing α-synuclein) and abnormal protein degradation all play a key role in disease progression. Because loss of dopamine in the striatum causes motor dysfunction in Parkinson's disease, dopamine supplementation can be used to alleviate motor symptoms but this is only a temporary solution as the efficacy diminishes with age and as the disease progresses. There are no known therapies that halt or reduce the progression of the disease, largely because the cause of Parkinson's disease remains enigmatic.

Parkinson's disease also causes symptoms in other parts of the nervous system. Constipation and gastrointestinal (GI) problems are often some of the earliest symptoms, well before the presence of dopamine dysfunction, and post mortem studies in Parkinson's disease patients identified protein accumulation in the enteric nervous system of the GI tract [1]. This 'Braak's hypothesis' suggests protein accumulation in enteric neurons spreads in a retrograde manner to the brain through the dorsal motor nucleus of the vagus and triggers Parkinson's disease. Braak observed in post mortem tissue that patients with pre-symptomatic Parkinson's disease had protein aggregation in the peripheral nervous system but not the central nervous system [1]. Protein aggregation ascended into the central nervous system and correlated with the development of motor dysfunction. This observation shows that the topographic ascending lesion pattern resembles a falling row of dominos and prompts the question; does Parkinson's disease originate outside the central nervous system?

Recent evidence supports the hypothesis that GI abnormalities, which precede central nervous system changes, trigger Parkinson's disease. For example, mice expressing mutant α-synuclein in gut enteric neurons exhibited extensive GI dysfunction followed by motor abnormalities [2]. Moreover, low doses of rotenone, a compound found in pesticides that causes Parkinson's-like conditions, produced GI disturbances and enteric neuronal α-synuclein aggregates in rats before neuronal protein aggregation [3, 4]. These studies, taken together with the early GI disturbances in humans, clearly implicate the GI system in the pathogenesis of Parkinson's disease.

The stomach and intestines comprise the GI 'digestive' system, which produces a number of hormones to aid energy metabolism, digestion and nutrient uptake into the circulation. Despite the fact that evidence suggests GI dysfunction triggers Parkinson's disease, little is known about gastrointestinal hormones in Parkinson's disease. This chapter examines how gut hormones influence the nigrostriatal dopamine system.

2. Ghrelin

Ghrelin is best known as a key modulator of energy homeostasis, with critical roles in appetite, adipocyte metabolism and glucose homeostasis [5-7]. These effects are mediated by ghrelin activating the growth hormone secretagogue receptor (GHSR)[8], a seven-transmembrane G-protein-coupled receptor [9] expressed in the brain, heart, lung, pancreas, intestine and adipose tissue [8, 10].

Pro-ghrelin mRNA is highly expressed in the stomach but is also found in the duodenum, jejunum, ileum, colon and pancreas [8]. Pro-ghrelin is acylated in the stomach by ghrelin o-acyltransferase (GOAT) with a medium-chain fatty acid (usually n-octanoic acid) added to serine-3 [11, 12]. Once ghrelin is acylated, it is transported to the golgi apparatus where it is cleaved to form 28 amino-acid mature ghrelin [13]. Both acyl and des-acyl ghrelin are secreted from the stomach into the circulation via the gastric vein [14] with des-acyl ghrelin being dominant in the blood [14].

Within the brain, abundant GHSR expression is found not only in the hypothalamus, reflecting the importance in energy metabolism, but also in many regions outside the hypothalamus [15]. Indeed, the substantia nigra pars compacta (SNpc) houses significant GHSR expression and the GHSR co-localizes with tyrosine hydroxylase (TH) (a dopaminergic marker) neurons, suggesting that ghrelin may play an important functional role in this nucleus. We showed recently that ghrelin binds to dopamine neurons in the SNpc and elicits action potential firing in identified dopamine neurons [16]. Moreover ghrelin increases TH expression (an enzyme involved in dopamine biosynthesis) in the midbrain, and increased dopamine turnover in the dorsal striatum – the innervation site of nerve terminals from dopamine cells in the SNpc [16]. Ghrelin also activates neighbouring dopamine neurons in the ventral tegmental area (VTA) and increases dopamine turnover in the ventral striatum [17], also known as the nucleus accumbens – the innervation site of nerve terminals from dopamine neurons in the VTA. Thus, ghrelin regulates dopamine neuronal function in the SNpc in a manner that suggests a neuroprotective effect against dopaminergic degeneration, as seen in Parkinson's disease.

We used transgenic mice models to show that ghrelin prevents neurodegeneration in SNpc dopamine neurons. For example, using the mitochondrial toxin MPTP, which selective kills dopamine neurons in the SNpc, we demonstrated that ghrelin knockout mice displayed greater SNpc dopamine cell loss and greater dopamine loss in the striatum. GHSR knockout mice also showed a greater dopamine cell loss in the SNpc and dopamine concentration in the striatum. However, re-expression of the GHSR on dopamine neurons only, using a cre/lox method, completely prevents the greater loss of dopamine neurons in the SNpc and dopamine concentration in the striatum [17]. These results conclusively demonstrate that ghrelin signaling in the SNpc, via the GHSR, restricts SNpc dopamine cell degeneration in mouse models of Parkinson's disease.

Moreover, i.p. ghrelin injection restricts dopamine cell loss in the SNpc and dopamine loss in the striatum *in vivo* [16, 18, 19], providing proof-of-principle data that ghrelin treatment to humans may alleviate symptoms of Parkinson's disease and prevent the development/progression of Parkinson's disease. Ghrelin reduces apoptosis *in vivo* and *in vitro* and attenuates MPTP-induced caspase 3 activity by regulating Bcl-2 and Bax [18, 20]. Bcl-2 and Bax are mitochondrial apoptotic signaling molecules suggesting that ghrelin exerts an influence on mitochondrial function. Ghrelin also reduced microglial activation in the SNpc after MPTP-induced dopamine cell death [19], which participates in the pathogenesis of Parkinson's disease. A recent study shows that apoptosis in degenerating cells produces a caspase-dependent signal that activates microglia [21], therefore it remains unknown as to whether the microglial activation is a direct effect of ghrelin or an indirect effect of greater caspase-mediated apoptotic cell death. However, studies show that ghrelin reduces pro-inflammatory markers such as tumor necrosis factor-α and interleukin 1β [19], produces anti-inflammatory effects in the periphery [22-24] and in a central hemorrhage model of brain damage [25]. These studies indicate that ghrelin probably has at least some direct effect on microglial activation but also an indirect effect via caspase-mediated signaling [21]. The neuroprotective effects of ghrelin involve enhanced mitochondrial function in SNpc dopamine neurons. For example, ghrelin treatment maintains mitochondrial biogenesis in dopamine neurons after MPTP-induced degeneration [16]. Uncoupling protein-2 (UCP2) is the key mitochondrial target through which ghrelin prevents degeneration. Ghrelin injections restrict dopamine neuronal degeneration after MPTP treatment in UCP2 wild type but not UCP2 knockout mice, highlighting the critical importance of UCP2 to prevent degeneration [16]. The neuroprotective effects of ghrelin on MPTP-induced nigrostriatal dopamine dysfunction included UCP2-dependent mitochondrial respiration, suppression of ROS production and mitochondrial biogenesis [16]. The critical role of UCP2 is supported by previous studies demonstrating that UCP2 is critical for nigrostriatal dopamine function [26] and protects against MPTP-induced degeneration [27-29].

Ghrelin is a hormone that is most well studied for its role in food intake and body weight regulation [6, 7]. Within the hypothalamus ghrelin initiates food intake by activating NPY neurons in the arcuate nucleus [5]. Activation of the ghrelin receptor (GHSR) increases AMPK activity, mitochondrial biogenesis and respiration, and drives food intake [30]. Furthermore, inhibition of AMPK prevents the ability of ghrelin to increase food intake [31]. AMPK is an integrator of cellular energy status and responds to metabolic stress by promoting pathways that favor energy production (fatty acid oxidation, glucose uptake) over energy (ATP) consumption [32]. AMPK activation also promotes mitochondrial biogenesis and function in peripheral and neuronal tissues [33-36], and because of this, we hypothesized that ghrelin mediates neuroprotection in the SNpc by increasing AMPK activity. Indeed, we recently demonstrated that increasing AMPK in the brain prevents MPTP-induced neurodegeneration [37]. We used a dietary approach to chronically activate

AMPK by feeding mice a normal chow diet containing 1% guanidinopropionic acid (GPA) before examining SNpc TH neurodegeneration in a mouse model of Parkinson's disease. GPA is a creatine analogue that inhibits creatine kinase activity, reduces intracellular phosphate levels and thereby robustly increases AMPK activity [33, 38]. Further, GPA stimulates AMPK-dependent mitochondrial biogenesis [35] through increased PGC1 alpha in muscle tissue [39]. In this study we showed that orally administered GPA protects SNpc TH neurons by directly increasing AMPK activity in these neurons. We used design-based stereology to show that GPA regulates TH cell number, cell volume and mitochondrial number and morphology within SNpc TH neurons while decreasing degeneration. In particular, GPA prevented a MPTP-induced decrease of TH cell number in the SNpc and partially retained dopamine levels in the striatum. We speculate that elevated AMPK activity confers the neuroprotective effects of GPA by regulating mitochondrial biogenesis and function. Robust pAMPK staining in TH neurons with and without MPTP indicates that GPA directly enhances AMPK function in SNpc TH neurons. The ability of GPA to activate AMPK in the brain is consistent with previous reports showing that GPA increases AMPK activity in peripheral tissues, such as muscle [33, 35, 40, 41]. Because ghrelin activates AMPK in the hypothalamus to drive food intake and AMPK activity in dopamine neurons reduces degeneration [42], we hypothesize that ghrelin prevents degeneration by increasing AMPK activity in the SNpc. This hypothesis requires further experimental proof.

It is interesting to note that calorie restriction (i.e. negative energy balance) increases plasma ghrelin and calorie restriction has profound beneficial effects on lifespan, neuroprotection, cognition and mood [43-51]. Cultured cells treated with serum from calorie-restricted rats display mitochondrial biogenesis, enhanced bioenergetic capacity and reduced ROS production [52]. These results suggest that the effects of calorie restriction are mediated by a humeral factor affecting mitochondrial metabolism. Indeed, ghrelin levels are increased during calorie restriction in mice, rats and humans [53-57] and ghrelin improved mitochondrial function by regulating ROS, respiration [16, 30], enzyme activity [58] and gene expression [59]. Therefore, ghrelin may underpin many of the enhanced neuronal functions during calorie restriction including neuroprotection [60]. While this hypothesis still needs experimental proof, recent studies support this concept. For example, calorie restriction did not produce a normal anti-anxiety effect in GHSR knockout mice [56] and GOAT knockout mice, which have no acyl ghrelin, were unable to maintain blood glucose levels during calorie restriction. These results show that ghrelin mediates anti-anxiety and glucose homeostasis in calorie restricted mice. Based on this, we hypothesized that ghrelin will mediate the neuroprotective effects of calorie restriction in MPTP mouse models of Parkinson's disease.

In contrast to calorie restriction, plasma ghrelin levels are decreased in obesity in mice and humans [61-63]. Recent evidence also associates obesity with Parkinson's disease in humans [64-66] and obesity is predicted to decrease lifespan in the future [67]. Indeed, obesity increases the susceptibility to MPTP-induced nigrostriatal dysfunction [68], causes reactive gliosis and exacerbates chemically-induced neurodegeneration [69]. Given that ghrelin protects against degeneration in mouse models of Parkinson's disease, we hypothesized that lower ghrelin levels in obesity contribute to dopamine degeneration in the SNpc [16].

The animal studies described above highlight the promise for ghrelin therapy in human Parkinson's disease patients. In Parkinson's disease, patients show delayed gastric emptying and other gastrointestinal symptoms [70, 71], which may be related to disturbed ghrelin secretion in Parkinson's disease, as ghrelin affects gastroprotection and gut motility [72-75].

In order to determine ghrelin levels in Parkinson's disease patients, Unger et al. measured postprandial ghrelin in 20 healthy controls and 39 Parkinson's disease patients. Their results show that Parkinson's disease patients had significantly reduced postprandial acyl ghrelin levels relative to controls [76]. An additional study also showed that Parkinson's disease patients exhibit a paradoxical relationship between BMI and ghrelin concentrations. In normal people, high plasma ghrelin correlates with low BMI, however Parkinson's disease patients show that the lower the BMI, the lower the plasma ghrelin concentration [77]. These two studies clearly demonstrate that Parkinson's disease patients have impaired ghrelin secretion and highlight a potential therapeutic application for ghrelin in Parkinson's disease.

Indeed, ghrelin is a unique hormone with potentially diverse therapeutic applications in Parkinson's disease. First, ghrelin could improve gastrointestinal dysfunction in Parkinson's disease. Second, ghrelin could prevent further nigral degeneration by acting directly on dopamine cells in the SNpc. Third, because weight loss is a common symptom of Parkinson's disease, exogenous ghrelin could help maintain normal energy homeostasis by promoting appetite and weight gain. Fourth, depression is a common symptom of Parkinson's disease and ghrelin positively affects mood and reduces anxiety [56]. Fifth, Parkinson's disease patients occasionally display learning and memory deficits and ghrelin enhances learning and memory by activating synaptic plasticity in the hippocampus [78]. These observations strongly suggest ghrelin has multiple beneficial effects on Parkinson's disease patients and no predictable side effects. Future studies should test the clinical efficacy of ghrelin treatment in Parkinson's disease patients, especially since many patients experience uncontrolled weight loss and impaired appetite regulation. This highlights the therapeutic potential of ghrelin in Parkinson's disease patients to maintain appetite and energy balance, and prevent further degeneration.

3. Glucagon like peptide 1 (GLP1)

GLP1 is a hormone produced by the proglucagon gene expressed in L cells predominantly in the lower gut (distal intestine and colon) but it is also found at lower levels in the pancreas and brain. Other proglucagon products include glucagon, glicentin, glucagon like peptide 2 and oxyntomodulin. GLP1 is a well-known satiety signal that is released into the bloodstream in response to ingested nutrients, such as fats and sugars. GLP1 inhibits food intake in several species including humans and is also a promising target to restrict diabetes since it accentuates glucose-dependent insulin release, inhibits glucagon and increases pancreatic β-cell growth [79]. GLP1 acts on the GLP1R, which is expressed in the gut, pancreas, brainstem, hypothalamus, thalamus, hippocampus and vagal afferent nerves [80-82]. The presence of the GLP1R in the brain indicates that GLP1 could have effects on neuronal function. Indeed, activation of the GLP1R promotes cell survival and plasticity including enhanced learning, protection from apoptotic cell death and from oxidative insults [83-89]. In contrast, treatment with GLP1R antagonists or studies with GLP1R knockout mice all demonstrate impaired synaptic plasticity as well as impaired learning, cognition and memory [85, 87]. These observations directly suggest that GLP1 has neuroprotective effects. For example, both central and peripheral GLP1 enhances synaptic plasticity in mice [87] and the GLP1 agonist exendin-4 increases neurogenesis in the hypothalamus [90] and stimulates both neurons and glia from neural progenitor cells in vitro and in vivo [91]. Moreover exendin-4 activates human neuronal cell differentiation and proliferation [92, 93] in vitro. Clearly, the ability to increase neurogenesis implicates GLP1 as

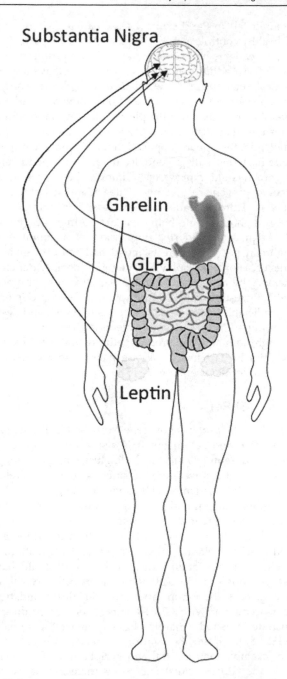

Fig. 1. Metabolic hormones directly target dopamine neurons in the substantia nigra. Ghrelin, glucagon-like peptide 1 (GLP1) and leptin receptors are all present in the substantia nigra suggesting a direct action of these hormones on dopamine neuronal function

a potential therapeutic agent that combats degeneration and facilitates regeneration in neurological disorders such as Parkinson's disease.

Recent animal studies show that GLP1 is an excellent therapeutic target to treat Parkinson's disease. For example, exendin-4 treatment for 2 weeks reduces amphetamine-induced circling behavior in 6-OHDA lesioned rats and reduced TH cell death in the SNpc [91]. The GLP1-induced neuroprotection was ascribed to neurogenesis in the subventricular zone and an increase in neural stem cells in the medial striatum. Harkavyi et al, also found similar results using two different Parkinson's disease models [94]. Exendin-4 reduced circling behavior in both 6-OHDA and lipopolysaccharide (LPS) models of Parkinson's disease. Consistent with these behavioural experiments, exendin-4 attenuated striatal dopamine loss and TH cell loss in the SNpc [94]. This study underscores the therapeutic potential of GLP1, as it showed that exendin arrests degeneration even after established nigral lesions. Li et al, detected GLP1R mRNA in both primary cortical neurons and ventral mesencephalic dopamine neurons [95]. Both GLP1 and exendin-4 prevent hypoxia and 6-OHDA-induced cell death in cells from GLP1R wild type but not GLP1R knockout mice. *In vivo*, exendin-4 protected dopamine neurons against degeneration, preserved dopamine levels and improved motor function in the MPTP mouse model of Parkinson's disease [95]. In order to characterize the neuroprotective properties of GLP1, Li et al overexpressed GLP1R in human neuroblastoma SH-SY5Y cells. Both Exendin-4 and GLP stimulated cell proliferation and cell viability by 2-fold after 24 hours and prevented hypoxia and 6-OHDA-induced cell death [93]. Exendin-4 and GLP1 ameliorated caspase 3 activity, decreased pro-apoptotic Bax and increase anti-apoptotic Bcl-2 proteins. Protein kinase A and PI3K pathways mediated the neuroprotective functions of GLP1R signaling although MAPK also played a minor role [93].

Exendin-4 has strong anti-inflammatory properties and GLP1 inhibits LPS-induced cytokine release [96, 97] and the anti-inflammatory effect of GLP1 could be mediated by promoting adipokines that target the brain to reduce neuroinflammation and improve neuroprotection [98] or by a direct effect as glia (and neurons) express the GLP1R [96]. Indeed, Kim et al, illustrated that systemic exendin-4 injection restricted the loss of dopamine neurons in the SNpc and dopamine fibers in the striatum by deactivating microglia in these regions [99]. Microglia are well described to exacerbate degeneration [21] by increasing pro-inflammatory cytokines, thus reduced microglial activation by exendin-4 in the nigrostriatal pathway suppresses degeneration. These studies highlighted above demonstrate the utility of activating GLP1R to treat Parkinson's disease. Indeed, research shows that activating GLP1R restricts degeneration not only in Parkinson's disease but also in models of Alzheimer's disease [100] and stroke [95]. The GLP1R agonist, exendin-4, provides the most attractive therapeutic potential as it has a much longer half-life than GLP1 itself (hours vs. minutes). Given that GLP1R activation with exendin-4 in animal studies provides significant neuroprotection in different models of Parkinson's disease, future studies are required to translate these findings into a clinical application. The ability of GLP1R activation to increase neurogenesis may provide long lasting protection against ongoing degeneration in Parkinson's disease patients. However, GLP1 suppresses food intake and this is an unwanted side effect in Parkinson's disease patients. Future studies need to address and circumvent these issues.

4. Leptin

Although leptin is predominantly secreted from adipose tissue and is not a gut hormone, it is pertinent to add a section on leptin and Parkinson's disease, as leptin is also an important

Figure 2

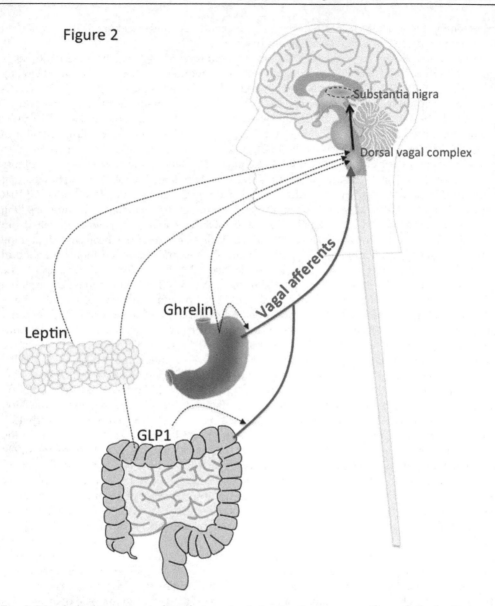

Fig. 2. Metabolic hormones indirectly target substantia nigra neurons through the brainstem. Ghrelin, glucagon-like peptide 1 and leptin receptors are present in the dorsal vagal complex. Vagal afferents from the stomach and intestines are also present in the dorsal vagal complex. Braak's hypothesis states that dopamine dysfunction is a product of retrograde degeneration from the gut (stomach/intestines), through the brainstem (dorsal vagal complex). Ghrelin and GLP1 may promote healthy gut function and thereby restrict retrograde degeneration. This circuit highlights the complicated and integrated manner in which metabolic hormones directly and indirectly regulate higher brain function

metabolic hormone. Leptin is best known for the hypothalamic regulation of energy homeostasis, including suppressing appetite and increasing energy expenditure [101]. However, significant leptin receptor expression exists outside the hypothalamus including in midbrain dopamine neurons [102] relevant to Parkinson's disease. The first indication that leptin plays a neuroprotective role came from in vitro studies. Lu et al showed that leptin prevents MPP+-induced cell death in SH-SY5Y cells through the phosphatidylinositol 3 kinase (PI3K) pathway but not the STAT3 or MAPK pathway [103]. Leptin also protects the nigrostriatal dopaminergic system from 6-hydroxydopamine (6-OHDA) induced degeneration *in vivo* [104]. 6-OHDA treatment caused a significant loss of dopamine neurons in the SNpc and dopamine concentration in the striatum that was reversed with leptin pretreatment. The 6-OHDA model offers an additional advantage over the MPTP mouse model as it allows a quantifiable measure of motor dysfunction. These studies showed that leptin decreased apomorphine-induced asymmetrical rotations contralateral to the side of 6-OHDA injections. Leptin pretreatment attenuated key apoptotic markers such as activated caspase 9 and activated caspase 3, DNA fragmentation and cytochrome C release. ERK1/2 phosphorylation mediated the anti-apoptotic effects of leptin by recruiting pCREB in cultured dopamine neurons. pCREB is an important transcription factor in dopamine neurons that induces neuroprotection by increasing BDNF expression and leptin increased BDNF in this study.

There are conflicting reports about plasma leptin concentrations in Parkinson's disease patients. Fiszer et al reported patients with weight loss had reduced plasma leptin concentrations [77] whereas Aziz et al observed no difference in the total levels of leptin or diurnal variation [105]. These results indicate that unintended weight loss in Parkinson's disease patients is unlikely to be due to abnormal serum leptin concentrations. Current human studies have only measured plasma leptin in relation to weight loss, future studies should also examine the effect on disease progression, as animal studies highlighted above suggest that leptin may have neuroprotective effects on SNpc dopamine neurons.

5. Conclusion

Gastrointestinal dysfunction, such as constipation, is a common symptom of Parkinson's disease that is observed well before any motor dysfunction caused by dopaminergic degeneration in the nigrostriatal pathway. Recent evidence suggests that Parkinson's disease may even start in the gastrointestinal tract. According to the 'Braak's' hypothesis, protein aggregation in enteric neurons spreads in a retrograde manner to the brain through the dorsal motor nucleus of the vagus and triggers Parkinson's disease [1]. In support of this theory, mutant α-synuclein in gut enteric neurons caused gastrointestinal (GI) dysfunction followed by motor abnormalities [2] and rotenone treatment, a compound found in pesticides that causes Parkinson's-like conditions, caused enteric neuronal α-synuclein accumulation and GI dysfunction in rats before neuronal protein aggregation [3, 4]. These studies, taken together with the early GI disturbances in humans, clearly implicate the GI system in the pathogenesis of Parkinson's disease. This chapter highlights recent work on two important gut hormones, ghrelin and GLP1, that also regulate nigrostriatal dopamine function. It is interesting to note that both hormones influence gut function, neuronal metabolism, appetite and peripheral energy metabolism, suggesting a novel link between neurodegeneration and energy metabolism. Future studies are required to translate promising results in animal studies into clinical therapies.

6. Acknowledgements

This work was supported by a Monash Fellowship, Monash University, Australia, an Australia Research Council Future Fellowship and NHMRC grants (NHMRC 546131, 1011274) to ZBA.

7. References

[1] Braak H, Rub U, Gai WP, Del Tredici K. Idiopathic Parkinson's disease: possible routes by which vulnerable neuronal types may be subject to neuroinvasion by an unknown pathogen. J Neural Transm. 2003 May;110(5):517-36.

[2] Kuo YM, Li Z, Jiao Y, Gaborit N, Pani AK, Orrison BM, et al. Extensive enteric nervous system abnormalities in mice transgenic for artificial chromosomes containing Parkinson disease-associated alpha-synuclein gene mutations precede central nervous system changes. Hum Mol Genet. 2010 May 1;19(9):1633-50.

[3] Drolet RE, Cannon JR, Montero L, Greenamyre JT. Chronic rotenone exposure reproduces Parkinson's disease gastrointestinal neuropathology. Neurobiol Dis. 2009 Oct;36(1):96-102.

[4] Pan-Montojo F, Anichtchik O, Dening Y, Knels L, Pursche S, Jung R, et al. Progression of Parkinson's disease pathology is reproduced by intragastric administration of rotenone in mice. PLoS One. 2010;5(1):e8762.

[5] Andrews ZB. Central mechanisms involved in the orexigenic actions of ghrelin. Peptides. 2011 May 17.

[6] Briggs DI, Andrews ZB. A Recent Update on the Role of Ghrelin in Glucose Homeostasis. Curr Diabetes Rev. 2011 May 4.

[7] Briggs DI, Andrews ZB. Metabolic status regulates ghrelin function on energy homeostasis. Neuroendocrinology. 2011;93(1):48-57.

[8] Kojima M, Hosoda H, Date Y, Nakazato M, Matsuo H, Kangawa K. Ghrelin is a growth-hormone-releasing acylated peptide from stomach. Nature. 1999 Dec 9;402(6762):656-60.

[9] Howard AD, Feighner SD, Cully DF, Arena JP, Liberator PA, Rosenblum CI, et al. A receptor in pituitary and hypothalamus that functions in growth hormone release. Science. 1996 Aug 16;273(5277):974-7.

[10] Guan XM, Yu H, Palyha OC, McKee KK, Feighner SD, Sirinathsinghji DJ, et al. Distribution of mRNA encoding the growth hormone secretagogue receptor in brain and peripheral tissues. Brain Res Mol Brain Res. 1997 Aug;48(1):23-9.

[11] Yang J, Brown MS, Liang G, Grishin NV, Goldstein JL. Identification of the acyltransferase that octanoylates ghrelin, an appetite-stimulating peptide hormone. Cell. 2008 Feb 8;132(3):387-96.

[12] Gutierrez JA, Solenberg PJ, Perkins DR, Willency JA, Knierman MD, Jin Z, et al. Ghrelin octanoylation mediated by an orphan lipid transferase. Proc Natl Acad Sci U S A. 2008 Apr 29;105(17):6320-5.

[13] Zhu X, Cao Y, Voogd K, Steiner DF. On the processing of proghrelin to ghrelin. J Biol Chem. 2006 Dec 15;281(50):38867-70.

[14] Murakami N, Hayashida T, Kuroiwa T, Nakahara K, Ida T, Mondal MS, et al. Role for central ghrelin in food intake and secretion profile of stomach ghrelin in rats. J Endocrinol. 2002 Aug;174(2):283-8.

[15] Zigman JM, Jones JE, Lee CE, Saper CB, Elmquist JK. Expression of ghrelin receptor mRNA in the rat and the mouse brain. J Comp Neurol. 2006 Jan 20;494(3):528-48.

[16] Andrews ZB, Erion D, Beiler R, Liu ZW, Abizaid A, Zigman J, et al. Ghrelin promotes and protects nigrostriatal dopamine function via a UCP2-dependent mitochondrial mechanism. J Neurosci. 2009 Nov 11;29(45):14057-65.

[17] Abizaid A, Liu ZW, Andrews ZB, Shanabrough M, Borok E, Elsworth JD, et al. Ghrelin modulates the activity and synaptic input organization of midbrain dopamine neurons while promoting appetite. J Clin Invest. 2006 Dec;116(12):3229-39.

[18] Jiang H, Li LJ, Wang J, Xie JX. Ghrelin antagonizes MPTP-induced neurotoxicity to the dopaminergic neurons in mouse substantia nigra. Exp Neurol. 2008 Aug;212(2):532-7.

[19] Moon M, Kim HG, Hwang L, Seo JH, Kim S, Hwang S, et al. Neuroprotective effect of ghrelin in the 1-methyl-4-phenyl-1,2,3,6-tetrahydropyridine mouse model of Parkinson's disease by blocking microglial activation. Neurotox Res. 2009 May;15(4):332-47.

[20] Dong J, Song N, Xie J, Jiang H. Ghrelin antagonized 1-methyl-4-phenylpyridinium (MPP(+))-induced apoptosis in MES23.5 cells. J Mol Neurosci. 2009 Feb;37(2):182-9.

[21] Burguillos MA, Deierborg T, Kavanagh E, Persson A, Hajji N, Garcia-Quintanilla A, et al. Caspase signalling controls microglia activation and neurotoxicity. Nature. 2011 Apr 21;472(7343):319-24.

[22] Huang CX, Yuan MJ, Huang H, Wu G, Liu Y, Yu SB, et al. Ghrelin inhibits post-infarct myocardial remodeling and improves cardiac function through anti-inflammation effect. Peptides. 2009 Dec;30(12):2286-91.

[23] Chow KB, Cheng CH, Wise H. Anti-inflammatory activity of ghrelin in human carotid artery cells. Inflammation. 2009 Dec;32(6):402-9.

[24] Theil MM, Miyake S, Mizuno M, Tomi C, Croxford JL, Hosoda H, et al. Suppression of experimental autoimmune encephalomyelitis by ghrelin. J Immunol. 2009 Aug 15;183(4):2859-66.

[25] Ersahin M, Toklu HZ, Erzik C, Cetinel S, Bangir D, Ogunc AV, et al. The Anti-Inflammatory and Neuroprotective Effects of Ghrelin in Subarachnoid Hemorrhage-Induced Oxidative Brain Damage in Rats. J Neurotrauma. 2010 Mar 5;27(6):1143-55.

[26] Andrews ZB, Rivera A, Elsworth JD, Roth RH, Agnati L, Gago B, et al. Uncoupling protein-2 promotes nigrostriatal dopamine neuronal function. European Journal of Neuroscience. 2006;24(1):32-6.

[27] Andrews ZB, Diano S, Horvath TL. Mitochondrial uncoupling proteins in the CNS: in support of function and survival. Nature Reviews Neuroscience. 2005;6(11):829-40.

[28] Andrews ZB, Horvath B, Barnstable CJ, Elsworth J, Yang L, Beal MF, et al. Uncoupling protein-2 is critical for nigral dopamine cell survival in a mouse model of Parkinson's disease.[erratum appears in J Neurosci. 2005 Feb 23;25(8):table of contents]. Journal of Neuroscience. 2005;25(1):184-91.

[29] Conti B, Sugama S, Lucero J, Winsky-Sommerer R, Wirz SA, Maher P, et al. Uncoupling protein 2 protects dopaminergic neurons from acute 1,2,3,6-methyl-phenyl-tetrahydropyridine toxicity. J Neurochem. 2005 Apr;93(2):493-501.

[30] Andrews ZB, Liu ZW, Walllingford N, Erion DM, Borok E, Friedman JM, et al. UCP2 mediates ghrelin's action on NPY/AgRP neurons by lowering free radicals. Nature. 2008 Jul 30;454(7206):846-51.

[31] Lopez M, Lage R, Saha AK, Perez-Tilve D, Vazquez MJ, Varela L, et al. Hypothalamic fatty acid metabolism mediates the orexigenic action of ghrelin. Cell Metab. 2008 May;7(5):389-99.

[32] Steinberg GR, Kemp BE. AMPK in Health and Disease. Physiol Rev. 2009 Jul;89(3):1025-78.

[33] Bergeron R, Ren JM, Cadman KS, Moore IK, Perret P, Pypaert M, et al. Chronic activation of AMP kinase results in NRF-1 activation and mitochondrial biogenesis. Am J Physiol Endocrinol Metab. 2001 Dec;281(6):E1340-6.

[34] Jager S, Handschin C, St-Pierre J, Spiegelman BM. AMP-activated protein kinase (AMPK) action in skeletal muscle via direct phosphorylation of PGC-1alpha. Proc Natl Acad Sci U S A. 2007 Jul 17;104(29):12017-22.

[35] Zong H, Ren JM, Young LH, Pypaert M, Mu J, Birnbaum MJ, et al. AMP kinase is required for mitochondrial biogenesis in skeletal muscle in response to chronic energy deprivation. Proc Natl Acad Sci U S A. 2002 Dec 10;99(25):15983-7.

[36] Dasgupta B, Milbrandt J. Resveratrol stimulates AMP kinase activity in neurons. Proc Natl Acad Sci U S A. 2007 Apr 24;104(17):7217-22.

[37] Horvath TL, Erion DM, Elsworth JD, Roth RH, Shulman GI, Andrews ZB. GPA protects the nigrostriatal dopamine system by enhancing mitochondrial function. Neurobiol Dis. 2011 Mar 13.

[38] Reznick RM, Shulman GI. The role of AMP-activated protein kinase in mitochondrial biogenesis. J Physiol. 2006 Jul 1;574(Pt 1):33-9.

[39] Williams DB, Sutherland LN, Bomhof MR, Basaraba SA, Thrush AB, Dyck DJ, et al. Muscle-specific differences in the response of mitochondrial proteins to beta-GPA feeding: an evaluation of potential mechanisms. Am J Physiol Endocrinol Metab. 2009 Jun;296(6):E1400-8.

[40] Reznick RM, Zong H, Li J, Morino K, Moore IK, Yu HJ, et al. Aging-associated reductions in AMP-activated protein kinase activity and mitochondrial biogenesis. Cell Metab. 2007 Feb;5(2):151-6.

[41] Chaturvedi RK, Adhihetty P, Shukla S, Hennessy T, Calingasan N, Yang L, et al. Impaired PGC-1alpha function in muscle in Huntington's disease. Hum Mol Genet. 2009 Aug 15;18(16):3048-65.

[42] Horvath TL, Diano S, Tschop M. Ghrelin in hypothalamic regulation of energy balance. Curr Top Med Chem. 2003;3(8):921-7.

[43] Colman RJ, Anderson RM, Johnson SC, Kastman EK, Kosmatka KJ, Beasley TM, et al. Caloric restriction delays disease onset and mortality in rhesus monkeys. Science. 2009 Jul 10;325(5937):201-4.

[44] Maswood N, Young J, Tilmont E, Zhang Z, Gash DM, Gerhardt GA, et al. Caloric restriction increases neurotrophic factor levels and attenuates neurochemical and behavioral deficits in a primate model of Parkinson's disease. Proc Natl Acad Sci U S A. 2004 Dec 28;101(52):18171-6.

[45] Contestabile A. Benefits of caloric restriction on brain aging and related pathological States: understanding mechanisms to devise novel therapies. Curr Med Chem. 2009;16(3):350-61.

[46] Komatsu T, Chiba T, Yamaza H, Yamashita K, Shimada A, Hoshiyama Y, et al. Manipulation of caloric content but not diet composition, attenuates the deficit in learning and memory of senescence-accelerated mouse strain P8. Exp Gerontol. 2008 Apr;43(4):339-46.

[47] Carter CS, Leeuwenburgh C, Daniels M, Foster TC. Influence of calorie restriction on measures of age-related cognitive decline: role of increased physical activity. J Gerontol A Biol Sci Med Sci. 2009 Aug;64(8):850-9.

[48] Halagappa VK, Guo Z, Pearson M, Matsuoka Y, Cutler RG, Laferla FM, et al. Intermittent fasting and caloric restriction ameliorate age-related behavioral deficits in the triple-transgenic mouse model of Alzheimer's disease. Neurobiol Dis. 2007 Apr;26(1):212-20.

[49] Abbott JD, Kent S, Levay EA, Tucker RV, Penman J, Tammer AH, et al. The effects of calorie restriction olfactory cues on conspecific anxiety-like behaviour. Behav Brain Res. 2009 Aug 12;201(2):305-10.

[50] Mantis JG, Fritz CL, Marsh J, Heinrichs SC, Seyfried TN. Improvement in motor and exploratory behavior in Rett syndrome mice with restricted ketogenic and standard diets. Epilepsy Behav. 2009 Jun;15(2):133-41.

[51] Levay EA, Govic A, Penman J, Paolini AG, Kent S. Effects of adult-onset calorie restriction on anxiety-like behavior in rats. Physiol Behav. 2007 Dec 5;92(5):889-96.

[52] Lopez-Lluch G, Hunt N, Jones B, Zhu M, Jamieson H, Hilmer S, et al. Calorie restriction induces mitochondrial biogenesis and bioenergetic efficiency. Proc Natl Acad Sci U S A. 2006 Feb 7;103(6):1768-73.

[53] Yukawa M, Cummings DE, Matthys CC, Callahan HS, Frayo RS, Spiekerman CF, et al. Effect of aging on the response of ghrelin to acute weight loss. J Am Geriatr Soc. 2006 Apr;54(4):648-53.

[54] Redman LM, Veldhuis JD, Rood J, Smith SR, Williamson D, Ravussin E. The effect of caloric restriction interventions on growth hormone secretion in nonobese men and women. Aging Cell. 2010 Feb;9(1):32-9.

[55] Barazzoni R, Zanetti M, Stebel M, Biolo G, Cattin L, Guarnieri G. Hyperleptinemia prevents increased plasma ghrelin concentration during short-term moderate caloric restriction in rats. Gastroenterology. 2003 May;124(5):1188-92.

[56] Lutter M, Sakata I, Osborne-Lawrence S, Rovinsky SA, Anderson JG, Jung S, et al. The orexigenic hormone ghrelin defends against depressive symptoms of chronic stress. Nat Neurosci. 2008 Jul;11(7):752-3.

[57] Zhao TJ, Liang G, Li RL, Xie X, Sleeman MW, Murphy AJ, et al. Ghrelin O-acyltransferase (GOAT) is essential for growth hormone-mediated survival of calorie-restricted mice. Proc Natl Acad Sci U S A. 2010 Apr 20;107(16):7467-72.

[58] Barazzoni R, Zhu X, Deboer M, Datta R, Culler MD, Zanetti M, et al. Combined effects of ghrelin and higher food intake enhance skeletal muscle mitochondrial oxidative capacity and AKT phosphorylation in rats with chronic kidney disease. Kidney Int. 2010 Jan;77(1):23-8.

[59] Barazzoni R, Bosutti A, Stebel M, Cattin MR, Roder E, Visintin L, et al. Ghrelin regulates mitochondrial-lipid metabolism gene expression and tissue fat distribution in liver and skeletal muscle. Am J Physiol Endocrinol Metab. 2005 Jan;288(1):E228-35.

[60] Andrews ZB. The extra-hypothalamic actions of ghrelin on neuronal function. Trends Neurosci. 2011 Jan;34(1):31-40.

[61] Briggs DI, Enriori PJ, Lemus MB, Cowley MA, Andrews ZB. Diet-induced obesity causes ghrelin resistance in arcuate NPY/AgRP neurons. Endocrinology. 2010;151(10):4745-55.

[62] Briggs DI, Lemus MB, Kua E, Andrews ZB. Diet-induced obesity attenuates fasting-induced hyperphagia. J Neuroendocrinol. 2011 Apr 25.

[63] Tschop M, Weyer C, Tataranni PA, Devanarayan V, Ravussin E, Heiman ML. Circulating ghrelin levels are decreased in human obesity. Diabetes. 2001 Apr;50(4):707-9.

[64] Abbott RD, Ross GW, White LR, Nelson JS, Masaki KH, Tanner CM, et al. Midlife adiposity and the future risk of Parkinson's disease. Neurology. 2002 Oct 8;59(7):1051-7.

[65] Hu G, Jousilahti P, Bidel S, Antikainen R, Tuomilehto J. Type 2 diabetes and the risk of Parkinson's disease. Diabetes Care. 2007 Apr;30(4):842-7.

[66] Hu G, Jousilahti P, Nissinen A, Antikainen R, Kivipelto M, Tuomilehto J. Body mass index and the risk of Parkinson disease. Neurology. 2006 Dec 12;67(11):1955-9.

[67] Olshansky SJ, Passaro DJ, Hershow RC, Layden J, Carnes BA, Brody J, et al. A potential decline in life expectancy in the United States in the 21st century. N Engl J Med. 2005 Mar 17;352(11):1138-45.

[68] Choi JY, Jang EH, Park CS, Kang JH. Enhanced susceptibility to 1-methyl-4-phenyl-1,2,3,6-tetrahydropyridine neurotoxicity in high-fat diet-induced obesity. Free Radic Biol Med. 2005 Mar 15;38(6):806-16.

[69] Sriram K, Benkovic SA, Miller DB, O'Callaghan JP. Obesity exacerbates chemically induced neurodegeneration. Neuroscience. 2002;115(4):1335-46.

[70] Goetze O, Wieczorek J, Mueller T, Przuntek H, Schmidt WE, Woitalla D. Impaired gastric emptying of a solid test meal in patients with Parkinson's disease using 13C-sodium octanoate breath test. Neurosci Lett. 2005 Mar 3;375(3):170-3.

[71] Unger MM, Hattemer K, Moller JC, Schmittinger K, Mankel K, Eggert K, et al. Real-time visualization of altered gastric motility by magnetic resonance imaging in patients with Parkinson's disease. Mov Disord. 2010 Apr 15;25(5):623-8.

[72] Brzozowski T, Konturek PC, Konturek SJ, Kwiecien S, Drozdowicz D, Bielanski W, et al. Exogenous and endogenous ghrelin in gastroprotection against stress-induced gastric damage. Regulatory peptides. 2004 Aug 15;120(1-3):39-51.

[73] Brzozowski T, Konturek PC, Sliwowski Z, Drozdowicz D, Kwiecien S, Pawlik M, et al. Neural aspects of ghrelin-induced gastroprotection against mucosal injury induced by noxious agents. Journal of physiology and pharmacology : an official journal of the Polish Physiological Society. 2006 Nov;57 Suppl 6:63-76.

[74] Shimizu Y, Chang EC, Shafton AD, Ferens DM, Sanger GJ, Witherington J, et al. Evidence that stimulation of ghrelin receptors in the spinal cord initiates propulsive activity in the colon of the rat. J Physiol. 2006 Oct 1;576(Pt 1):329-38.

[75] Shafton AD, Sanger GJ, Witherington J, Brown JD, Muir A, Butler S, et al. Oral administration of a centrally acting ghrelin receptor agonist to conscious rats triggers defecation. Neurogastroenterol Motil. 2009 Jan;21(1):71-7.

[76] Unger MM, Moller JC, Mankel K, Eggert KM, Bohne K, Bodden M, et al. Postprandial ghrelin response is reduced in patients with Parkinson's disease and idiopathic REM sleep behaviour disorder: a peripheral biomarker for early Parkinson's disease? J Neurol. 2010 Dec 24.

[77] Fiszer U, Michalowska M, Baranowska B, Wolinska-Witort E, Jeske W, Jethon M, et al. Leptin and ghrelin concentrations and weight loss in Parkinson's disease. Acta Neurol Scand. 2009 Dec 17.

[78] Diano S, Farr SA, Benoit SC, McNay EC, da Silva I, Horvath B, et al. Ghrelin controls hippocampal spine synapse density and memory performance. Nature Neuroscience. 2006;9(3):381-8.

[79] Drucker DJ. The biology of incretin hormones. Cell metabolism. 2006 Mar;3(3):153-65.

[80] Drucker DJ. Enhancing the action of incretin hormones: a new whey forward? Endocrinology. 2006 Jul;147(7):3171-2.

[81] Turton MD, O'Shea D, Gunn I, Beak SA, Edwards CM, Meeran K, et al. A role for glucagon-like peptide-1 in the central regulation of feeding. Nature. 1996 Jan 4;379(6560):69-72.

[82] Campos RV, Lee YC, Drucker DJ. Divergent tissue-specific and developmental expression of receptors for glucagon and glucagon-like peptide-1 in the mouse. Endocrinology. 1994 May;134(5):2156-64.

[83] Cabou C, Campistron G, Marsollier N, Leloup C, Cruciani-Guglielmacci C, Penicaud L, et al. Brain glucagon-like peptide-1 regulates arterial blood flow, heart rate, and insulin sensitivity. Diabetes. 2008 Oct;57(10):2577-87.

[84] Drucker DJ. Glucagon-like peptides: regulators of cell proliferation, differentiation, and apoptosis. Molecular endocrinology. 2003 Feb;17(2):161-71.

[85] During MJ, Cao L, Zuzga DS, Francis JS, Fitzsimons HL, Jiao X, et al. Glucagon-like peptide-1 receptor is involved in learning and neuroprotection. Nat Med. 2003 Sep;9(9):1173-9.

[86] Greig NH, Mattson MP, Perry T, Chan SL, Giordano T, Sambamurti K, et al. New therapeutic strategies and drug candidates for neurodegenerative diseases: p53 and TNF-alpha inhibitors, and GLP-1 receptor agonists. Annals of the New York Academy of Sciences. 2004 Dec;1035:290-315.

[87] McClean PL, Gault VA, Harriott P, Holscher C. Glucagon-like peptide-1 analogues enhance synaptic plasticity in the brain: a link between diabetes and Alzheimer's disease. Eur J Pharmacol. 2010 Mar 25;630(1-3):158-62.

[88] Perry TA, Greig NH. A new Alzheimer's disease interventive strategy: GLP-1. Curr Drug Targets. 2004 Aug;5(6):565-71.

[89] Stoffers DA, Kieffer TJ, Hussain MA, Drucker DJ, Bonner-Weir S, Habener JF, et al. Insulinotropic glucagon-like peptide 1 agonists stimulate expression of homeodomain protein IDX-1 and increase islet size in mouse pancreas. Diabetes. 2000 May;49(5):741-8.

[90] Belsham DD, Fick LJ, Dalvi PS, Centeno ML, Chalmers JA, Lee PK, et al. Ciliary neurotrophic factor recruitment of glucagon-like peptide-1 mediates neurogenesis, allowing immortalization of adult murine hypothalamic neurons. The FASEB journal : official publication of the Federation of American Societies for Experimental Biology. 2009 Dec;23(12):4256-65.

[91] Bertilsson G, Patrone C, Zachrisson O, Andersson A, Dannaeus K, Heidrich J, et al. Peptide hormone exendin-4 stimulates subventricular zone neurogenesis in the adult rodent brain and induces recovery in an animal model of Parkinson's disease. J Neurosci Res. 2008 Feb 1;86(2):326-38.

[92] Luciani P, Deledda C, Benvenuti S, Cellai I, Squecco R, Monici M, et al. Differentiating effects of the glucagon-like peptide-1 analogue exendin-4 in a human neuronal cell model. Cell Mol Life Sci. 2010 Nov;67(21):3711-23.

[93] Li Y, Tweedie D, Mattson MP, Holloway HW, Greig NH. Enhancing the GLP-1 receptor signaling pathway leads to proliferation and neuroprotection in human neuroblastoma cells. J Neurochem. 2010 Jun;113(6):1621-31.

[94] Harkavyi A, Abuirmeileh A, Lever R, Kingsbury AE, Biggs CS, Whitton PS. Glucagon-like peptide 1 receptor stimulation reverses key deficits in distinct rodent models of Parkinson's disease. J Neuroinflammation. 2008;5:19.

[95] Li Y, Perry T, Kindy MS, Harvey BK, Tweedie D, Holloway HW, et al. GLP-1 receptor stimulation preserves primary cortical and dopaminergic neurons in cellular and rodent models of stroke and Parkinsonism. Proceedings of the National Academy of Sciences of the United States of America. 2009 Jan 27;106(4):1285-90.

[96] Iwai T, Ito S, Tanimitsu K, Udagawa S, Oka J. Glucagon-like peptide-1 inhibits LPS-induced IL-1beta production in cultured rat astrocytes. Neurosci Res. 2006 Aug;55(4):352-60.

[97] Li Y, Cao X, Li LX, Brubaker PL, Edlund H, Drucker DJ. beta-Cell Pdx1 expression is essential for the glucoregulatory, proliferative, and cytoprotective actions of glucagon-like peptide-1. Diabetes. 2005 Feb;54(2):482-91.

[98] Kim Chung le T, Hosaka T, Yoshida M, Harada N, Sakaue H, Sakai T, et al. Exendin-4, a GLP-1 receptor agonist, directly induces adiponectin expression through protein kinase A pathway and prevents inflammatory adipokine expression. Biochem Biophys Res Commun. 2009 Dec 18;390(3):613-8.

[99] Kim S, Moon M, Park S. Exendin-4 protects dopaminergic neurons by inhibition of microglial activation and matrix metalloproteinase-3 expression in an animal model of Parkinson's disease. J Endocrinol. 2009 Sep;202(3):431-9.

[100] Qin Z, Sun Z, Huang J, Hu Y, Wu Z, Mei B. Mutated recombinant human glucagon-like peptide-1 protects SH-SY5Y cells from apoptosis induced by amyloid-beta peptide (1-42). Neurosci Lett. 2008 Oct 31;444(3):217-21.

[101] Gautron L, Elmquist JK. Sixteen years and counting: an update on leptin in energy balance. The Journal of clinical investigation. 2011 Jun 1;121(6):2087-93.

[102] Hommel JD, Trinko R, Sears RM, Georgescu D, Liu ZW, Gao XB, et al. Leptin receptor signaling in midbrain dopamine neurons regulates feeding. Neuron. 2006 Sep 21;51(6):801-10.

[103] Lu J, Park CS, Lee SK, Shin DW, Kang JH. Leptin inhibits 1-methyl-4-phenylpyridinium-induced cell death in SH-SY5Y cells. Neurosci Lett. 2006 Oct 30;407(3):240-3.

[104] Weng Z, Signore AP, Gao Y, Wang S, Zhang F, Hastings T, et al. Leptin protects against 6-hydroxydopamine-induced dopaminergic cell death via mitogen-activated protein kinase signaling. J Biol Chem. 2007 Nov 23;282(47):34479-91.

[105] Aziz NA, Pijl H, Frolich M, Roelfsema F, Roos RA. Leptin, adiponectin, and resistin secretion and diurnal rhythmicity are unaltered in Parkinson's disease. Mov Disord. 2011 Mar;26(4):760-1.

Part 2

Prion Diseases

3

The Effects of Trimethylamine N-Oxide on the Structural Stability of Prion Protein

Barbara Yang, Kuen-Hua You,
Shing-Chuen Wang, Hau-Ren Chen and Cheng-I Lee
Department of Life Science, National Chung Cheng University
Taiwan,
ROC

1. Introduction

Transmissible spongiform encephalopathies (TSEs) are diseases that affect the central nervous system in both humans and animals. TSEs can be ascribed to conformational conversion of prion protein (PrP). "Prion" stands for "proteinaceous infectious particle", which was discovered in the disease-transmitting material of infectious brain tissues and named by Prusiner (Prusiner 1982). The normal, cellular form of PrP (PrP^C) is a α-helix-rich glycoprotein attached to the outer cell surface by a glycophosphatidyl inositol linkage. The biological role of PrP^C remains ambiguous. Since Cu^{2+} is unique among divalent metal ions in its ability to bind to PrP^C in the octarepeat region (four copies of the repeat ProHisGlyGlyGlyTrpGlyGln) in the N-terminal domain (Whittal et al. 2000), the prion protein has been suggested to play a role in maintaining cellular copper concentration and signal transduction (Brown et al. 1998; Mouillet-Richard et al. 2000). PrP^C is non-infectious, whereas the abnormal and infectious, Scrapie isoform of PrP (PrP^{Sc}) has been considered to be the major infectious component of the genetic, sporadic and transmissible fatal neuro degenerative prion diseases that affect both human and animals (Prusiner 1998). PrP^{Sc} is rich in β-sheet structures and it has a pronounced tendency to misfold and to subsequently aggregate into highly stable and insoluble amyloid plaques. This PrP^{Sc} plagess are resistant to digestion by proteinase K, whereas PrP^C is sensitive to digestion by proteinase K (Prusiner 1998). PrP^{Sc} is responsible for many diseases in humans, including Kuru, Gerstmann-Sträussler-Scheinker disease (GSS), fatal familial insomnia (FFI), Creutzfeldt-Jakob disease (CJD) and the BSE-related, variant Creutzfeldt-Jakob disease (vCJD) (Horwich & Weissman 1997; Prusiner 1997; Will et al. 1996). The infectious nature of these fatal diseases differ from other infectious diseases in that the pathogen is a proteinaceous particle rather than typical pathogens, such as viruses, bacteria and fungi. Therefore, a "protein-only" hypothesis has been proposed (Griffith 1967; Prusiner 1998). A protein designated as "protein X" has been proposed to be involved in structural conversion of PrP^C into PrP^{Sc} (Telling et al. 1995) in the protein-only model. After decades of study on prion proteins, protein X has not been identified. Thus, the mechanism of how PrP^C is converted into PrP^{Sc} remains ambiguous.

The structure of prion proteins has been studied in human (Calzolai & Zahn 2003; Donne et al. 1997; Zahn et al. 2000), hamster (James et al. 1997) and mouse sequences (Gossert et al.

2005; Riek et al. 1996). The structure of truncated mouse PrP (121-231) has been solved and reveals a α-helical protein containing 52% of α-helical and 3% of β-sheet structures (PDB code: 1AG2, (Riek et al. 1996)). Furthermore, NMR structure of hamster prion 90-231 reveals a flexible N-terminus and a structured C-terminal fragment (125-228) containing 43% of α-helical and 6% of β-sheet structures (PDB code: 1B10, (James et al. 1997)). The high flexibility of the N-terminus was confirmed in recombinant full-length hamster prion protein PrP 29-231 (Donne et al. 1997). The representative NMR structure of mouse prion is shown in Figure 1.

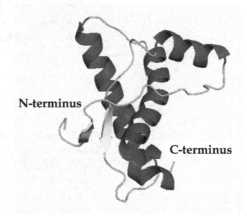

Fig. 1. The NMR structure of mouse prion protein (PDB code: 1AG2, (Riek et al. 1996)). The α-helical structures are represented by red ribbons, and the antiparallel β-sheet structure is colored in yellow. This figure was produced using the PyMol graphic package

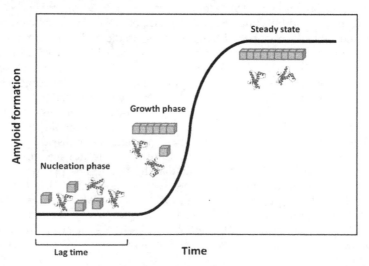

Fig. 2. Representative curve of nuclei-dependent polymerization model for amyloid formation

The formation of amyloid fibrils can be described by the polymerization model (Tsong & Baldwin 1972) illustrated in Figure 2. In this nucleation-dependent polymerization model, the conversion of proteins into nuclei that subsequently serve as seeds for amyloid fibrils is the rate-limiting step. Therefore, amyloid formation has a lag phase in which nucleation from protein monomers takes place. The spectroscopic signal for detecting amyloid fibrils is very weak during this nucleation phase, but the signal will enhance significantly during the fast polymerization catalyzed by the nuclei in the growth phase. Finally, the signal remains constant at a steady stateas that the ordered amyloid fibrils and protein monomers are at equilibrium.

In previous studies of recombinant PrP, a partially folded intermediate of PrP 90-231 has been suggested (Apetri et al. 2004; Kuwata et al. 2002; Nicholson et al. 2002). These partially unfolded states can potentially initiate amyloid formation (Abedini & Raleigh 2009; Chiti & Dobson 2009). Consequently, extensive works on the interaction of samll molecules and PrP have been conducted in order to find pharmacological chaperones that can stabilize the structure of PrP^C (Nicoll et al. 2010). Chemical chaperones is an important target in the developments of therapies for prion disease. In the study of protein folding, osmolyte is a well-know factor that acts as a chemical chaperone to assist proteins to fold. Furthermore, cellular osmolarity can be changed by the ion-transportations. An increase in intracellular osmolarity caused by ion-transoprtation resulting astrocyte dysfunction in neurological disorders has been reviewed (Seifert et al. 2006). Therefore, it is essential to study osmolytes that affect folding of prion proteins. The chemical structure of the osmolyte trimethylamine N-oxide (TMAO) is illustrated in Figure 3 that TMAO is a zwitterionic compound at neutral pH, but is positively charged below pH 4.7 (Lin & Timasheff 1994). TMAO is a well known protective osmolyte that can increase structural stability of proteins against chemical or temperature-induced denaturation (Baskakov et al. 1998; Bolen & Baskakov 2001; Celinski & Scholtz 2002; Gursky 1999; Qu et al. 1998). TMAO has an extraordinary ability to force thermodynamically unstable proteins to fold (Baskakov & Bolen 1998). In contrast, TMAO destabilizes proteins at low pH (Singh et al. 2005).

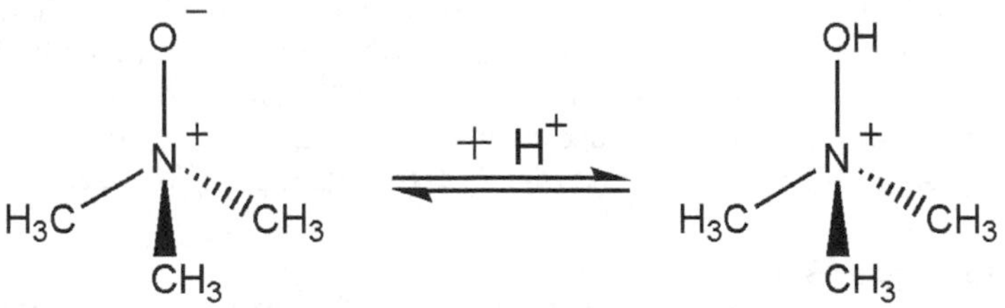

Fig. 3. Chemical structure of zwitterionic TMAO in equilibrium with its cationic form

A previous study by Tatzel and co-workers indicated that TMAO and the organic solvent dimethylsulfoxide (DMSO) prevent scrapie formation *in vitro* (Tatzelt et al. 1996). This study suggests a potential stratagy for preventing PrP^{Sc} by stabilizing the conformation of PrP^C. In contrast, later studies indicated that TMAO destabilized the α-helical conformation of full-length human prion at neutral pH at high temperature (Nandi et al. 2006) and human prion proteins at low pH (Granata et al. 2006). The structure of α-helix-rich prion protein is destabilized and the prion protein is converted to β-sheet structured oligomeric species (Nandi et al. 2006).

In this study, we examined the effect of TMAO on conformational stability in full-length mouse prion proteins (MoPrPs) and their structural conversion to amyloid fibrils. A possible mechanism of TMAO on fibril formation is proposed based on the nucleation-dependent polymerization model.

2. Materials and methods

We characterized TMAO-induced structural change in MoPrP by circular dichroism spectroscopy and 8-anilino-1-naphthalenesulfonic acid (ANS)-binding fluorescence assay, and compared the effect of TMAO on the formation of amyloid fibrils by thioflavin T (ThT) binding assay and transmission electron microscopy (TEM).

Chemicals used in this work were purchased from Sigma Chemcial Co. (St. Louis, Missouri, USA), and used without further purification.

2.1 Protein expression and purification

Plasmid pET101 encoding mouse prion (23-231) was transformed into competent *E. coli* BL21 (DE3) and expressed in the form of inclusion bodies. The protein was purified on a Ni-sepharose column according to a previously described procedure (Bocharova et al. 2005). The purity of the isolated protein was confirmed by SDS-PAGE. The correct native conformation, containing mainly α-helical structures, was confirmed by circular dichroism spectroscopy.

2.2 Far-UV circular dichroism spectroscopy

Far-UV circular dichroism spectra of mouse prion was recorded with a J-815 (Jasco, Japan) spectropolarimeter equipped with a Peltier temperatue control system (model PTC 423). For measurements in the far-UV region, a quartz cell with a path length of 0.1 cm was used in nitrogen atmosphere. For protein samples, the concentration of MoPrP was kept constant at 10 μM in 10 mM 2-(*N*-morpholino)ethanesulfonic acid (MES, pH 6.0). Far-UV circular dichroism spectra between 200 and 250 nm were recorded. An accumulation of five scans with a scan speed of 50 nm per minute was performed at 20 °C. The thermal-induced denaturation of proteins was conducted by heating protein solutions at the rate of 1 °C/min, and measuring the molar ellipticity at 222 nm every 0.5 °C. The reading of molar ellipticity at 222 nm in accordance with temperature change was normalized for further analysis. The data were analyzed with Origin 6.0 from OriginLab (Northampton, Massachusetts, USA).

2.3 ANS fluorescence assay

ANS solution was added into 10 μM of TMAO-incubated MoPrP in 10 mM MES (pH 6.0) to a final concentration of 100 μM. For each sample, two fluorescence emission spectra were collected by a F-4500 fluorometer (Hitachi, Japan) with excitation either at 295 nm or 385 nm, respectively.

2.4 Fibril formation

Fibril conversion was conducted at 20 μM protein in the solution containing 2 M guanidine hydrochloride (GdnHCl) and 50 mM MES (pH 6) at 37 °C as described in a previous study on mouse prion fibrils (Bocharova et al. 2005). At the end of the experiments, the fibril samples were dialyzed against 20 mM sodium acetate (pH 5.5) for further experiments.

2.5 ThT fluorescence assay of fibril conversion

Aliquots withdrawn during the time course of incubation at 37 °C were diluted into 5 mM sodium acetate buffer (pH 5.5) to a final sample concentration of 0.5 μM. ThT solution was added to a final concentration of 10 μM. For each sample, two emission spectra were collected by a F-4500 fluorometer (Hitachi, Japan) equipped with a 150 W Xenon lamp. The fluorescence spectra were recorded from 470 to 550 nm with excitation wavelength of 450 nm. The maximum fluorescence emission at 482 nm was determined. The reported fluorescence readings were average values for two measurements.

2.6 TEM

The aliquotes of mouse prion fibril samples were stained with 2% tungsten phosphoric acid onto carbon-coated 200-mesh copper grids. The samples were adsorbed onto copper grids for 30 sec and subsequently washed with PBS and mQH$_2$O. The samples were air-dried before imaging. The TEM images were collected by a H-7100 TEM (Hitachi, Japan). The analysis of fibril length and width was carried out on WICF ImageJ software (National Institutes of Health).

3. Results and discussion

We characterized the effect of the osmolyte TMAO on the structure of MoPrP by far-UV circular dichroism spectroscopy and ANS-binding fluorescence assay. Furthermore, we tested the effect of TMAO on amyloid fibril formation. The prion fibrils grown at different concentrations of TMAO were analyzed by TEM.

3.1 Secondary structure and protein stability

We collected far-UV circular dichroism spectra for MoPrP at pH 6.0 at 20 °C. As shown in Figure 4, MoPrP has the typical feature of α-helical conformation as indicated by the circular dichroic signals at 208 nm and 222 nm. In prior investigations of TMAO and its effects on MoPrP structure, circular dichroism spectra of MoPrP in 2 M TMAO were recorded every hour. These spectra collected within 6 hours are very similar (data not shown). Since the extension of incubation does not affect the structural features of MoPrP, the following spectroscopic experiments were conducted without prolonged incubation.

3.1.1 TMAO causes unfolding and destabilizes MoPrP

We investigated the addition of TMAO in the range of 0.5 ~ 2 M and its effect on MoPrP using circular dichroism spectroscopy. The results are presented in Figure 4A. Osmolyte TMAO exhibits substantial interference below 205 nm. Therefore, the interfering circular dichroic signal was removed from the plot. In the absence of TMAO, MoPrP has clear circular dichroic feature of α-helical conformation at 208 and 222 nm. After addition of 0.5 M and 1.0 M TMAO, the circular dichroic signal indicative of α-helix structure at 208 nm decreased slightly, while the signal at 222 nm remained generally unchanged. Significantly, addition of 1.5 M and 2.0 M weakens the entire α-helical conformation. The unfolding of α-helical structure has been reported with similar work performed at low pH (Granata et al. 2006). Consistently, the significant unfolding of prion proteins is carried out at > 1.0 M TMAO as illustrated in Figure 4B. Differently, the dichroic signal at 208 nm is affected by TMAO more severely than that at 222 nm. The dichroic signal at 208 nm dominants the dichroic curve of α-helix in the absence of TMAO, but this signal is largely weakened by the addition of TMAO. The dichroic curve of TMAO-affected partially folded α-helical structure observed in this work is not identical to the curves observed in the similar work performed at high temperature (Nandi et al. 2006). These results indicated that TMAO affect the structure of prion proteins differently under different conditions. At neutral pH, TMAO is zwitterionic, but it becomes cationic at low pH. Full-length prion protein includes polybasic N-terminal region 23-30 which is essential for effective folding into the native cellular conformation (Ostapchenko et al. 2008). Therefore, the differentiation of TMAO-induced conformational change at different pH values can be partially, if not all, ascribed to the interaction between TMAO and the polybasic N-terminal region.

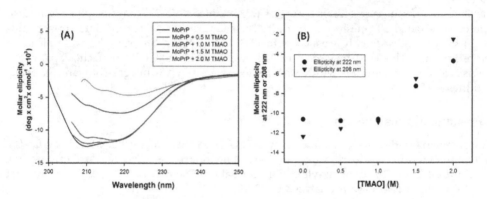

Fig. 4. (A) Far-UV circular dichroism spectra of 10 μM MoPrP measured after the addition of TMAO. (B) Comparison of mollar ellipticity at 222 nm and 208 nm in various concentration of TMAO

TMAO is known to increase the melting temperature of various proteins (Arakawa & Timasheff 1985). Therefore, in addition to the conformation change, the structural stability of MoPrP in the presence of TMAO was examined with thermal-induced denaturation monitored by the molar ellipticity at 222 nm. The molar ellipticity was normalized to represent the fraction of unfolded proteins as presented in Figure 5.

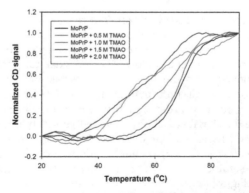

Fig. 5. Thermal-induced denaturation of MoPrP monitored the circular dichroic signal at 222 nm

The curves of heat-induced denaturation can be described by a cooperative two-state model of denaturation in which proteins are transited between natively folded states and denatured unfolded states. By monitoring the circular dichroic signal at 222 nm, the natively folded MoPrP has the minimum intensity, whereas fully unfolded proteins has the maximum readings. These denaturation curves can be analyzed based on the Gibbs-Helmholtz equation:

$$\Delta G_U^\circ(T) = \Delta H^\circ(T_m)(1 - \frac{T}{T_m}) - \Delta G_p^\circ[(T_m - T) + T\ln(\frac{T}{T_m})] \tag{1}$$

Based on the above equation, the melting temperature (T_m) of MoPrP can be determine. In the absence of TMAO, the T_m of MoPrP is 68.63 °C. Addition of 0.5 M TMAO does not affect the thermal-denaturation curve significantly, as the T_m value was calculated to be 68.19 °C. In the presence of 1.0 ~ 1.5 M TMAO, the thermal-denaturation curve shifted toward low temperature significantly, as MoPrP starts to denature at ~32 °C. In contrast to the denaturation curve collected in the absence of TMAO, the thermal-denaturation curves of MoPrP treated with ≥ 1.0 M TMAO are not typical of cooperative two-state unfolding. These curves implies that TMAO changes the unfolding pathway, and that more intermediates are present at high concentration of TMAO.

3.2 TMAO-induced conformational change within the native state

The hydrophobic dye ANS has been widely used to detect the conformational changes in proteins, as ANS preferentially binds to hydrophobic protein surfaces. The binding of ANS to hydrophobic area causes significant increase in the fluorescence emission of ANS. Therefore, we detected ANS fluorescence emission upon excitation at at 385 nm to detect the change of hydrophobicity of MoPrP as presented in Figure 6. Clearly, ANS-bound MoPrP emits fluorescence at 470 nm and 495 nm upon excitation at 385 nm which indicates the presence of two distinct ANS-binding pockets. Addition of 0.5 M TMAO weakens the fluorescence emission of ANS slightly, but addition of 1.0 ~ 2.0 M TMAO substantially increased ANS fluorescence. The increase of ANS emission at 470 nm is more pronounced than the fluorescence at 495 nm. It indicates that the hydrophobicity represents by 470 nm is more sensitive to TMAO than the other one at 495 nm. Overall, this result indicates that TMAO increases hydrophobic surface at two distinct sites in MoPrP.

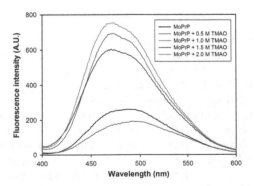

Fig. 6. Fluorescence of ANS in the absence and in the presence of TMAO upon excitation at 385 nm

In addition to the change of hydrophobicity in MoPrP, we detected ANS fluorescence emission upon excitation at 295 nm to study the TMAO-induced conformational change. Excitation at 295 nm excites tryptophan (Trp) and ANS at the same time, but this excitation causes the energy transfer from Trp (donor) in the N-terminus to ANS (acceptor). As the energy transfer efficiency (E) is determined by the distance of donor-acceptor (r) in the relation of E α r^{-6}, the fluorescence spectra with excitation at 295 nm provide the distance information between Trp and ANS-bound residues. As illustrated in Figure 7, in the absence of TMAO, MoPrP has fluorescence emission at 350 nm and 485 nm arising from Trp and ANS-binding, respectively. Upon the addition of TMAO, the energy in Trp transfers to MoPrP-bound ANS efficiently that the signal of Trp at 350 nm is completely abolished, and the fluorescence of ANS is significantly enhanced. The fluorescence spectra of ANS in the presence of TMAO illustrate a strong peak at 408 nm, a medium, broad peak at ~460 nm and a weak, broad peak at ~490 nm overlapped with the broad peak at 460 nm. The fluorescence at 490 nm is a typical emission of ANS-binding as observed in Figure 6. This weak signal at 490 nm could be ascribed to MoPrP-bound ANS molecules that do not accept energy from Trp efficiently. As the addition of TMAO causes the peaks at 408 nm and at 460 nm to increase at different degrees, it is predicted that there are two distinct hydrophobic pockets near the N-terminal region but away from Trp with different distances.

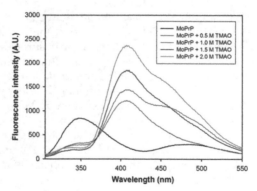

Fig. 7. Fluorescence of ANS in the absence and in the presence of TMAO upon excitation at 295 nm

3.2 Fibril conversion in TMAO

Partially unfolded MoPrP can potentially initiate formation of amyloid fibrils (Abedini & Raleigh 2009; Chiti & Dobson 2009). In 2 M GdnHCl, MoPrP is about half folded and is readily converted into amyloid fibrils (Breydo et al. 2005). Formation of amyloid fibrils can be monitored by ThT-binding fluorescence because the fluorescence of ThT is greatly enhanced when ThT binds to β-sheet rich structures, which are the main structures found in the amyloid fibrils (LeVine 1999). Therefore, the intensity of ThT-binding fluorescence represents the amount of amyloid fibrils converted from protein monomers in the absence of TMAO. As illustrated in Figure 8, the kinetics of fibril conversion shows sigmoidal curves. The MoPrP starts to form amyloid fibrils after 6 hours of incubation as monitored by ThT-binding fluorescence. The prion fibrils grow rapidly such that the maximum ThT fluorescence reached ~400 after 8 hours of amyloid fibril conversion. In the presence of 0.5

or 1.0 M of TMAO, the amyloid fibrils grow very well such that the maximum values of ThT fluorescence are higher in comparison to those in the absence of TMAO. When the concentration of TMAO is increased to 1.5 M and above, MoPrP rarely converts to amyloid fibrils as indicated by low ThT-binding fluorescence.

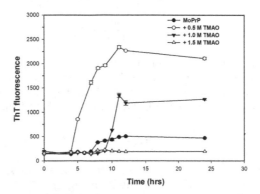

Fig. 8. Kinetic traces for amyloid fibril formation from MoPrP monitored by ThT-binding fluorescence in the presence of 2 M GdnHCl and various concentrations of TMAO at pH 6.0 at 37 °C. The fluorescence readings were average values of two measurements

The quantity of prion fibrils judged by the maximum ThT fluorescence in the presence of TMAO is presented in Figure 9A. Clearly, addition of 0.5 and 1.0 M TMAO promotes amyloid formation as the reading of ThT-fluorescence is greatly enhanced in comparison to that in the absence of TMAO. In contrast, when the concentration of TMAO was increased further, the fibril conversion was inhibited. It is interesting to observe enhancement of fibril conversion by TMAO at ≤ 1.0 M. This result is consistent with previous work performed on α-synuclein that 1.0 M TMAO yields large amount of fibril whereas 2.0 and 3.0 M of TMAO inhibits the fibril formation (Uversky et al. 2001).

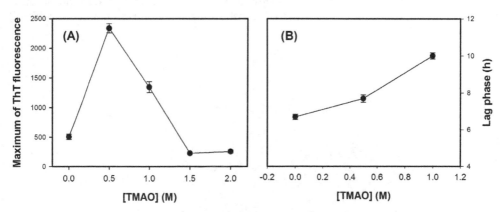

Fig. 9. (A)The quantity of amyloid fibrils converted from MoPrP monitored by the maximum of ThT-binding fluorescence measured two times, and (B) the calculated lag phase of fibril conversion in the absence and in the presence of TMAO

The formation of amyloid fibrils in the presence of 0 ~ 1.5 M TMAO follows the nucleation-dependent polymerization model as illustrated in Figure 2. According to this nucleation-dependent polymerization model, the lag phase of amyloid formation from MoPrP can be determined by fitting the time-dependent changes in the ThT fluorescence (F) over time (t) of the reaction as shown in the following equation (Bocharova et al. 2005):

$$F = F_0 + \frac{\Delta F}{1 + \exp[k(t_m - t)]} \tag{2}$$

Where F_0 is the minimum level of ThT fluorescence during the lag phase, ΔF is the difference of ThT fluorescence between the maximum level (steady state) and the minimum level (lag phase), k is the rate constant of fibril growth (h^{-1}), and t_m is the observed time at the midpoint of transition. The lag time (t_l) of fibril formation can be calculated as:

$$t_l = t_m - \frac{2}{k} \tag{3}$$

According to these two equations, the lag time for fibril formation in the presence of 0, 0.5 and 1.0 M TMAO was determined as presented in Figure 9B. Previous work on fibril conversion from α-synuclein in the presence of TMAO reported acceleration of amyloid formation in a wide range of TMAO concentration (1.0 ~ 3.0 M) due to osmolyte-induced stabilization of the partially folded intermediate (Uversky et al. 2001). Similarly, TMAO stabilizes some partially folded intermediates. However, these partially folded intermediates slightly disfavour the nucleation reaction resulting in slight extension of the nucleation phase and also the following growth phase.

3.3 Morphology of prion fibrils grown with TMAO
Variation of conditions for fibril formation from the identical protein can yield different morphology. For example, Makarava and Baskakov have observed curved and straight fibrils from the same mouse prion protein and identical solvent conditions but different in the shaking speed (Makarava & Baskakov 2008). Therefore, we investigated the morphology of mouse prion fibrils by electron microscopy. In our experiment, for mature mouse prion fibrils grown in 2 M GdnHCl, the length is mostly longer than 500 nm, and the width is about 20 nm as illustrated in Figure 10.

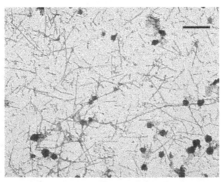

Fig. 10. TEM image of mature prion fibrils grown in 2 M GdnHCl at pH 6.0 at 37 °C. The scale bar represents 500 nm

The growth phase of fibril conversion in the absence of TMAO is very short, whereas this elongation process takes longer in the addition of TMAO. To compare the morphology of prion fibrils during elongation in the absence and in the presence of TMAO, we collected TEM images of fibril samples in the middle point of growth phase. As illustrated in Figure 11, the prion fibrils grown in the absence of TMAO are long and straight, whereas fibrils converted in the presence of TMAO look like short rods.

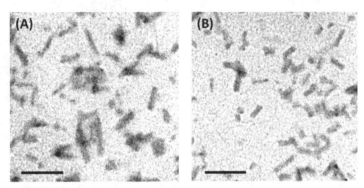

Fig. 11. TEM images of mouse prion fibrils at the middle point of growth phase (A) in the absence of TMAO and (B) in the presence of 1.0 M TMAO. The scale bar represents 200 nm

Oligomers, protofibrils and mature fibrils involved in the formation of amyloid fibrils are typically distinguished by the length and width of the fibrils. Therefore, we statistically compared the length and the width of prion fibrils converted in the absence and in the presence of 0.5 M and 1.0 M TMAO. As illustrated in Figure 12A, in the absence of TMAO, the fibril length is populated in two groups including one normal distribution between 60 ~ 180 nm and an elongation at > 180 nm. Prion fibrils with the addition of 0.5 M TMAO are normally distributed between 20 ~ 160 nm and the most populated length is 80 ~ 120 nm. Increasing TMAO to 1.0 M shortens the prion fibrils, so that the fibril length ranges from 20 to 140 nm with the most populated length being 40 ~ 60 nm. The average length of prion fibrils is 144 nm in the absence of TMAO. Addition of TMAO shortens the average length of prion fibrils to 92 and 61 nm in the presence of 0.5 M and 1.0 M, respectively. In contrast to the fibril length, the width of prion fibrils is similar as illustrated in Figure 12B, and the average of the width is 19 nm regardless the presence of TMAO.

The structural effect of osmolyte TMAO on prion proteins and fibril conversion has been investigated extensively in this work. At pH 6.0, 20 °C, the α-helical conformation of MoPrP is unfolded by TMAO. When the concentration of TMAO is low at ≤ 1.0 M, the degree of unfolding is small and the fibril conversion takes place on the mostly folded α-helical structures. In contrast to low concentration of TMAO, high concentration of TMAO at >1.0 M largely unfolds the α-helix and this unfolding inhibits amyloid formation completely. In other words, low concentration of TMAO decellarates the prion nucleation represented by lag phase in nucleation-dependent polymerization model, whereas TMAO enhances the growth of prion fibrils. This contrast effect indicates that the structural requirement of prion proteins in nucleation and in fibril elongation is different. The importance of partial unfolding of prion in amyloid formation has been suggested (Apetri et al. 2004; Kuwata et al. 2002; Nicholson et al. 2002). The structure of partially folded prion protein that initiates amyloid formation remains unclear. Our recent computational simulation proposed that the

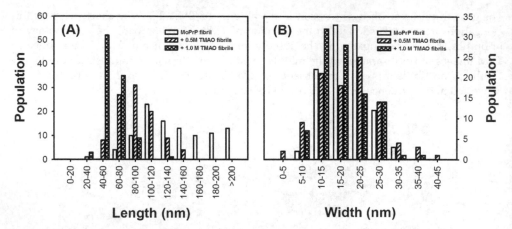

Fig. 12. Histrogram of length and width of prion fibrils measured on 100 fibrils in the absence and in the presence of 0.5 M and 1.0 M TMAO

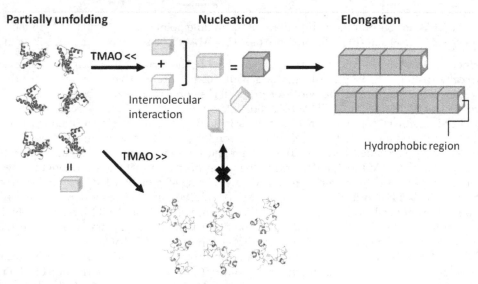

Fig. 13. A scheme illustrating the proposed effect of TMAO based on nucleation-dependent polymerization model

denatured state of prion protein is partially folded with α-helical conformation (Lee & Chang 2010). In prion nucleation, high α-helical conformation is preferred and intermolecular β-sheet interactions occur between prion monomers (Lee et al. 2010). This interaction of intermolecular β-sheets is most likely the initiation of nucleation. This intermolecular interaction might be correlated with a double-layered filament within one fibril as observed by atomic force microscopy (Anderson et al. 2006). When the α-helical structure is mostly lost and the intermolecular interaction is largely weakened, the amyloid formation can not take place due to failure of nucleation as illustrated in Figure 13. After nuclei are formed as fibril seeds, the elongation requires stable interactions between nuclei and proteins. As amyloid fibrils have been proposed to have hydrophobic interior (Buchete & Hummer 2007; Carroll et al. 2006), the area of the hydrophobic surface is important in fibril elongation. The hydrophobicity at the ANS-binding pockets that accept energy from Trp is induced significantly by TMAO, and the high hydrophobicity promotes hydrophobic interactions of nuclei and proteins to form the hydrophobic interior. Notably, in the presence of low concentration of TMAO, the amount of fibrils is significantly increased, but the fibril length is shortened in the middle of growth phase. This phenomenon could be due to adjustment of interaction between nuclei under high hydrophobicity as judged by long growth phase in the presence of TMAO. Taking togther these findings, a certain amount of α-helical conformation seems to be required in the structural conversion of prion proteins in nucleation, and hydrophobic interaction is essential in fibril elongation.

4. Conclusion

In this study, we have investigated the structural effect of osmolytes TMAO on MoPrP proteins and the features of mouse prion fibrils. Low concentration of TMAO alters α-helical structures resulting deceleration of nucleation serving as fibril seeds, but TMAO enhances hydrophobicity promoting fibril growth. High concentration of TMAO inhibits amyloid formation completely by inducing loss of α-helical conformation. This study provides more information in the details of molecular structure and interaction in amyloid formation. These findings are essential in further search for therapeutic therapies for prion disease.

5. Acknowledgment

We are grateful to National Science Council for financial support (Project 100-2321-B-194-001). We also thank Dr. Raymond Chung for editing the manuscript. Usage of PyMol graphics packages and WICF ImageJ software is gratefully acknowledged.

6. References

Abedini, A. and Raleigh, D. P. (2009). A role for helical intermediates in amyloid formation by natively unfolded polypeptides? *Phys Biol*, 6, 1, 15005.

Anderson, M., Bocharova, O. V., Makarava, N., et al. (2006). Polymorphism and ultrastructural organization of prion protein amyloid fibrils: an insight from high resolution atomic force microscopy. *J Mol Biol*, 358, 2, 580-596.

Apetri, A. C., Surewicz, K. and Surewicz, W. K. (2004). The effect of disease-associated mutations on the folding pathway of human prion protein. *J Biol Chem*, 279, 17, 18008-18014.

Arakawa, T. and Timasheff, S. N. (1985). The stabilization of proteins by osmolytes. *Biophys J*, 47, 3, 411-414.

Baskakov, I. and Bolen, D. W. (1998). Forcing thermodynamically unfolded proteins to fold. *J Biol Chem*, 273, 9, 4831-4834.

Baskakov, I., Wang, A. and Bolen, D. W. (1998). Trimethylamine-N-oxide counteracts urea effects on rabbit muscle lactate dehydrogenase function: a test of the counteraction hypothesis. *Biophys J*, 74, 5, 2666-2673.

Bocharova, O. V., Breydo, L., Salnikov, V. V., et al. (2005). Copper(II) inhibits in vitro conversion of prion protein into amyloid fibrils. *Biochemistry*, 44, 18, 6776-6787.

Bocharova, O. V., Breydo, L., Salnikov, V. V., et al. (2005). Synthetic prions generated in vitro are similar to a newly identified subpopulation of PrPSc from sporadic Creutzfeldt-Jakob disease. *Protein Sci*, 14, 5, 1222-1232.

Bolen, D. W. and Baskakov, I. V. (2001). The osmophobic effect: natural selection of a thermodynamic force in protein folding. *J Mol Biol*, 310, 5, 955-963.

Breydo, L., Bocharova, O. V., Makarava, N., et al. (2005). Methionine oxidation interferes with conversion of the prion protein into the fibrillar proteinase K-resistant conformation. *Biochemistry*, 44, 47, 15534-15543.

Brown, D. R., Schmidt, B. and Kretzschmar, H. A. (1998). Effects of copper on survival of prion protein knockout neurons and glia. *J Neurochem*, 70, 4, 1686-1693.

Buchete, N. V. and Hummer, G. (2007). Structure and dynamics of parallel beta-sheets, hydrophobic core, and loops in Alzheimer's A beta fibrils. *Biophys J*, 92, 9, 3032-3039.

Calzolai, L. and Zahn, R. (2003). Influence of pH on NMR structure and stability of the human prion protein globular domain. *J Biol Chem*, 278, 37, 35592-35596.

Carroll, A., Yang, W., Ye, Y., et al. (2006). Amyloid fibril formation by a domain of rat cell adhesion molecule. *Cell Biochem Biophys*, 44, 2, 241-249.

Celinski, S. A. and Scholtz, J. M. (2002). Osmolyte effects on helix formation in peptides and the stability of coiled-coils. *Protein Sci*, 11, 8, 2048-2051.

Chiti, F. and Dobson, C. M. (2009). Amyloid formation by globular proteins under native conditions. *Nat Chem Biol*, 5, 1, 15-22.

Donne, D. G., Viles, J. H., Groth, D., et al. (1997). Structure of the recombinant full-length hamster prion protein PrP(29-231): the N terminus is highly flexible. *Proc Natl Acad Sci U S A*, 94, 25, 13452-13457.

Gossert, A. D., Bonjour, S., Lysek, D. A., et al. (2005). Prion protein NMR structures of elk and of mouse/elk hybrids. *Proc Natl Acad Sci U S A*, 102, 3, 646-650.

Granata, V., Palladino, P., Tizzano, B., et al. (2006). The effect of the osmolyte trimethylamine N-oxide on the stability of the prion protein at low pH. *Biopolymers*, 82, 3, 234-240.

Griffith, J. S. (1967). Self-replication and scrapie. *Nature*, 215, 5105, 1043-1044.

Gursky, O. (1999). Probing the conformation of a human apolipoprotein C-1 by amino acid substitutions and trimethylamine-N-oxide. *Protein Sci*, 8, 10, 2055-2064.

Horwich, A. L. and Weissman, J. S. (1997). Deadly conformations--protein misfolding in prion disease. *Cell*, 89, 4, 499-510.

James, T. L., Liu, H., Ulyanov, N. B., et al. (1997). Solution structure of a 142-residue recombinant prion protein corresponding to the infectious fragment of the scrapie isoform. *Proc Natl Acad Sci U S A*, 94, 19, 10086-10091.

Kuwata, K., Li, H., Yamada, H., et al. (2002). Locally disordered conformer of the hamster prion protein: a crucial intermediate to PrPSc? *Biochemistry*, 41, 41, 12277-12283.

Lee, C. I. and Chang, N. Y. (2010). Characterizing the denatured state of human prion 121-230. *Biophys Chem*, 151, 1-2, 86-90.

Lee, S., Antony, L., Hartmann, R., et al. (2010). Conformational diversity in prion protein variants influences intermolecular beta-sheet formation. *EMBO J*, 29, 1, 251-262.

LeVine, H., 3rd (1999). Quantification of beta-sheet amyloid fibril structures with thioflavin T. *Methods Enzymol*, 309, 274-284.

Lin, T. Y. and Timasheff, S. N. (1994). Why do some organisms use a urea-methylamine mixture as osmolyte? Thermodynamic compensation of urea and trimethylamine N-oxide interactions with protein. *Biochemistry*, 33, 42, 12695-12701.

Makarava, N. and Baskakov, I. V. (2008). The same primary structure of the prion protein yields two distinct self-propagating states. *J Biol Chem*, 283, 23, 15988-15996.

Mouillet-Richard, S., Ermonval, M., Chebassier, C., et al. (2000). Signal transduction through prion protein. *Science*, 289, 5486, 1925-1928.

Nandi, P. K., Bera, A. and Sizaret, P. Y. (2006). Osmolyte trimethylamine N-oxide converts recombinant alpha-helical prion protein to its soluble beta-structured form at high temperature. *J Mol Biol*, 362, 4, 810-820.

Nicholson, E. M., Peterson, R. W. and Scholtz, J. M. (2002). A partially buried site in homologous HPr proteins is not optimized for stability. *J Mol Biol*, 321, 2, 355-362.

Nicoll, A. J., Trevitt, C. R., Tattum, M. H., et al. (2010). Pharmacological chaperone for the structured domain of human prion protein. *Proc Natl Acad Sci U S A*, 107, 41, 17610-17615.

Ostapchenko, V. G., Makarava, N., Savtchenko, R., et al. (2008). The polybasic N-terminal region of the prion protein controls the physical properties of both the cellular and fibrillar forms of PrP. *J Mol Biol*, 383, 5, 1210-1224.

Prusiner, S. B. (1982). Novel proteinaceous infectious particles cause scrapie. *Science*, 216, 4542, 136-144.

Prusiner, S. B. (1997). Prion diseases and the BSE crisis. *Science*, 278, 5336, 245-251.

Prusiner, S. B. (1998). Prions. *Proc Natl Acad Sci U S A*, 95, 23, 13363-13383.

Qu, Y., Bolen, C. L. and Bolen, D. W. (1998). Osmolyte-driven contraction of a random coil protein. *Proc Natl Acad Sci U S A*, 95, 16, 9268-9273.

Riek, R., Hornemann, S., Wider, G., et al. (1996). NMR structure of the mouse prion protein domain PrP(121-321). *Nature*, 382, 6587, 180-182.

Seifert, G., Schilling, K. and Steinhauser, C. (2006). Astrocyte dysfunction in neurological disorders: a molecular perspective. *Nat Rev Neurosci*, 7, 3, 194-206.

Singh, R., Haque, I. and Ahmad, F. (2005). Counteracting osmolyte trimethylamine N-oxide destabilizes proteins at pH below its pKa. Measurements of thermodynamic parameters of proteins in the presence and absence of trimethylamine N-oxide. *J Biol Chem*, 280, 12, 11035-11042.

Tatzelt, J., Prusiner, S. B. and Welch, W. J. (1996). Chemical chaperones interfere with the formation of scrapie prion protein. *EMBO J*, 15, 23, 6363-6373.

Telling, G. C., Scott, M., Mastrianni, J., et al. (1995). Prion propagation in mice expressing human and chimeric PrP transgenes implicates the interaction of cellular PrP with another protein. *Cell*, 83, 1, 79-90.

Tsong, T. Y. and Baldwin, R. L. (1972). A sequential model of nucleation-dependent protein folding: kinetic studies of ribonuclease A. *J Mol Biol*, 63, 3, 453-469.

Uversky, V. N., Li, J. and Fink, A. L. (2001). Trimethylamine-N-oxide-induced folding of alpha-synuclein. *FEBS Lett*, 509, 1, 31-35.

Whittal, R. M., Ball, H. L., Cohen, F. E., et al. (2000). Copper binding to octarepeat peptides of the prion protein monitored by mass spectrometry. *Protein Sci*, 9, 2, 332-343.

Will, R. G., Ironside, J. W., Zeidler, M., et al. (1996). A new variant of Creutzfeldt-Jakob disease in the UK. *Lancet*, 347, 9006, 921-925.

Zahn, R., Liu, A., Luhrs, T., et al. (2000). NMR solution structure of the human prion protein. *Proc Natl Acad Sci U S A*, 97, 1, 145-150.

4

Computational Studies of the Structural Stability of Rabbit Prion Protein Compared to Human and Mouse Prion Proteins

Jiapu Zhang

Centre in Informatics and Applied Optimization & Graduate School of Sciences,
Informatics Technology and Engineering, University of Ballarat,
Mount Helen, VIC 3353
Australia

1. Introduction

Prion diseases are invariably fatal and highly infectious neurodegenerative diseases affecting humans and animals. The neurodegenerative diseases such as Creutzfeldt-Jakob disease, variant Creutzfeldt-Jakob diseases, Gerstmann-Sträussler-Scheinker syndrome, Fatal Familial Insomnia, Kuru in humans, scrapie in sheep, bovine spongiform encephalopathy (or 'mad-cow' disease) and chronic wasting disease in cattle belong to prion diseases. By now there have not been some effective therapeutic approaches to treat all these prion diseases. In 2008, canine mammals including dogs (canis familials) were the first time academically reported to be resistant to prion diseases Polymenidoua et al. (2008). Rabbits are the mammalian species known to be resistant to infection from prion diseases from other species Vorberg et al. (2003). Horses were reported to be resistant to prion diseases too Perez et al. (2010). By now all the NMR structures of dog, rabbit and horse prion proteins had been released into protein data bank respectively in 2005, 2007 and 2010 Lysek et al. (2005); Perez et al. (2010); Wen et al. (2010a). Thus, at this moment it is very worth studying the NMR molecular structures of horse, dog and rabbit prion proteins to obtain insights into their immunity prion diseases.

The author found that dog and horse prion proteins have stable molecular dynamical structures whether under neutral or low pH environments, but rabbit prion protein has stable molecular dynamical structures only under neutral pH environment. Under low pH environment, the stable α-helical molecular structures of rabbit prion protein collapse into β-sheet structures. This article focuses the studies on rabbit prion protein (within its C-terminal NMR, X-ray and Homology molecular structured region RaPrP^C (120-230)), compared with human and mouse prion proteins (HuPrP^C (125-228) and MoPrP^C (124-226) respectively). The author finds that some salt bridges contribute to the structural stability of rabbit prion protein under neutral pH environment.

As we all know, the disease infectious prions PrP^{Sc} are rich in β-sheets (about 43% β-sheet) Griffith (1967) and the normal cellular prions PrP^C are predominant in α-helices (42% α-helix, 3% β-sheet) Pan et al. (1993). Prion diseases are believed caused by the conversion of normal PrP^C to abnormally folded PrP^{Sc}, and prion diseases are so-called protein 'structural conformational' diseases. Thus, we may study the molecular structures of prion proteins to obtain some insights of prion diseases. Human prion diseases include the Creutzfeldt-Jakob disease, variant Creutzfeldt-Jakob diseases, Gerstmann-Sträussler-Scheinker syndrome, Fatal Familial Insomnia, and Kuru. The NMR solution structure of the human prion protein (1QLX.pdb) was released into the PDB bank (www.pdb.org) in 1999 and last modified in 2009 Zahn et al. (2000). Mice are popular experimental laboratory animals and the NMR structure of mouse prion protein (1AG2.pdb) was released into the PDB bank in 1997 and last modified in 2009 Riek et al. (1996). Rabbits, dogs and horses were reported to be resistant to prion diseases Perez et al. (2010); Polymenidoua et al. (2008); Vorberg et al. (2003) and by the end of 2010 their NMR structures (2FJ3.pdb, 1XYK.pdb, and 2KU4.pdb respectively) were completed to release into the PDB bank Lysek et al. (2005); Perez et al. (2010); Wen et al. (2010a). The X-ray structure of rabbit prion protein (3O79.pdb) was released into PDB bank in 2010 too Khan et al. (2010). At this moment it is very worth studying these molecular structures of horse, dog, rabbit, human and mouse prion proteins to reveal some secrets of prion diseases. The author found that dog and horse prion proteins have stable molecular dynamical structures whether under neutral or low pH environments Zhang and Liu (2011); Zhang (2011a), but rabbit prion protein has stable molecular dynamical structures only under neutral pH environment Zhang (2010); Zhang and Liu (2011); Zhang (2011a;b). Under low pH environment, among all the prion proteins above-mentioned only for the rabbit prion protein, its stable α-helical molecular structures collapse into β-sheet structures Zhang (2010); Zhang and Liu (2011); Zhang (2011a;b). The conversion of disease PrP^{Sc} from normal PrP^C is just involving 'conformational change' from predominantly α-helical protein to one rich in β-sheet structure. This article specially focuses on the rabbit prion protein to obtain some insights into the immunity of rabbits to prion diseases.

For the rabbit prion protein, we have its NMR and X-ray structures (2FJ3.pdb and 3O79.pdb respectively). Early in 2004, Epa Zhang et al. (2006) made molecular modeling of a homology structure (denoted 6EPA.pdb) for rabbit prion protein RaPrP^C(120-229), which was constructed using the NMR structure of the human prion protein (1QLX.pdb) as the template. Besides all these structures of rabbit prion protein, the knowledge on their conformational evolution/dynamics is considered essential to understand rabbit prion and the molecular modeling (MM) and molecular dynamics (MD) approach takes advantage beyond the experimental limit. In Section 2, this article first briefly reviews the main MD results of the homology MM structure Zhang et al. (2006) at 500 K and of the wild-type NMR structure at 450 K Zhang (2011b), compared with the MD of the wild-type NMR structures of human (HuPrP^C (125-228), 1QLX.pdb) and mouse (MoPrP^C (124-226), 1AG2.pdb) prion proteins. Section 3 will present the wild-type NMR rabbit, human and mouse MD comparisons at 350 K. Because the X-ray structure 3O79.pdb was produced differently from the NMR structure 2FJ3.pdb and the Homology structure 6EPA.pdb, we will not do their MD comparisons; however, in Section 4, we will give detailed sequence and structure alignment analysis of all these three rabbit prion structures compared with human and mouse wild-type structures. Section 5 gives some concluding remarks on rabbit prion protein and prion diseases.

2. MD reviews on the 500 K homology rabbit prion protein and the 450 K NMR rabbit prion protein

2.1 The homology rabbit prion protein at 500 K Zhang et al. (2006)

Zhang et al.   Zhang et al. (2006) studied the MD of RaPrP^C(120-229) homology structure (6EPA.pdb). The MD simulations used Amber 8 Case et al. (2004) PMEMD program, with explicit water at different temperatures and pH values. The simulation conditions are listed in Table 1 of Zhang et al. (2006). The RMSD (root mean square deviation) and radius of gyration results are shown in Fig.s 2-3 of Zhang et al. (2006), where we may see that rabbit prion protein has more stable structural dynamical behavior compared to the human and mouse prion proteins at 500 K under neutral pH environment. This is also shown in Fig. 4 of Zhang et al. (2006) of snapshots for human, mouse and rabbit prion proteins at 5ns, 10ns, 15ns, 20ns, 25ns, and 30ns respectively. Fig. 4 of Zhang et al. (2006) shows that the helices of HuPrP and MoPrP were unfolded but RaPrP still keeps the helical structures at 500 K under neutral pH environment. The performance of RaPrP also shows that 500 K is a not a very bad temperature chosen for theoretical research for RaPrP. Under low pH environment at 500 K, these helical structures of RaPrP were unfolded. One of the reasons of the rabbit prion protein unfolding is due to the remove of the salt bridges such as N177-R163 (Fig. 5 of Zhang et al. (2006)). We may see in Fig. 5 of Zhang et al. (2006) the salt bridge / hydrogen bond between Arginine 163 and Aspartic acid 177 is conserved through a large part of the simulations and contributes to the protein stability of rabbit prion protein structure. Simulations at low pH value, where this salt bridge is absent, show RMSD and radius of gyration values for the rabbit prion protein to be of the same magnitude as the human and mouse prion proteins.

2.2 The NMR rabbit prion protein at 450 K Zhang (2011b)

Zhang Zhang (2011b) did the MD studies on the NMR rabbit prion protein RaPrP^C(124-228) (2FJ3.pdb) at 450 K under both neutral and low pH environments for the simulations of 20 ns. Zhang Zhang (2011b) found that "the secondary structures under low pH environment at 450 K have great differences between rabbit prion protein and human and mouse prion proteins: the α-helices of rabbit prion protein were completely unfolded and began to turn into β-sheets but those of human and mouse prion proteins were not changed very much. These results indicate the C-terminal region of RaPrP^C has lower thermostability than that of HuPrP^C and MoPrP^C. Under the low pH environment, the salt bridges such as D177-R163, D201-R155 were removed (thus the free energies of the salt bridges changed the thermostability) so that the structure nearby the central helices 1Ữ3 was changed for rabbit prion protein" Zhang (2011b). The author continued his MD simulations for another 10 ns. The secondary structures for the MD simulations of 30 ns (Fig. 1) shows the same conclusion as that of Zhang (2011b).

We may say that the salt bridges such as D177-R163, N201-R155 contribute to the structural stability of wild-type rabbit prion protein (Fig. 1). At 450 K, whether in neutral or in low pH environments, the α-helical secondary structures of dog prion protein have not changed for the long 30 ns' simulations Zhang and Liu (2011); at 350 K, horse prion protein has the same molecular structural dynamics Zhang (2011a) during the 30 ns' long simulations.

Fig. 1. Secondary structures of rabbit, human and mouse prion proteins (from up to down) at 450 K under neutral and low (from left to right) pH environments (red: α-helix, pink: π-helix, yellow: 3_{10}-helix, green: β-bridge, blue: β-sheet, purple: Turn, Black: Bend; x-axis: time (0-30 ns), y-axis: residue numbers).

3. 350 K

350 K might be a practical temperature for some experimental laboratory works. Zhang Zhang (2011c) did MD simulations for wild-type rabbit, dog and horse prion NMR structures at 350 K. The findings of 350 K are: "dog and horse prion proteins have stable molecular structures whether under neutral or low pH environments. Rabbit prion protein has been found having stable molecular structures under neutral pH environment, but without structural stability under low pH environment. Under low pH environment, the salt bridges such as D177-R163 were broken and caused the collapse of the stable α-helical molecular structures". Here the MD simulations are done for wild-type human and mouse prion proteins in the use of the same Materials and Methods as in Zhang (2011c).

Seeing Fig. 2, we know that at 350 K human and mouse prion proteins have stable molecular structures whether under neutral or low pH environments.

Clearly the following salt bridges play an important role to the NMR structural stability of rabbit prion protein: (1) GLU210-ARG207-GLU206-LYS203 (99.78%, 88.85%, 82.74%, H3-H3), GLU210-HIS176 (74.31%, H3-H2), GLU206-HIS176 (57.10%, H3-H2), ARG207-HIS176 (0.52%, H3-H2), ASP177-ARG163 (19.54%, H2-S2); (2) ARG150-ASP146-ARG147-ASP143 (91.38%, 100%, 86.43%, H1-H1), HIS139-ARG150 (50.96%), HIS139-ASP146 (92.62%); (3) ASP201-ARG155 (10.07%, H3-H1), ASP201-ARG150 (2.61%, H3-H1), ASP201-ARG147

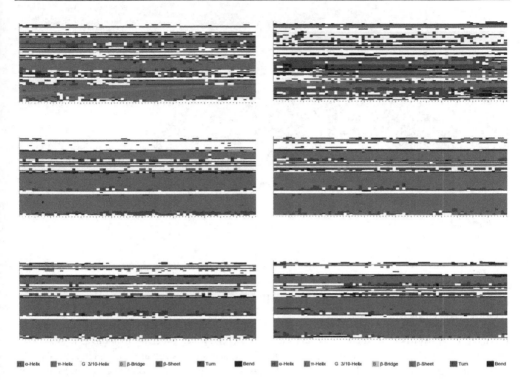

Fig. 2. Secondary structures of rabbit, human and mouse prion proteins (from up to down) at 350 K under neutral to low pH environments (from left to right) (X-axis: 0 ns - 30 ns (from left to right), Y-axis: residue numbers 124 - 228 / 125 - 228 / 124 - 226 (from up to down)).

(0.01%, H3-H1), ASP201-HIS186 (0.50%, H3-H2); and(4) ARG155-ASP201 (10.07%, H1-H3), TYR156-HIS186 (H1-H2, 71.69%), ARG155-GLU151 (20.70%, H1-H1), ARG155-GLU195 (0.06%, H1-H1), where H1, H2, H3 denote the α-helix 1, 2, 3 respectively, S1, S2 denote the β-strand 1 and 2 respectively, and '%' denotes the percentage during the whole simulation of 30 ns. Compared with human, mouse, dog and horse NMR prion proteins, rabbit NMR prion protein has some special salt bridges which contribute to its structural stability at 350 K during the simulation of 30 ns (Fig. 3) (human, mouse, dog and horse NMR prion proteins have not these salt bridges).

4. Alignment analyses

We make the sequence alignment of PrP from horse, dog, rabbit, human and mouse protein (Fig. 4).

In Fig. 4, "*" means that the residues in that column are identical in all sequences in the alignment, ":" means that conserved substitutions have been observed, "." means that semi-conserved substitutions are observed, the RED color takes place at small (small+ hydrophobic (incl.aromatic-Y)) residues, the BLUE color takes place at acidic residues, the MAGENTA color takes place at Basic-H residues,GREEN color takes place at

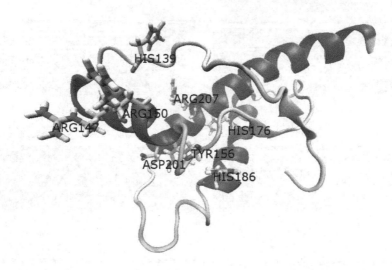

Fig. 3. Some special salt bridges ARG207-HIS176, TYR156-HIS186, HIS139-ARG150, ASP201-ARG147, ASP201-ARG150, ASP201-HIS186, ARG155-GLU151 of wild-type NMR rabbit prion protein at 350 K.

Hydroxyl+sulfhydryl+amine+G residues, and Grey color takes place at unusual amino/imino acids etc.. For the structural domain, in Fig. 4 we can see some special residues listed in Table 1 for horse, dog, human and mouse prion proteins, which might contribute to characters of each structure respectively. Rabbits differ from horses, dogs, humans and mice at: S173 (N174

Horse	S167 (others are D), Y222 (others are S), Q226 (others are Y), V241 (others are I), F245 (others are S)
Dog	L129 (others are M), S165 (others are P), N170 (others are S), S173 (others are N), V244 (others are I)
Human	I138 (immunities are L), S143 (others are N), H155 (others are Y), M166 (others are V), I183 (immunities are V), E219 (others are Q), S230 (immunities are A)
Mouse	I183 (immunities are V), V215 (others are I), D217 (others are Q), S230 (immunities are A)

Table 1. Alignment analysis of special residues for HoPrP, DoPrP, HuPrP, and MoPrP.

for horse, T174 for dogs, N174 for humans and mice), Q219 (K220 for horses and humans, R220 for dogs and mice), A224 (F225 for horses, Y225 for dogs, humans and mice), L232 (I233 for dogs, V233 for horse, humans and mice), and G228 (others are S229). For rabbits, at positions 89 and 97 the residues are special from all others (G89 (others are N90), S97 (others are N98)). These special residues are illuminated in Fig. 5. Some recent researches are focusing on the loop between β2 and α2, i.e. PrP(164-171) Apostol et al. (2011); Fernandez-Funez et al. (2011); Khan et al. (2010); Perez et al. (2010); Wen et al. (2010a;b); we may see in Fig. 5 that the immune animals horses, dogs and rabbits have some residues in this loop different from humans and mice.

Lastly, we illuminate the figure (Fig. 6) of rabbit prion protein, including the homology, NMR and X-ray structures (6EPA.pdb, 2FJ3.pdb, and 3O79.pdb respectively). We superpose the homology structure onto the NMR structure and find the RMSD value is 3.2031669 angstroms.

CLUSTAL 2.1 multiple sequence alignment

```
          901234567890123456789012345678901234567890  1234567890123456789012345 67
HorsePrP  MVKSHVGGWILVLFVATWSDVGLCKKRPKPGG-WNTGGSRYPGQGSPGGNRYPPQGGGGW  59
DogPrP    MVKSHIGSWILVLFVAMWSDVGLCKKRPKPGGGWNTGGSRYPGQGSPGGNRYPPQGGGGW  60
RabbitPrP --MAHLGYWMLLLFVATWSDVGLCKKRPKPGGGWNTGGSRYPGQSSPGGNRYPPQGGG-W  57
HumanPrP  --MANLGCWMLVLFVATWSDLGLCKKRPKPGG-WNTGGSRYPGQGSPGGNRYPPQGGGGW  57
MousePrP  --MANLGYWLLALFVTMWTDVGLCKKRPKPGG-WNTGGSRYPGQGSPGGNRYPPQGG-TW  56
          : ::* *:* ***: *:*:*********** *********** .*********** *
```

```
          89012345678901234567890123456789012 34  567890123456789012345 6
HorsePrP  GQPHGGGWGQPHGGGWGQPHGGGWGQPHGGGWGQGG-SHGQWNKPSKPKTNMKHVAGAA  118
DogPrP    GQPHGGGWGQPHGGGWGQPHGGGWGQPHGGGWGQGG-THSQWNKPSKPKTNMKHVAGAA  119
RabbitPrP GQPHGGGWGQPHGGGWGQPHGGGWGQPHGGG-WGQGG-THNQWGKPSKPKTSMKHVAGAA  115
HumanPrP  GQPHGGGWGQPHGGGWGQPHGGGWGQPHGGG-WGQGGGTHSQWNKPSKPKTNMKHMAGAA  116
MousePrP  GQPHGGGWGQPHGGSWGQPHGGSWGQPHGGG-WGQGGGTHNQWNKPSKPKTNLKHVAGAA  115
          **************.*******.*********.***** :*.**.*******.*:*:****
```

```
          119        130       140       150       160       170
          789012345678901234567890123456789012345678901234567890123456
HorsePrP  AAGAVVGGLGGYMLGSAMSRPLIHFGNDYEDRYYRENMYRYPNQVYYRPVSEYSNQNNFV  178
DogPrP    AAGAVVGGLGGYLLGSAMSRPLIHFGNDCEDRYYRENMYRYPNQVYYRSVDQYNNQSTFV  179
RabbitPrP AAGAVVGGLGGYMLGSAMSRPLIHFGNDYEDRYYRENMYRYPNQVYYRPVDQYSNQNSFV  175  --1
HumanPrP  AAGAVVGGLGGYMLGSAMSRPIIHFGSDYEDRYYRENMHRYPNQVYYRPVDQYSNQNNFV  176
MousePrP  AAGAVVGGLGGYMLGSAMSRPMIHFGNDWEDRYYRENMYRYPNQVYYRPVDQYSNQNNFV  175
          *************.*******.:****.* *********.**********..::*.**..**
```

```
          180       190       200       210       220       231
          789012345678901234567890123456789012345678901234567  8901234
HorsePrP  HDCVNITVKQHTVTTTTKGENFTETDVKIMERVVEQMCITQYQKEYEAFQQ--RGASVVL  236
DogPrP    HDCVNITVKQHTVTTT-KGENFTETDIKMMERVVEQMCITQYQRESEAYYQ--RGASVIL  236
RabbitPrP HDCVNITVKQHTVTTTTKGENFTETDIKIMERVVEQMCITQYQQESQAAYQ--RAAGVLL  233  --1
HumanPrP  HDCVNITIKQHTVTTTTKGENFTETDVKMMERVVEQMCITQYERESQAYYQ--RGSSMVL  234
MousePrP  HDCVNITIKQHTVTTTTKGENFTETDVKMMERVVEQMCVTQYQKESQAYYDGRRSSSTVL  235
          *******:*********  **********:*:**********:***::*  :*  :  *.:. :*
```

```
          567890123456789123
HorsePrP  FSSPPVVLLIFFLIFLIVG  255
DogPrP    FSSPPVILLVSFLIFLIVG  255
RabbitPrP FSSPPVILLISFLIFLIVG  252
HumanPrP  FSSPPVILLISFLIFLIVG  253
MousePrP  FSSPPVILLISFLIFLIVG  254
          ******.**. ********
```

Fig. 4. Horse, dog, rabbit, human and mouse prion protein sequence alignment.

Similarly, we superpose the X-ray structure onto the NMR structure and we get their RMSD value is 2.7918559 angstroms. This implies the homology structure 6EPA.pdb made in 2004 by Epa Zhang et al. (2006) is as effective as the X-ray structure 3O79.pdb released recently on date 2010-11-24 (last modified on 2011-02-02).

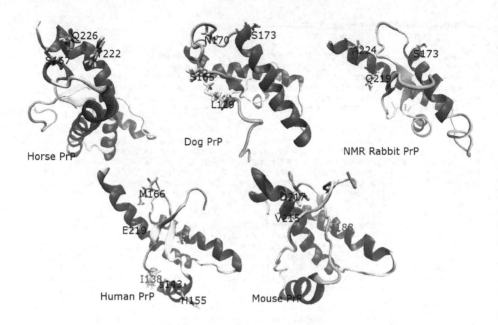

Fig. 5. Special residues owned only by HoPrP, DoPrP, RaPrP, HuPrP, and MoPrP respectively.

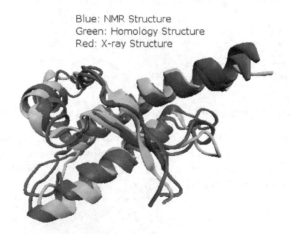

Fig. 6. Rabbit prion protein NMR, homology and X-ray structures (2FJ3.pdb, 6EPA.pdb, and 3O79.pdb).

5. Conclusion

To really reveal the secrets of prion diseases is very hard. Prion proteins have two regions: unstructured region and structured region. Rabbits, horses, and dogs were reported having immunity to prion diseases. Fortunately, by the end of 2010 all the NMR molecular structures of rabbit, horse, and dog prion proteins had been released into PDB bank already; for rabbit prion protein, its X-ray structure was also released into PDB bank in the end of 2010. Prion diseases are 'structural conformational' diseases. This paper timely presents a clue to reveal some secrets in the view of the dynamics of prion molecular structures. MD results of the author nearly in the passing 10 years show to us a common conclusion: under low pH environment at many levels of temperatures with different starting MD velocities, rabbit prion protein always unfolds its α-helical structures into β-sheet structures. Prion diseases are just caused by the conversion from predominant α-helices of PrP^C into rich β-sheets of PrP^{Sc}. Hence, we should furthermore study rabbits, horses and dogs, compared with humans and mice in order to reveal some secrets of prion diseases; for us, it is a long shot but certainly worth pursuing.

6. Acknowledgments

This research is supported by a Victorian Life Sciences Computation Initiative (http://www.vlsci.org.au) grant number VR0063 on its Peak Computing Facility at the University of Melbourne, an initiative of the Victorian Government. The author appreciates kind invitations and acceptance of this paper.

7. References

Apostol M.I., Wiltzius J.J.W., Sawaya M.R., Cascio D., Eisenberg D., 2011. Atomic structures suggest determinants of transmission barriers in mammalian prion disease. Biochem. 50, 2456–2463.

Case D.A., Darden T.A., Cheatham T.E., Simmerling III C.L., Wang J., Duke R.E., Luo R., Merz K.M., Wang B., Pearlman D.A., Crowley M., Brozell S., Tsui V., Gohlke H., Mongan J., Hornak V., Cui G., Beroza P., Schafmeister C., Caldwell J.W., Ross W.S., Kollman P.A., 2004. AMBER 8, University of California, San Francisco.

Fernandez-Funez P., Zhang Y., Sanchez-Garcia J., Jensen K., Zou W.Q., Rincon-Limas D.E., 2011. Pulling rabbits to reveal the secrets of the prion protein. Commun. Integr. Biol. 4(3), 262-266.

Griffith J.S., 1967. Self-replication and scrapie. Nature 215, 1043—1044.

Khan M.Q., Sweeting B., Mulligan V.K., Arslan P.E., Cashman N.R., Pai E.F., Chakrabartty A., 2010. Prion disease susceptibility is affected by beta-structure folding propensity and local side-chain interactions in PrP. Proc. Natl. Acad. Sci. USA 107: 19808-19813.

Lysek D.A., Schorn C., Nivon L.G., Esteve-Moya V., Christen B., Calzolai L., von Schroetter C., Fiorito F., Herrmann T., Guntert P., Wuthrich K., 2005. Prion protein NMR structures of cats, dogs, pigs, and sheep. Proc. Natl. Acad. Sci. USA 102, 640-645.

Nisbet R.M., Harrison C.F., Lawson V.A., Masters C.L., Cappai R., Hill A.F., 2010. Residues surrounding the glycosylphosphatidylinositol anchor attachment site of PrP modulate prion infection: insight from the resistance of rabbits to prion disease. J. Virol. 84 (13), 6678–6686.

Pan K.M., Baldwin M., Nguyen J., Gasset M., Serban A., Groth D., Mehlhorn I., Huang Z.W., Fletterick R., Cohenu F.E., Prusiner S.B., 1993. Conversion of alpha-helices into beta-sheets features in the formation of the scrapie prion proteins. Proc. Natl. Acad. Sci. USA 90(23), 10962-10966.

Perez D.R., Damberger F.F., Wuthrich K., 2010. Horse prion protein NMR structure and comparisons with related variants of the mouse prion protein. J. Mol. Biol. 400(2), 121-128.

Polymenidoua M., Trusheimb H., Stallmacha L., Moosa R., Julius J.A., Mielea G., Lenzbauerb C., Aguzzia A., 2008. Canine MDCK cell lines are refractory to infection with human and mouse prions. Vaccine 26(21), 2601-2614.

Riek R., Hornemann S., Wider G., Billeter M., Glockshuber R., Wuthrich K., 1996. NMR structure of the mouse prion protein domain PrP(121-321). Nature 382, 180-182.

Tabrett C.A., Harrison C.F., Sshmidt B., Bellingham S.A., Hardy T., Sanejouand Y.H., Hill A.F., Hogg P.J., 2010. Changing the solvent accessibility of the prion protein disulfide bond markedly influences its trafficking and effect on cell function. Biochem. J. 428, 169–182.

Vorberg I., Martin H.G., Eberhard P., Suzette A.P., 2003. Multiple amino acid residues within the rabbit prion protein inhibit formation of its abnormal isoform. J. Virol. 77, 2003–2009.

Wen Y., Li J., Yao W., Xiong M., Hong J., Peng Y., Xiao G., Lin D.H., 2010. Unique structural characteristics of the rabbit prion protein. J. Biol. Chem.285: 31682-31693.

Wen Y., Li J., Xiong M.Q., Peng Y., Yao W.M., Hong J., Lin D.H., 2010. Solution structure and dynamics of the I214V mutant of the rabbit prion protein. PLoS ONE 5(10), e13273.

Zahn R., Liu A., Luhrs T., Riek R., Von Schroetter C., Garcia F.L., Billeter M., Calzolai L., Wider G. Wuthrich K., 2000. NMR solution structure of the human prion protein. Proc. Natl. Acad. Sci. USA 97(1), 145-150.

Zhang J.P., 2010. Studies on the structural stability of rabbit prion probed by molecular dynamics simulations of its wild-type and mutants. J. Theor. Biol. 264(1), 119—122.

Zhang J.P., Liu D.D.W., 2011. Molecular dynamics studies on the structural stability of wild-type dog prion protein. J. Biomol. Struct. Dyn. 28(6), 861-869.

Zhang J.P., 2011. The structural stability of wild-type horse prion protein. J. Biomol. Struct. Dyn., in press.

Zhang J.P., 2011. Comparison studies of the structural stability of rabbit prion protein with human and mouse prion proteins. J. Theor. Biol. 269(1), 88—95.

Zhang J.P., 2011. The nature of the infectious agents: PrP models of resistant species to prion diseases (dog, rabbit and horses). Book Chapter In: Prions and Prion Diseases: New Developments (J.M. Verdier Eds.), NOVA Publishers, 2011. arXiv:1106.4628v1.

Zhang J.P., Varghese J.N., Epa V.C., 2006. Studies on the conformational stability of the rabbit prion protein. CSIRO Preventative Health National Research Flagship Science Retreat, Aitken Hill, Melbourne, 12—15 September 2006, Poster in Excellence (last document of webpage http://sites.google.com/site/jiapuzhang/).

Part 3

Motor Neuron Diseases

5

Modeling Spinal Muscular Atrophy in Mouse: A Disease of Splicing, Stability, and Timing

Thomas W. Bebee and Dawn S. Chandler
The Center for Childhood Cancer at the Research Institute at
Nationwide Children's Hospital, Columbus, Ohio;
The Department of Pediatrics, The Ohio State University, Columbus, Ohio;
United States of America

1. Introduction

Proximal spinal muscular atrophy (SMA) is a progressive neurodegenerative disease associated with the loss of alpha motor neurons in the lumbar spinal cord. The loss of these motor neurons leads to the progressive atrophy of the associated proximal muscles, eventual respiratory distress, and death. SMA occurs in about 1 in 6,000 to 10,000 live births and is a leading genetic cause of infant mortality (Burnett et al. 2009). SMA is subdivided into several groupings based on disease onset, severity, and outcome. The most severe form of SMA is referred to as type 0, or embryonic SMA, wherein patients are born with severe muscle atrophy and have expected lifespans of less than 6 months. The most common type of SMA is type I, which is characterized by disease onset within 6 months and mortality by age 2. Children with SMA type I often fail to sit unaided or walk, have difficulty breathing, and often require respiratory assistance. SMA type II children experience disease onset between 6 to 18 months and will not gain the ability to walk. Two forms of SMA are characterized by disease onset later in life and have unaltered life expectancies: juvenile and adult onset SMA, or type III and IV, respectively. Juvenile onset SMA type III is distinguished by disease onset after the age of 2, but there is variability of onset that can extend to early teen years. Type III children are often able to walk, and the ability to remain ambulatory throughout life can further subdivide this juvenile onset SMA. The least severe form of SMA is adult onset SMA type IV. This form of SMA does not emerge until the adult years and often presents with difficulty in performing previously attainable activities, such as climbing stairs (Zerres et al. 1995; Zerres et al. 1997; Zerres et al. 1997).

In SMA disease progression, the inability to achieve normal motor function is often the primary indication of disease. The level of motor function decline in SMA disease progression can be measured by the loss of functional motor units in SMA patients. In severe forms of SMA, there is a rapid loss of motor neurons innervating proximal muscles. This measure of reduced motor units can be observed by evaluating the Compound Motor Action Potential (CMAP) and Motor Unit Number Estimation (MUNE). The total number of innervated motor units is reduced in SMA disease as measured by these two tests and is correlated with age, severity of disease, and disease progression (Swoboda et al. 2005). The loss of motor neurons early in the onset of disease argues for the significance of motor neurons in disease, although additional components of the disease may provide for the rapid degeneration of SMA patients in late disease. Respiratory weakness is a common feature of both severe and milder forms of SMA. Children with type I or II SMA will often require respiratory assistance by way of Bi-level Positive Airway Pressure (BiPAP) (Bach et al. 2003), just as less severe forms of SMA also exhibit respiratory weakness that may require assistive breathing and respiratory therapy. While SMA is most directly associated with motor neuron loss, neuronal defects in sensory neurons are also observed in severe SMA patients (Rudnik-Schoneborn et al. 2003). A new emerging component of SMA is cardiac involvement in a subset of severe SMA patients, such as congenital cardiac defects and bradycardia (Bach et al. 2003; Rudnik-Schoneborn et al. 2008).

2. Genetic cause of SMA, reduced levels of SMN protein

The decreased level of the crucial Survival Motor Neuron (SMN) protein is the cause of SMA disease. The low levels of SMN protein are due to the loss of the essential Survival Motor Neuron-1 (*SMN1*) gene located on chromosome 5q13. SMA patients have lost *SMN1* by mutation or deletion, and the functional loss of *SMN1* is the disease locus of SMA (Lefebvre et al. 1995). In mice, the loss of the homologous *Smn* gene results in embryonic lethality (Schrank et al. 1997; Hsieh-Li et al. 2000); however, humans carry a duplication of the *SMN1* gene, *SMN2*, which encodes the same SMN protein. All SMA patients are genetically comprised of *SMN1* gene loss (mutation or deletion) with variable copy numbers of *SMN2* (Lefebvre et al. 1995; Lefebvre et al. 1997; McAndrew et al. 1997). The copy number of *SMN2* inversely correlates with the severity of SMA, where higher copy numbers of *SMN2* increase SMN protein and, therefore, decrease the severity of disease (Lefebvre et al. 1997; McAndrew et al. 1997). SMA patients that have 1-2 copies of *SMN2* are often associated with severe SMA type I, and SMA patients with higher *SMN2* copy number exhibit SMA type II-IV (Lefebvre et al. 1997).

The incomplete compensation for the loss of *SMN1* by *SMN2* is due to the inefficient splicing of the *SMN2* pre-mRNA (Lefebvre et al. 1995; Lorson et al. 1999). The altered splicing is due primarily to a single silent C>T point mutation in exon 7 that reduces recognition of exon 7 by the splicing machinery (Lorson et al. 1999). The functional role of the C>T mutation in exon 7 skipping can be explained by two models. The first model describes the loss of a putative exon splicing enhancer for SF2/ASF (SRSF1), where reduced binding of SF2/ASF (SRSF1) is associated with *SMN2* exon 7 skipping (Lorson et al. 2000; Cartegni et al. 2002; Cartegni et al. 2006). The second model is explained by the generation of an exonic splicing silencer for hnRNP A1 (Kashima et al. 2003; Kashima et al. 2007). Both of these models functionally explain the alteration in the recognition of exon 7 via the C>T point mutation that generates transcripts lacking exon 7 (ΔX7) from *SMN2*. The complex splicing regulation of *SMN* exon 7 beyond the critical C>T mutation has been recently reviewed (Bebee et al. 2010; Singh et al. 2011).

SMA is a disease associated with reduced splicing efficiency of SMN encoding transcripts. Furthermore, the significance of reduced SMN protein in normal cellular maintenance is underscored by the importance of *SMN* in splicing. SMN is crucial for splicing, as the SMN protein is the primary scaffolding protein involved in the maturation of the core splicing factors, or U snRNPs (Fischer et al. 1997; Liu et al. 1997; Pellizzoni et al. 1999; Meister et al. 2001; Pellizzoni et al. 2002). The SMN protein, in complex with several other components, comprises the SMN complex (Paushkin et al. 2002). The SMN complex loads the heptameric Sm ring (Raker et al. 1996) onto the Sm site of U snRNPs, completing the processing of the splicing core components for function in canonical splicing of nascent transcripts (Fischer et al. 1997; Liu et al. 1997). In SMA, the SMN protein levels are reduced due to loss of *SMN1*, and the primary product of *SMN2* is the SMNΔ7 protein produced by the transcripts lacking exon 7 (Lefebvre et al. 1995; Lefebvre et al. 1997). The SMNΔ7 protein is unstable and exhibits reduced protein function (Wang et al. 2001; Cho et al. 2010). However, a portion of *SMN2* transcripts encode full-length SMN protein sufficient for birth, but insufficient for motor neuron maintenance. The ability of *SMN2* to generate full-length transcripts provides for potential therapeutic intervention by increasing transcription or correcting the splicing of *SMN2* to increase the pools of SMN to levels consistent with normal development.

3. Genetic modeling of SMA in mouse

The duplication event of *SMN1* that generated *SMN2* occurred late in evolutionary history, and thus, mice carry only a single *Smn* gene homologous to *SMN1* (Bergin et al. 1997; Rochette et al. 2001). After identification of the gene responsible for SMA disease, efforts to model the human disease in mice began by generating null alleles of the mouse *Smn* gene (Summarized in Table 1). Null alleles of the *Smn* gene were generated by replacing exon 2 or 7 with reporter cassettes, and from these experiments the Smn gene was found to be essential as *Smn* -/- mice were embryonic lethal at the eight cell stage post fertilization (Schrank et al. 1997; Hsieh-Li et al. 2000). The requirement of SMN for survival is congruent with the function of SMN in maturation of the splicing machinery as an essential function for viability in eukaryotes. Mice heterozygous for the *Smn* null alleles have normal lifespans and do not exhibit haploinsufficiency; however, they do develop a mild form of SMA with muscle weakness and motor neuron loss later in life (Jablonka et al. 2000; Monani et al. 2000).

SMA is a disease of reduced SMN protein, and although the loss of Smn represents the loss of *SMN1* seen in SMA patients, this does not fully model the genetics of SMA. To more closely recapitulate the etiology of SMA, bac transgenes that included *SMN2* were introduced into the *Smn* null mice (Hsieh-Li et al. 2000; Monani et al. 2000). The *SMN2* in the bac transgenes exhibit splicing defects similar to *SMN2*, as exon 7 is primarily skipped and low SMN expression is seen. The level of SMN protein generated from the *SMN2* transgenes was sufficient to correct the embryonic lethality in *Smn* null mice. The rescue by *SMN2* in *Smn* null mice is in accordance with the observation that all SMA patients have *SMN2* present. Moreover, increased copy numbers of *SMN2* led to variable severities of SMA that stratify human SMA disease. Mice with 2 copies of *SMN2* ("Line89") exhibited severe SMA with an average lifespan of 4-6 postnatal days, but an increase of the *SMN2* copy number to 8 rescued the Line89 mice from SMA disease (Monani et al. 2000). Mice generated using a second *Smn* null allele (disruption of *Smn* exon 7) in combination with an *SMN2* bac transgene, termed the Taiwanese or Hsieh-Li mice, generated mice that exhibited severe to mild SMA. Hsieh-Li mice with 2 copies of *SMN2* survived 1 week and mice with 4 copies of *SMN2* had normal survival but developed peripheral necrosis (Hsieh-Li et al. 2000). A simplified crossing scheme of these mice now allows for independent generation of both the severe mice that survive 10 days, as well as the mild mice with normal survival (Riessland et al. 2010).

In severe SMA mouse models, reduced SMN protein, loss of anterior horn lumbar motor neurons, and muscle atrophy lead to the observed reduction in survival of 6-10 days (Hsieh-Li et al. 2000; Monani et al. 2000). Interestingly, the lifespan of the severe Line89 mouse was extended to PND13.5 by transgenic over-expression of the SMNΔ7 transcript (Le et al. 2005).

Genotype	Phenotype and Notes	Shorthand	References
Smn-/-	Embryonic lethal at preimplantation (8 cell stage). Smn exon 2 knockout.	Smn knockout	Schrank 1997
Smn+/-	Grossly normal with normal lifespan in the heterozygous Smn exon 2 knockout mice. Motor neuron loss in spinal cord: 40% at 6 months, 54% at 12 months.	Line89 het carrier	Jablonka 2000
Smn-/-; SMN2(2Hung)+/+	Bac transgene (115 kb) including human SMN2, SERF1 and part of NAIP genes; rescues embryonic lethality of Smn-/- (HPRT knockout of Smn exon 7). Variable SMN2 copy number, with increasing copy number lessening disease severity (Type I-III).	Taiwanese or Hsieh-Li	Hsieh-Li 2000
Smn-/-; SMN2(89Ahmb)+/+	Transgene containing SMN2 (35.5 kb); rescues Smn-/- (exon 2 null allele) embryonic lethality. 2 copies of SMN2 in the mice have severe SMA and die postnatally with mean survival PND4-6. Motor neuron loss PND5. Eight copies of SMN2 rescue SMA phenotype.	Line89	Monani 2000
SmnF7/Δ7; NSE-Cre	Cre-mediated Smn exon 7 excision in neurons. Mice develop a SMA like pathology with progressive motor neuron loss (cell body number and axon number) in the lumbar spinal cord, muscle atrophy, and have a mean survival of 25 days.	F7 or exon 7 floxed	Frugier 2000, Cifuentes-Diaz 2002
SmnF7/Δ7; HSA-Cre	Cre-mediated Smn exon 7 loss in skeletal muscle. Muscle cell death and dystrophy-like pathology, with a mean survival of 33 days.	F7 or exon 7 floxed	Cifuentes-Diaz 2001
Smn-/-; SMN2(89Ahmb)+/+; SMN1(A2G)+/-	Heterozygous expression of SMN1 A2G patient mutation transgene increase survival of Line89 mice to ~227 days, but is dependent upon SMN2 (2 copies). Reduced motor neuron number in spinal cord (29%) and facial nucleus (19%) at 3.5 months. ~25% reduction in spinal motor axon by 5 months, muscle atrophy, and axonal sprouting in gastrocnemius and triceps. Homozygous A2G are phenotypically normal.	A2G	Monani 2003

Table 1. Mouse models of SMA. (continues on next page)

Genotype	Phenotype and Notes	Shorthand	References
SmnF7/F7; Alfp-Cre	Cre-mediated Smn exon 7 excision in hepatocytes is embryonic lethal at E18.5.	F7 or exon 7 floxed	Vitte 2004
Smn-/-; SMN2(89Ahmb)+/+; SMNΔ7+/+	Expression of the SMNΔ7 transgene in Line89 mice extend survival to ~13.5 days. Motor neuron loss by PND9, weight and motor deficits, and muscle atrophy.	SMNΔ7	Le 2005
Smn-/-; SMN2(89Ahmb)+/+; SMN1(A111G)+/-	Transgene of SMN1 A111G patient mutation rescues Line89 mice. Survival is normal but requires SMN2 (2 copies). Gastrocnemius muscle hypertrophy at 10 months and rescued the deficits in snRNP assembly seen in the Line89 mice.	A111G	Workman 2009
Smn2B/-	Mutation of exonic enhancer in Smn exon 7 leads to low Smn protein levels and mean survival of 28 days. Muscle weakness and atrophy, and reduced motor neurons at PND21.	2B	Bowerman 2009, Bowerman 2010
Smn-/-; SMN2(N11)+/-; SMN2(N46)+/-	Mice with three copies of SMN2 from N11(one copy) and N46 (two copies) alleles have a mean survival of 14-16 days. Muscle atrophy and motor neuron loss by PND15. Respiratory deficits and NMJ defects in diaphragm.	3 copy SMN2	Michaud 2010
SmnF7/-; SMN2(89Ahmb)+/+; Olig2-Cre	Cre-mediated Smn exon 7 excision in motor neuron progenitor cells that also express basal SMN from SMN2. 70% survival to 12 months, motor neuron loss in spinal cord, muscle atrophy, and reduced sensory neuron innervation and number in DRG.	Olig2-Cre SMA	Park 2010
SmnC>T	Smn gene carrying the SMN2 exon 7 C>T mutation induces exon 7 skipping and reduces Smn protein. Mild SMA disease onset at 60 days associated with hind limb weakness, reduced activity and rearing, and muscle hypertrophy in gastrocnemius. Normal survival.	Smn C>T	Gladman 2010

Table 1. (continued) Mouse models of SMA

The mechanism of life extension in this severe SMA mouse model is not easily understood but begs the question of whether the SMNΔ7 protein has a functional role in normal development and/or neuroprotection. Another transgene that modified the survival of the severe Line89 mice is the SMN1 A2G mutation. The A2G transgene alone was unable to rescue the *Smn* null mice; however, survival extension through expression of the A2G transgene was contingent upon expression of SMN from the *SMN2* transgene. The transgenic A2G mouse develops mild SMA early in life, though survival is near 1 year and the mice with SMA pathology can appear normal until disease progression late in life. The A2G mice are associated with motor neuron defects such as motor neuron loss, branching, neurofilament accumulation, and failure to respond to repeated stimuli (Monani et al. 2003; Kariya et al. 2008). The milder SMA phenotype may be explained by the partial ability of the A2G mutant SMN protein to bind to normal full-length SMN. This binding is greater than that of the SMNΔ7 protein, arguing the potential for partial rescue of SMN complex formation in the A2G SMA mouse model (Monani et al. 2003).

SMA mouse models that carry the *SMN2* gene can be used to evaluate the expression and splicing of *SMN2* in tissues otherwise inaccessible in SMA patients, such as the central nervous system (CNS). Furthermore, the effect of disease progression and therapies targeting correction of *SMN2* can also be evaluated in mice that have the *SMN2* bac transgenes. The short lifespan of the severe SMA mouse models also allows for rapid evaluation of treatments aimed at increasing SMN, as changes in survival can readily be addressed in the short-lived mice. However, the short lifespan of these SMA models does not allow for therapeutic intervention at later time-points in development and SMA disease. Further attempts to modulate the lifespan of the severe SMA by simply titrating the copy number of *SMN2* in mice have proven difficult. One group generated two *SMN2* transgenic lines that harbor 1 or 2 copies of *SMN2* per allele (lines N11 and N46). When combined to generate a 3 copy *SMN2* mouse, the survival was extended to PND14-16 with some outlier longer lived mice (Michaud et al. 2010). This average survival is similar to the SMNΔ7 mice and is accompanied by severe muscle weakness and atrophy late in disease, motor neuron loss by PND13, abnormal EMG, and NMJ defects. These mice also exhibit respiratory deficiencies associated with reduced volume and frequency. Additional allelic series of mice have been generated harboring alterations in the *Smn* gene and *SMN* hybrid alleles to titrate SMN protein levels in mice (These mice can be found on the Jackson Laboratories web site http://jaxmice.jax.org/list/ra1733.html).

Successful generation of SMA mouse models was achieved through the loss of Smn protein using *Smn* null alleles in combination with transgenic expression of SMN from *SMN2* and other SMN transgenes. However, to simplify the genetics of modeling SMA in mice, it would be desirable to place both the gene loss and modifier expression in the same locus. The cosegregation of these two genetic events would allow for regulation of transcription and splicing in the endogenous genetic locus. The *Smn* C>T allele was engineered by introducing the *SMN2* exon 7 C>T mutation in the murine *Smn* gene. The *Smn* C>T mouse mimics the genetics of SMA patients, and recapitulates the splicing defect of *SMN2*, wherein exon 7 is skipped due to the C>T mutation. These mice exhibit reduced total *Smn* protein and a mild SMA phenotype characterized by hind limb weakness and inactivity consistent with type III SMA (Gladman et al. 2010). A second *Smn* C>T allele has been engineered (*Smn* C-T-Neo); however, this allele harbors the exon 7 C>T mutation with the neo cassette in intron 7 and additional sequences at the 5′ end of exon 8. The splicing pattern of this mouse allele is primarily exon 7 skipped transcripts, and as such, produces very low Smn protein levels leading to embryonic lethality. The *Smn* C-T-Neo mouse has been used as an inducible *Smn* allele as the low Smn protein levels can be increased by the removal of the neo cassette; however, this must be done early in embryonic development (E7.5) or the embryo will be resorbed (Hammond et al. 2010).

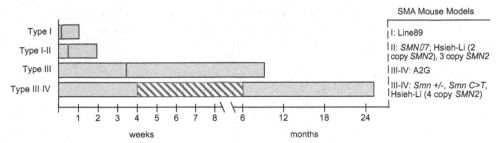

Fig. 1. SMA mouse models: survival and disease onset. Graphical representations of mean survivals of SMA mouse models types I-IV are shown by grey bars. Time scale is in weeks 0-8 and in months 6-24. A red line indicates the disease onset of SMA phenotype. For the mild SMA mouse models, a red-hashed box indicates variable onset in the listed SMA mouse models (i.e.: *Smn* +/- is 6 months, *Smn* C>T is 8 weeks, and Hsieh-Li (4 copy *SMN2*) has tail necrosis starting at 4 weeks)

Mutations in the mouse exon splicing enhancer for Tra2beta (2B) in exon 7 produces high levels of skipped transcripts in the absence of the C>T mutation (DiDonato et al. 2001). The mutation in the Tra2Beta enhancer is not associated with SMA mutations, and though it does induce exon 7 skipping, it does not recapitulate the splicing defect of *SMN2*. A mouse with the Tra2beta mutation in *Smn* (*Smn2B*-Neo) has low Smn protein levels that are associated with reduced size at two weeks, a lifespan of one month, and motor neuron loss late in disease progression (Bowerman et al. 2009; Bowerman et al. 2010). *Smn* alleles that genetically simplify and model SMA disease provide for evaluation of Smn protein reduction in SMA disease progression and can be used in evaluating therapeutic regimes for SMA. In choosing the appropriate mouse model to test therapeutics the survival and disease onset will be crucial considerations (graphically represented in Fig. 1).

4. Addressing the tissue specificity and timing of SMN expression in mouse models of SMA

The requirement for SMN expression in survival and motor neuron maintenance was evident in the genetic modelling of SMA in mice. However, the spatial and temporal requirement for SMN expression in tissues affected by SMA was not initially evaluated. To evaluate the requirement of SMN in specific tissues for SMA disease pathology, the deletion (Table 1) and expression of SMN in specific tissues (Table 2) has been tested in mice. An inducible *Smn* allele in which exon 7 is flanked by loxP sites (F7 allele) can replicate the loss of exon 7 (Frugier et al. 2000). This model has been utilized to knockout *Smn* exon 7 in a variety of tissues such as neurons, muscles, and liver by tissue specific Cre expression. The removal of exon 7 by Cre recombinase is irreversible and is associated with cell death in the target tissue being tested (Frugier et al. 2000; Cifuentes-Diaz et al. 2001; Vitte et al. 2004). The loss of full-length SMN through use of the inducible F7 *Smn* allele in neurons lead to neuronal cell death and mice exhibiting SMA pathology associated with motor neuron loss, whereas loss in muscle leads to a muscular dystrophy-like phenotype in the absence of motor neuron loss (Frugier et al. 2000; Cifuentes-Diaz et al. 2001). In an inverse experiment, increased expression of SMN was isolated to either neurons or muscle by tissue specific promoters in the severe Line89 mice. Rescue of the SMA phenotype was observed in neuronal expression of SMN whereas muscle expression did not rescue the SMA disease (Gavrilina et al. 2008). Together, these studies argue that the expression of SMN is a requirement for basic cellular maintenance and that SMN expression in neurons can rescue the SMA phenotype.

The targeted excision of *Smn* exon 7 (F7) can remove Smn protein rather than reduce the levels, as is seen in SMA patients. To recapitulate the reduced levels of SMN protein, the F7 targeted deletion was used in motor neuron progenitor cells in conjunction with low levels of SMN generated by two copies of the *SMN2* transgene. SMN reduction restricted to motor neuron precursors resulted in a mild SMA pathology, survival rate of 70% at one year, reduced weight and muscle mass, and central and peripheral nerve dysfunction. This study reports a direct effect of reduced SMN protein levels in motor neurons leading to SMA pathology in mice. The reduced severity of SMA may be explained by the presence of normal levels of SMN in other cell types, which would also have reduced SMN protein levels in SMA disease (Park et al. 2010).

The evaluation of SMA mouse models has elucidated changes that occur early and late in disease progression. Thus, the timing of SMN replacement in disease may alter the therapeutic benefit of SMN replacement for disease correction. This consideration has been addressed in severe SMA mouse models in both genetic and therapy based experiments. Most drug treatment regimes require early administration to allow for survival extension and improvement of phenotype in severe mouse models of SMA, including prenatal treatment for Line89 mice (Riessland et al. 2010). Gene therapy using scAAV9 SMN expression argues that early postnatal expression of SMN in motor neurons is required for survival extension, with the greatest success at PND1. However, the rescue observed by systemic delivery of the viral vector required transduction of motor neurons in the CNS (Foust et al. 2010; Valori et al. 2010; Dominguez et al. 2011). Accordingly, the inability to rescue survival at later time-points may be a result of limited access to the CNS by the maturation of the blood brain barrier. The use of RNA molecules that mediate splicing correction can extend survival when administered early postnatally as well (Baughan et al. 2009; Coady et al. 2010; Passini et al. 2010). The ability of each of these therapeutic modalities requires access to the CNS and motor neurons for effective therapeutic benefit in SMA mouse models.

The use of genetic models of induced SMN expression can bypass the limitation of other therapeutic strategies to determine the therapeutic window in SMA mouse models. Genetic induction of *Smn* from embryonic lethal *Smn* hypomorphic alleles can prevent early embryonic lethality when induced early in utero (E7.5) (Hammond et al. 2010). Recently, genetic induction of SMN expression using a high expressing doxycycline inducible SMN transgene showed similar survival extension in the severe SMNΔ7 mice, comparable to that of scAAV9 SMN treatment (Foust et al. 2010; Le et al. 2011). In the doxycycline inducible SMN model, induction in embryos (E13.5) had the greatest survival extension to over 200 days, whereas neonatally treated (PND0-3) SMNΔ7 mice survived 86 days. Interestingly, the removal of doxycycline (i.e.: SMN over-expression ceased) at weaning (28 days) did not lend to rapid decline or death, arguing that lower levels of SMN expression may be sufficient later in life (Le et al. 2011). Together, these data argue for the requirement of early postnatal expression of SMN for therapeutic benefit in severe SMA mouse models, and SMN expression in motor neurons is required for considerable increase in mean lifespan. A still unresolved question is whether the same timing of SMN replacement will be required for treatment in milder SMA mouse models, or if a later therapeutic window exists. Some evidence offers that late treatment in mild SMA may be beneficial as the use of ASOs that correct *SMN2* splicing in the Hsieh-Li (4 copy *SMN2*) mouse can reduce tail necrosis seen in these mice (Hua et al. 2010).

Genotype	Phenotype and Notes	Shorthand	References
Smn-/-; *SMN2(89Ahmb)+/+;* *PrP92-SMN+/+*	SMN expression in neurons under the prion promoter (PrP) recues disease in Line89 mice.	Neuronal SMN	Gavrillina 2008
Smn-/-; *SMN2(89Ahmb)+/+;* *HAS63-SMN+/+*	SMN expression in muscle under the human skeletal actin (HAS) promoter does not rescue SMA disease in Line89 mice. Leaky expression in neurons can afford moderate rescue in Line89 mice.	Muscle SMN	Gavrillina 2008
Smn-/-; *SMN2(89Ahmb)+/+;* *SMNΔ7+/+;* *ROSA26rtTA+/+;* *Luci-TRE-SMN+/+*	Induction of SMN expression by doxycycline within 3 days. Embryonic (E13) and PND0 treatment extend survival, mean 100 days but can extend to 200 days, and corrects NMJ defects. Removal of doxycycline at 28 days exhibits continued survival and rescue of NMJ defects.	Doxycycline Inducible SMN	Le 2011
SmnC-T-Neo/C-T-Neo;CreEsr1 and Smn2B-Neo/2B-Neo;CreEsr1	Tamoxifen induced Cre-mediated excision of the neomycin cassette alters the hypomorphic *C-T-Neo* and *2B-Neo* alleles from ~5% SMN to ~30% and 16%, respectively. Early (E7.5) tamoxifen treatment can rescue to embryonic lethality and resorption of the *C-T-Neo* mouse early in embryonic development, though the ability to rescue animals to birth has not been shown.	Inducible *Smn* hypomorphic alleles	Hammond 2011
Smn +/+; Tg SMN2; CreERT2	Inducible SMN expression is under control of tamoxifen inducible Cre (CreERT2). Tamoxifen administration in embryonic (E13.5), neonatal (PND1.5), and weanling (4 week old) mice induces SMN expression. Ability to rescue survival has not yet assessed in SMA mouse models.	Tamoxifen Inducible SMN	Bebee 2011

Table 2. Inducible SMN mouse models

5. SMN snRNP function and splicing in SMA mouse models

The best-characterized function of SMN is the maturation of the core snRNPs required for splicing (Fig. 2). To test the effect of reduced SMN levels on snRNP assembly in SMA, the maturation of both major (U2) and minor (U12) snRNPs were assessed in severe Line 89 mice. In these severe mice, the reduction of SMN protein correlated with reduced maturation of a subset of snRNPs, especially the minor spliceosomal pathway U11 and U12 snRNPs (Gabanella et al. 2007). In the SMNΔ7 mice, reduced U4 snRNP maturation was also reduced in the brain and kidney. The relative levels of snRNAs in the SMNΔ7 mice were altered in disease progression, with the minor spliceosome again showing the greatest reduction at PND11 in the SMA mouse models (Zhang et al. 2008). To genetically evaluate perturbations of snRNP assembly in SMA disease, a transgene of the mild SMA mutation in *SMN1* (A111G) was expressed in Line89 mice. Expression of the A111G transgene extended survival to a normal lifespan with no observable phenotype, though the A111G mice showed signs of muscle hypertrophy in the gastrocnemius at 10 months of age. The survival extension was *SMN2* dependent as A111G failed to rescue the *Smn* -/- mice alone, arguing

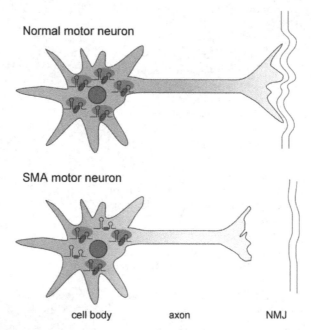

Fig. 2. SMN function in motor neurons. Normal and SMA motor neurons are depicted with blue shading corresponding to SMN protein levels. The SMN complex (blue oval) loads the Sm core (red circle) onto the Sm site (red box) of U snRNAs. In normal motor neurons sufficient SMN is present to form the mature U snRNPs, whereas SMA motor neurons lack sufficient SMN to mature all U snRNAs. Reduced SMN leads to motor neuron loss and dysfunction, which can be seen by immaturity of the NMJ and eventual loss of motor neurons by retraction of the axonal processes and cell death. While U snRNP maturation is the primary function of SMN, other functions of SMN in the axon or at the NMJ may still contribute to SMA pathology

for intragenic complementation between the SMN from *SMN2* and the mutant A111G SMN protein. Analysis of snRNP assembly in the severe Line89 mice also showed reduced U4 and minor spliceosomal snRNP maturation that was subsequently rescued by the expression of the A111G transgene (Workman et al. 2009).

The impact of SMN reduction in mice leads to reduced maturation and relative levels of snRNAs during SMA disease progression. The impact of the alteration in the maturation of the core splicing machinery on splicing in SMA disease was addressed in the severe mouse models of SMA at early and late stage disease. Evaluation of SMNΔ7 mice prior to disease (PND1) and early in disease (PND7) did not show differences in splicing, but later in disease progression (PND11 and 13), global splicing changes were observed using a splicing sensitive microarray (Zhang et al. 2008; Baumer et al. 2009). Major changes in splicing of neuronal and cellular damage genes were observed (Baumer et al. 2009). In the more severe Line89 mice, gene expression analysis in PND1 mice did not show major expression changes in the presymptomatic mice. However, genes involved in extracellular matrix, myelination, and cellular growth factors showed major changes in late disease progression at PND5 (Murray et al. 2010). These observations set SMA as a global splicing disease late in disease progression, which may account either for the effect of cellular stress on global splicing or a global alteration in snRNPs that contribute to disease in mouse models of SMA. While the importance of SMN protein in other non-snRNP associated neuronal functions in still under evaluation, it is clear that the reduction of SMN directly correlates with reduced maturation of snRNPs. As *SMN2* is itself improperly spliced, the potential for reduced exon 7 inclusion when SMN is low was evaluated using in vitro splicing assays. Extracts prepared from cells expressing low levels of SMN reduced inclusion of *SMN* exon 7, implicating a negative feedback loop effect of low SMN protein levels on exon 7 inclusion. This could be associated with the weak definition of exon 7, making the *SMN* transcript more susceptible to low levels of mature snRNPs required for canonical splicing (Jodelka et al. 2010).

6. Neurological manifestations in SMA mouse models

SMA is a disease of motor neurons, and as such mouse models of SMA have been evaluated for both the loss of motor neurons in the development of SMA disease, as well as other neurological manifestations in the SMA mouse models. Neuronal evaluation of the SMA mouse models has uncovered the timing of motor neuron loss and populations of neurons affected in the SMA mice. The neurological manifestations and major findings in the SMA mouse models have been outlined below.

The loss of motor neurons in SMA as observed in SMA patients was the first neuronal cell types evaluated in models of SMA mice. Histological analyses of motor neuron populations in the spinal cord of SMA mouse models have demonstrated that the loss of motor neurons is also seen during the progression of the disease in mice. Surprisingly, the loss of motor neurons in the spinal cord is a late marker of disease, occurring after a motor deficit is already observed and late in disease progression (Hsieh-Li et al. 2000; Jablonka et al. 2000; Monani et al. 2000; Monani et al. 2003; Le et al. 2005; Avila et al. 2007; Kariya et al. 2008; Bowerman et al. 2009; Michaud et al. 2010; Park et al. 2010; Riessland et al. 2010). The development of motor neurons was thus further analysed in the most severe mice (Line 89) during embryonic and neonatal development. In the Line89 mice the neuronal pathfinding and development of motor neurons appears normal in this SMA mouse model, although some abnormal axonal swelling were more pronounced in the SMA mouse model compared to control littermates (McGovern et al. 2008). The presence of motor function deficits in the SMA mouse models prior to motor neuron loss raised the question of whether motor neuron function was compromised. To evaluate the function of the motor neurons, both anatomical and electrophysiological analyses have been performed in severe and mild SMA mouse models. In severe and mild models of SMA, accumulation of neurofilament in the presynaptic termini of motor neurons, disorganization of the postsynaptic NMJ, reduced synaptic vesicle release, and motor neuron sprouting have been reported (Cifuentes-Diaz et al. 2001; Monani et al. 2003; Kariya et al. 2008; McGovern et al. 2008; Murray et al. 2008; Kong et al. 2009; Ling et al. 2010; Michaud et al. 2010; Park et al. 2010; Lee et al. 2011). The changes at the NMJ are also associated with expression of immature isoforms of both the acetylcholine receptor (AChR) and myosin heavy chain (MyHC) (Kariya et al. 2008; Lee et al. 2011). The loss of motor neurons and changes in expression of genes involved in myelination, growth factor signalling, and extracellular matrix are associated with late stage of disease in SMA mouse models (Murray et al. 2010). The susceptibility of motor neurons holds true from mouse to human, in addition the susceptibility can also differ in subpopulations of motor neurons in a single muscle such as the levator auris longus (LAL) muscle (Murray et al. 2008; Murray et al. 2010; Ruiz et al. 2010).

The defects observed in motor neuron function followed by loss of motor neurons late in disease raised the question of whether other neuronal populations were affected in the SMA mouse models. Defects in sensory neurons have been reported in SMA patients (Rudnik-Schoneborn et al. 2003), and the 3 copy *SMN2* mouse also exhibited latency in response to heat (Michaud et al. 2010). The potential for sensory neuron malfunction in SMA was further evaluated in the SMNΔ7 mouse model. A reduction in the input of sensory neurons to the motor neurons of the spinal cord as well as perturbation of the neuronal circuitry was evident as early as PND4 in the SMNΔ7 mice (Ling et al. 2010; Mentis et al. 2011). Furthermore, the reduction of sensory input into lumbar motor neurons was also observed in the Olig2-Cre mouse even when the sensory neurons did not have reduced SMN protein (Park et al. 2010). The reduction of SMN protein also has consequences for neuronal growth and development as evidenced by reduced neuronal numbers in the brain and eye of severe SMA mouse models Line89 and *Smn* 2B (Liu et al. 2010; Wishart et al. 2010). The modelling of SMA in mice have recapitulated the motor neuron loss as is seen in SMA patients, as well as identified neuronal populations affected by reduced SMN levels in the SMA mouse models.

7. Cardiac and pulmonary involvement

Reports of cardiac defects including congenital heart defects, bradycardia, left ventricular cardiomyopathy, and sympathetic-vagal imbalance have recently been reported in severe SMA mouse models (Bevan et al. 2010; Heier et al. 2010; Shababi et al. 2010). Evaluation of 63 severe SMA type I patients reported that 24% presented with severe bradycardia (Bach 2007). In the severe SMNΔ7 mouse model bradycardia was also present due to reduced autonomic innervation, and in turn increased vagal tone. Anatomical analysis of SMNΔ7 mice hearts was positive for dilated cardiomyopathy and reduced contractile function (Bevan et al. 2010; Heier et al. 2010). Therapies aimed at increasing SMN protein by treatment with scAAV9 SMN or TSA were able to improve heart function and survival in the treated SMNΔ7 mice (Bevan et al. 2010; Heier et al. 2010). A third group reported congenital defects present in the severe Line89 mice in the left ventricular septum and wall, but these abnormalities were not observed in the SMNΔ7 mice. However, fibrotic deposition and oxidative stress markers accumulated in the SMNΔ7 heart as disease progressed (Shababi et al. 2010). The collective effect of changes in the heart of SMA models decreases the functional output and implicates additional neuronal targets by way of autonomic neuronal dysfunction in SMA mouse models. As cardiac involvement has not been reported in most severe SMA patients, further analysis of patients to identify cardiac defects will be required to determine if cardiac treatment is a consideration for SMA patients.

Respiratory complications are common during SMA disease progression and are often associated with mortality in severe SMA. Long-term respiratory treatment is often requirement in both severe and mild SMA patients. The 3 copy *SMN2* mice appear normal at PND1 but have reduced numbers of innervated NMJ in the diaphragm at PND9, associated with reduced respiratory capacity starting at PND7 (Michaud et al. 2010). Similar structural defects at the NMJ in the diaphragm of SMA type I patients have also been reported (Kariya et al. 2008). Analysis of the most severe SMA mouse model (Line89) from E10.5 to PND2 for motor neuron developmental defects showed the diaphragm was not affected; however, intercostal muscle denervation was observed (Kariya et al. 2008; McGovern et al. 2008). The defects in motor neurons of the diaphragm and intercostal muscles may account for respiratory deficiency in mouse models of SMA, and may be a point of therapeutic intervention in SMA patients.

8. Therapeutic approaches in SMA treatment

The severity of SMA is directly associated with low SMN protein levels, thus the reintroduction of SMN would predict correction of the disease. The presence of *SMN2* in all SMA patients provides for a direct therapeutic target to increase SMN levels. Therapeutic approaches for increasing transcriptional activity of *SMN2*, splicing correction of *SMN2* exon 7, or stability of SMN protein are major considerations in development of SMA therapies. Additionally, increasing SMN levels by gene therapy or treating the disease pathology in an SMN independent manner are alternative approaches in SMA therapeutic development. Mouse models of SMA have enabled the evaluation of these therapeutic approaches in pre-clinical therapeutic regimes for treatment of SMA.

Small molecules or drugs were the first therapies evaluated for treatment of SMA in mouse models of SMA. Many of the initial drugs are FDA approved drugs and transcriptional activators, histone deacetylase (HDAC) inhibitors. These drugs increased SMN levels by transcriptional activity, splicing of *SMN2* exon 7, and/or SMN protein stability (Chang et al. 2001; Avila et al. 2007; Mattis et al. 2008; Narver et al. 2008; Tsai et al. 2008; Riessland et al. 2010; Mentis et al. 2011). Additional drugs have been used that target increased stability of SMN, read through of *SMN2* transcripts, incorporation of *SMN2* exon 7, as well as second-generation drugs that work via multiple mechanisms (Garbes et al. 2009; Hastings et al. 2009; Butchbach et al. 2010). These drugs improved SMN protein levels and SMA phenotype, and often the extension of survival observed in treatment of severe SMA mouse models was 30%. However, in current clinical trials in SMA patients, these therapies have proven ineffectual (Chen et al. 2010).

Drug correction of *SMN2* splicing underscores the importance of targeting the correction of *SMN2* splicing as a mode for increased SMN expression. The use of RNA based therapies aimed at increasing exon 7 inclusion can be achieved by sequestering a negatively acting sequence in the pre-mRNA and preventing it negative function (Singh et al. 2006; Hua et al. 2007; Williams et al. 2009; Hua et al. 2010; Passini et al. 2010), recruiting positively acting splicing factors to exon 7 (Baughan et al. 2009; Meyer et al. 2009; Voigt et al. 2010), blocking exon 8 inclusion (Dickson et al. 2008), or providing an RNA substrate used in the splicing reaction (trans-splicing) (Coady et al. 2010). These techniques have successfully increased exon 7 inclusion and SMN levels, and have improved survival and phenotype in SMA mouse models.

To reintroduce SMN, viral gene therapies that encode SMN can correct disease if SMN is expressed in the appropriate tissues and cell types. Self-complimentary adeno-associated virus serotype 9 (scAAV9) can transduce motor neurons in mice when administered early postnatally, and the expression of SMN in motor neurons can reduce disease pathology, as well as extend survival in the SMNΔ7 mouse model (Foust et al. 2010; Valori et al. 2010; Dominguez et al. 2011). The requirement for early expression of SMN using scAAV9 argues that SMN is required early postnatally for disease correction. However, the ability of the viral treatment to reach the spinal cord and motor neurons was reduced after PND5. The early therapeutic window outlined by scAAV9 treatment likely represents a limitation of viral gene therapy, and does not necessarily reflect the therapeutic window for SMN replacement.

Most SMA patients present with disease after motor neuron loss and motor function has already occurred. Treatment of the disease pathology may afford therapeutic intervention even in the absence of altering SMN levels. Cell based therapies to replace the lost motor neurons have initially been tested by transplanting normal cells that were programmed to mature into motor neurons. These cells were injected in the spinal cord, engrafted in the spinal cord, and can improve function and survival in the SMNΔ7 mice (Corti et al. 2008). Furthermore, increasing muscle mass by inhibiting myostatin with the antagonist follistatin can reduce muscle loss and improve function and survival, though transgenic overexpression of follistatin in SMNΔ7 mice failed to improve the survival of the mice (Rose et al. 2009; Sumner et al. 2009). As therapeutic development for SMA continues, the use of SMA mouse models will continue to be instrumental in pre-clinical testing of therapies for SMA.

9. Summary and conclusion

The modeling of SMA in mice has successfully recapitulated many components of SMA pathology associated with reduced levels of SMN protein. The use of these SMA mouse models has proven invaluable in further understanding the etiology of SMA disease, uncovering the neurological manifestations of SMA disease, and the importance of when and where SMN expression is required for correction of SMA pathology in mice. The use of mouse models of SMA to determine the pathological manifestations in SMA and testing therapeutic approaches continues as the need for therapies for this devastating disease remains.

10. Acknowledgements

This work was funded by the Association Francaise Contre les Myopathies (AFM) (14278 to D.S.C.) and by student fellowships from the Research Institute at Nationwide Children's Hospital and the Jeffrey J. Seilhamer Cancer Foundation (T.W.B.). We would like to thank Casey Gentis for editorial support in submission of this work.

11. References

Avila, A. M., B. G. Burnett, A. A. Taye, F. Gabanella, M. A. Knight, P. Hartenstein, Z. Cizman, N. A. Di Prospero, L. Pellizzoni, K. H. Fischbeck and C. J. Sumner (2007). "Trichostatin A increases SMN expression and survival in a mouse model of spinal muscular atrophy." *The Journal of clinical investigation* 117(3): 659-671.

Bach, J. R. (2007). "Medical considerations of long-term survival of Werdnig-Hoffmann disease." *American journal of physical medicine & rehabilitation / Association of Academic Physiatrists* 86(5): 349-355.

Bach, J. R., J. Vega, J. Majors and A. Friedman (2003). "Spinal muscular atrophy type 1 quality of life." *American journal of physical medicine & rehabilitation / Association of Academic Physiatrists* 82(2): 137-142.

Baughan, T. D., A. Dickson, E. Y. Osman and C. L. Lorson (2009). "Delivery of bifunctional RNAs that target an intronic repressor and increase SMN levels in an animal model of spinal muscular atrophy." *Human molecular genetics* 18(9): 1600-1611.

Baumer, D., S. Lee, G. Nicholson, J. L. Davies, N. J. Parkinson, L. M. Murray, T. H. Gillingwater, O. Ansorge, K. E. Davies and K. Talbot (2009). "Alternative splicing events are a late feature of pathology in a mouse model of spinal muscular atrophy." *PLoS genetics* 5(12): e1000773.

Bebee, T. W., J. T. Gladman and D. S. Chandler (2010). "Splicing regulation of the survival motor neuron genes and implications for treatment of spinal muscular atrophy." *Front Biosci* 15: 1191-1204.

Bergin, A., G. Kim, D. L. Price, S. S. Sisodia, M. K. Lee and B. A. Rabin (1997). "Identification and characterization of a mouse homologue of the spinal muscular atrophy-determining gene, survival motor neuron." *Gene* 204(1-2): 47-53.

Bevan, A. K., K. R. Hutchinson, K. D. Foust, L. Braun, V. L. McGovern, L. Schmelzer, J. G. Ward, J. C. Petruska, P. A. Lucchesi, A. H. Burghes and B. K. Kaspar (2010). "Early heart failure in the SMNDelta7 model of spinal muscular atrophy and correction by postnatal scAAV9-SMN delivery." *Human molecular genetics* 19(20): 3895-3905.

Bowerman, M., C. L. Anderson, A. Beauvais, P. P. Boyl, W. Witke and R. Kothary (2009). "SMN, profilin IIa and plastin 3: a link between the deregulation of actin dynamics and SMA pathogenesis." *Molecular and cellular neurosciences* 42(1): 66-74.

Bowerman, M., A. Beauvais, C. L. Anderson and R. Kothary (2010). "Rho-kinase inactivation prolongs survival of an intermediate SMA mouse model." *Human molecular genetics* 19(8): 1468-1478.

Burnett, B. G., T. O. Crawford and C. J. Sumner (2009). "Emerging treatment options for spinal muscular atrophy." *Current treatment options in neurology* 11(2): 90-101.

Butchbach, M. E., J. Singh, M. Thorsteinsdottir, L. Saieva, E. Slominski, J. Thurmond, T. Andresson, J. Zhang, J. D. Edwards, L. R. Simard, L. Pellizzoni, J. Jarecki, A. H. Burghes and M. E. Gurney (2010). "Effects of 2,4-diaminoquinazoline derivatives on SMN expression and phenotype in a mouse model for spinal muscular atrophy." *Hum Mol Genet* 19(3): 454-467.

Cartegni, L., M. L. Hastings, J. A. Calarco, E. de Stanchina and A. R. Krainer (2006). "Determinants of exon 7 splicing in the spinal muscular atrophy genes, SMN1 and SMN2." *Am J Hum Genet* 78(1): 63-77.

Cartegni, L. and A. R. Krainer (2002). "Disruption of an SF2/ASF-dependent exonic splicing enhancer in SMN2 causes spinal muscular atrophy in the absence of SMN1." *Nat Genet* 30(4): 377-384.

Chang, J. G., H. M. Hsieh-Li, Y. J. Jong, N. M. Wang, C. H. Tsai and H. Li (2001). "Treatment of spinal muscular atrophy by sodium butyrate." *Proceedings of the National Academy of Sciences of the United States of America* 98(17): 9808-9813.

Chen, T. H., J. G. Chang, Y. H. Yang, H. H. Mai, W. C. Liang, Y. C. Wu, H. Y. Wang, Y. B. Huang, S. M. Wu, Y. C. Chen, S. N. Yang and Y. J. Jong (2010). "Randomized, double-blind, placebo-controlled trial of hydroxyurea in spinal muscular atrophy." *Neurology* 75(24): 2190-2197.

Cho, S. and G. Dreyfuss (2010). "A degron created by SMN2 exon 7 skipping is a principal contributor to spinal muscular atrophy severity." *Genes & development* 24(5): 438-442.

Cifuentes-Diaz, C., T. Frugier, F. D. Tiziano, E. Lacene, N. Roblot, V. Joshi, M. H. Moreau and J. Melki (2001). "Deletion of murine SMN exon 7 directed to skeletal muscle leads to severe muscular dystrophy." *The Journal of cell biology* 152(5): 1107-1114.

Cifuentes-Diaz, C., T. Frugier, F. D. Tiziano, E. Lacene, N. Roblot, V. Joshi, M. H. Moreau and J. Melki (2001). "Deletion of murine SMN exon 7 directed to skeletal muscle leads to severe muscular dystrophy." *J Cell Biol* 152(5): 1107-1114.

Coady, T. H. and C. L. Lorson (2010). "Trans-splicing-mediated improvement in a severe mouse model of spinal muscular atrophy." *J Neurosci* 30(1): 126-130.

Corti, S., M. Nizzardo, M. Nardini, C. Donadoni, S. Salani, D. Ronchi, F. Saladino, A. Bordoni, F. Fortunato, R. Del Bo, D. Papadimitriou, F. Locatelli, G. Menozzi, S. Strazzer, N. Bresolin and G. P. Comi (2008). "Neural stem cell transplantation can ameliorate the phenotype of a mouse model of spinal muscular atrophy." *The Journal of clinical investigation* 118(10): 3316-3330.

Dickson, A., E. Osman and C. L. Lorson (2008). "A negatively acting bifunctional RNA increases survival motor neuron both in vitro and in vivo." *Human gene therapy* 19(11): 1307-1315.

DiDonato, C. J., C. L. Lorson, Y. De Repentigny, L. Simard, C. Chartrand, E. J. Androphy and R. Kothary (2001). "Regulation of murine survival motor neuron (Smn) protein levels by modifying Smn exon 7 splicing." *Human molecular genetics* 10(23): 2727-2736.

Dominguez, E., T. Marais, N. Chatauret, S. Benkhelifa-Ziyyat, S. Duque, P. Ravassard, R. Carcenac, S. Astord, A. Pereira de Moura, T. Voit and M. Barkats (2011). "Intravenous scAAV9 delivery of a codon-optimized SMN1 sequence rescues SMA mice." *Human molecular genetics* 20(4): 681-693.

Fischer, U., Q. Liu and G. Dreyfuss (1997). "The SMN-SIP1 complex has an essential role in spliceosomal snRNP biogenesis." *Cell* 90(6): 1023-1029.

Foust, K. D., X. Wang, V. L. McGovern, L. Braun, A. K. Bevan, A. M. Haidet, T. T. Le, P. R. Morales, M. M. Rich, A. H. Burghes and B. K. Kaspar (2010). "Rescue of the spinal muscular atrophy phenotype in a mouse model by early postnatal delivery of SMN." *Nat Biotechnol* 28(3): 271-274.

Frugier, T., F. D. Tiziano, C. Cifuentes-Diaz, P. Miniou, N. Roblot, A. Dierich, M. Le Meur and J. Melki (2000). "Nuclear targeting defect of SMN lacking the C-terminus in a mouse model of spinal muscular atrophy." *Human molecular genetics* 9(5): 849-858.

Gabanella, F., M. E. Butchbach, L. Saieva, C. Carissimi, A. H. Burghes and L. Pellizzoni (2007). "Ribonucleoprotein Assembly Defects Correlate with Spinal Muscular Atrophy Severity and Preferentially Affect a Subset of Spliceosomal snRNPs." *PLoS ONE* 2(9): e921.

Garbes, L., M. Riessland, I. Holker, R. Heller, J. Hauke, C. Trankle, R. Coras, I. Blumcke, E. Hahnen and B. Wirth (2009). "LBH589 induces up to 10-fold SMN protein levels by several independent mechanisms and is effective even in cells from SMA patients non-responsive to valproate." *Human molecular genetics* 18(19): 3645-3658.

Gavrilina, T. O., V. L. McGovern, E. Workman, T. O. Crawford, R. G. Gogliotti, C. J. DiDonato, U. R. Monani, G. E. Morris and A. H. Burghes (2008). "Neuronal SMN expression corrects spinal muscular atrophy in severe SMA mice while muscle-specific SMN expression has no phenotypic effect." *Hum Mol Genet* 17(8): 1063-1075.

Gladman, J. T., T. W. Bebee, C. Edwards, X. Wang, Z. Sahenk, M. M. Rich and D. S. Chandler (2010). "A humanized Smn gene containing the SMN2 nucleotide alteration in exon 7 mimics SMN2 splicing and the SMA disease phenotype." *Human molecular genetics* 19(21): 4239-4252.

Hammond, S. M., R. G. Gogliotti, V. Rao, A. Beauvais, R. Kothary and C. J. DiDonato (2010). "Mouse survival motor neuron alleles that mimic SMN2 splicing and are inducible rescue embryonic lethality early in development but not late." *PLoS ONE* 5(12): e15887.

Hastings, M. L., J. Berniac, Y. H. Liu, P. Abato, F. M. Jodelka, L. Barthel, S. Kumar, C. Dudley, M. Nelson, K. Larson, J. Edmonds, T. Bowser, M. Draper, P. Higgins and A. R. Krainer (2009). "Tetracyclines that promote SMN2 exon 7 splicing as therapeutics for spinal muscular atrophy." *Sci Transl Med* 1(5): 5ra12.

Heier, C. R., R. Satta, C. Lutz and C. J. DiDonato (2010). "Arrhythmia and cardiac defects are a feature of spinal muscular atrophy model mice." *Human molecular genetics* 19(20): 3906-3918.

Hsieh-Li, H. M., J. G. Chang, Y. J. Jong, M. H. Wu, N. M. Wang, C. H. Tsai and H. Li (2000). "A mouse model for spinal muscular atrophy." *Nat Genet* 24(1): 66-70.

Hua, Y., K. Sahashi, G. Hung, F. Rigo, M. A. Passini, C. F. Bennett and A. R. Krainer (2010). "Antisense correction of SMN2 splicing in the CNS rescues necrosis in a type III SMA mouse model." *Genes Dev* 24(15): 1634-1644.

Hua, Y., K. Sahashi, G. Hung, F. Rigo, M. A. Passini, C. F. Bennett and A. R. Krainer (2010). "Antisense correction of SMN2 splicing in the CNS rescues necrosis in a type III SMA mouse model." *Genes & development* 24(15): 1634-1644.

Hua, Y., T. A. Vickers, B. F. Baker, C. F. Bennett and A. R. Krainer (2007). "Enhancement of SMN2 exon 7 inclusion by antisense oligonucleotides targeting the exon." *PLoS biology* 5(4): e73.

Jablonka, S., B. Schrank, M. Kralewski, W. Rossoll and M. Sendtner (2000). "Reduced survival motor neuron (Smn) gene dose in mice leads to motor neuron degeneration: an animal model for spinal muscular atrophy type III." *Hum Mol Genet* 9(3): 341-346.

Jodelka, F. M., A. D. Ebert, D. M. Duelli and M. L. Hastings (2010). "A feedback loop regulates splicing of the spinal muscular atrophy-modifying gene, SMN2." *Human molecular genetics* 19(24): 4906-4917.

Kariya, S., G. H. Park, Y. Maeno-Hikichi, O. Leykekhman, C. Lutz, M. S. Arkovitz, L. T. Landmesser and U. R. Monani (2008). "Reduced SMN protein impairs maturation of the neuromuscular junctions in mouse models of spinal muscular atrophy." *Human molecular genetics* 17(16): 2552-2569.

Kashima, T. and J. L. Manley (2003). "A negative element in SMN2 exon 7 inhibits splicing in spinal muscular atrophy." *Nat Genet* 34(4): 460-463.

Kashima, T., N. Rao, C. J. David and J. L. Manley (2007). "hnRNP A1 functions with specificity in repression of SMN2 exon 7 splicing." *Human molecular genetics* 16(24): 3149-3159.

Kong, L., X. Wang, D. W. Choe, M. Polley, B. G. Burnett, M. Bosch-Marce, J. W. Griffin, M. M. Rich and C. J. Sumner (2009). "Impaired synaptic vesicle release and immaturity of neuromuscular junctions in spinal muscular atrophy mice." *The Journal of neuroscience : the official journal of the Society for Neuroscience* 29(3): 842-851.

Le, T. T., V. L. McGovern, I. E. Alwine, X. Wang, A. Massoni-Laporte, M. M. Rich and A. H. Burghes (2011). "Temporal requirement for high SMN expression in SMA mice." *Human molecular genetics*.

Le, T. T., L. T. Pham, M. E. Butchbach, H. L. Zhang, U. R. Monani, D. D. Coovert, T. O. Gavrilina, L. Xing, G. J. Bassell and A. H. Burghes (2005). "SMNDelta7, the major product of the centromeric survival motor neuron (SMN2) gene, extends survival in mice with spinal muscular atrophy and associates with full-length SMN." *Hum Mol Genet* 14(6): 845-857.

Lee, Y. I., M. Mikesh, I. Smith, M. Rimer and W. Thompson (2011). "Muscles in a mouse model of spinal muscular atrophy show profound defects in neuromuscular development even in the absence of failure in neuromuscular transmission or loss of motor neurons." *Developmental biology* 356(2): 432-444.

Lefebvre, S., L. Burglen, S. Reboullet, O. Clermont, P. Burlet, L. Viollet, B. Benichou, C. Cruaud, P. Millasseau, M. Zeviani and et al. (1995). "Identification and characterization of a spinal muscular atrophy-determining gene." *Cell* 80(1): 155-165.

Lefebvre, S., P. Burlet, Q. Liu, S. Bertrandy, O. Clermont, A. Munnich, G. Dreyfuss and J. Melki (1997). "Correlation between severity and SMN protein level in spinal muscular atrophy." *Nat Genet* 16(3): 265-269.

Ling, K. K., M. Y. Lin, B. Zingg, Z. Feng and C. P. Ko (2010). "Synaptic defects in the spinal and neuromuscular circuitry in a mouse model of spinal muscular atrophy." *PLoS ONE* 5(11): e15457.

Liu, H., D. Shafey, J. N. Moores and R. Kothary (2010). "Neurodevelopmental consequences of Smn depletion in a mouse model of spinal muscular atrophy." *J Neurosci Res* 88(1): 111-122.

Liu, Q., U. Fischer, F. Wang and G. Dreyfuss (1997). "The spinal muscular atrophy disease gene product, SMN, and its associated protein SIP1 are in a complex with spliceosomal snRNP proteins." *Cell* 90(6): 1013-1021.

Lorson, C. L. and E. J. Androphy (2000). "An exonic enhancer is required for inclusion of an essential exon in the SMA-determining gene SMN." *Human molecular genetics* 9(2): 259-265.

Lorson, C. L., E. Hahnen, E. J. Androphy and B. Wirth (1999). "A single nucleotide in the SMN gene regulates splicing and is responsible for spinal muscular atrophy." *Proceedings of the National Academy of Sciences of the United States of America* 96(11): 6307-6311.

Mattis, V. B., M. E. Butchbach and C. L. Lorson (2008). "Detection of human survival motor neuron (SMN) protein in mice containing the SMN2 transgene: applicability to preclinical therapy development for spinal muscular atrophy." *J Neurosci Methods* 175(1): 36-43.

McAndrew, P. E., D. W. Parsons, L. R. Simard, C. Rochette, P. N. Ray, J. R. Mendell, T. W. Prior and A. H. Burghes (1997). "Identification of proximal spinal muscular atrophy carriers and patients by analysis of SMNT and SMNC gene copy number." *Am J Hum Genet* 60(6): 1411-1422.

McGovern, V. L., T. O. Gavrilina, C. E. Beattie and A. H. Burghes (2008). "Embryonic motor axon development in the severe SMA mouse." *Hum Mol Genet* 17(18): 2900-2909.

Meister, G., D. Buhler, R. Pillai, F. Lottspeich and U. Fischer (2001). "A multiprotein complex mediates the ATP-dependent assembly of spliceosomal U snRNPs." *Nature cell biology* 3(11): 945-949.

Mentis, G. Z., D. Blivis, W. Liu, E. Drobac, M. E. Crowder, L. Kong, F. J. Alvarez, C. J. Sumner and M. J. O'Donovan (2011). "Early functional impairment of sensory-motor connectivity in a mouse model of spinal muscular atrophy." *Neuron* 69(3): 453-467.

Meyer, K., J. Marquis, J. Trub, R. Nlend Nlend, S. Verp, M. D. Ruepp, H. Imboden, I. Barde, D. Trono and D. Schumperli (2009). "Rescue of a severe mouse model for spinal muscular atrophy by U7 snRNA-mediated splicing modulation." *Human molecular genetics* 18(3): 546-555.

Michaud, M., T. Arnoux, S. Bielli, E. Durand, Y. Rotrou, S. Jablonka, F. Robert, M. Giraudon-Paoli, M. Riessland, M. G. Mattei, E. Andriambeloson, B. Wirth, M. Sendtner, J. Gallego, R. M. Pruss and T. Bordet (2010). "Neuromuscular defects and breathing disorders in a new mouse model of spinal muscular atrophy." *Neurobiology of disease* 38(1): 125-135.

Monani, U. R., M. T. Pastore, T. O. Gavrilina, S. Jablonka, T. T. Le, C. Andreassi, J. M. DiCocco, C. Lorson, E. J. Androphy, M. Sendtner, M. Podell and A. H. Burghes (2003). "A transgene carrying an A2G missense mutation in the SMN gene modulates phenotypic severity in mice with severe (type I) spinal muscular atrophy." *J Cell Biol* 160(1): 41-52.

Monani, U. R., M. Sendtner, D. D. Coovert, D. W. Parsons, C. Andreassi, T. T. Le, S. Jablonka, B. Schrank, W. Rossoll, T. W. Prior, G. E. Morris and A. H. Burghes (2000). "The human centromeric survival motor neuron gene (SMN2) rescues embryonic lethality in Smn(-/-) mice and results in a mouse with spinal muscular atrophy." *Hum Mol Genet* 9(3): 333-339.

Murray, L. M., L. H. Comley, D. Thomson, N. Parkinson, K. Talbot and T. H. Gillingwater (2008). "Selective vulnerability of motor neurons and dissociation of pre- and post-synaptic pathology at the neuromuscular junction in mouse models of spinal muscular atrophy." *Human molecular genetics* 17(7): 949-962.

Murray, L. M., S. Lee, D. Baumer, S. H. Parson, K. Talbot and T. H. Gillingwater (2010). "Pre-symptomatic development of lower motor neuron connectivity in a mouse model of severe spinal muscular atrophy." *Human molecular genetics* 19(3): 420-433.

Narver, H. L., L. Kong, B. G. Burnett, D. W. Choe, M. Bosch-Marce, A. A. Taye, M. A. Eckhaus and C. J. Sumner (2008). "Sustained improvement of spinal muscular atrophy mice treated with trichostatin A plus nutrition." *Annals of neurology* 64(4): 465-470.

Park, G. H., Y. Maeno-Hikichi, T. Awano, L. T. Landmesser and U. R. Monani (2010). "Reduced survival of motor neuron (SMN) protein in motor neuronal progenitors functions cell autonomously to cause spinal muscular atrophy in model mice expressing the human centromeric (SMN2) gene." *The Journal of neuroscience : the official journal of the Society for Neuroscience* 30(36): 12005-12019.

Park, G. H., Y. Maeno-Hikichi, T. Awano, L. T. Landmesser and U. R. Monani (2010). "Reduced survival of motor neuron (SMN) protein in motor neuronal progenitors functions cell autonomously to cause spinal muscular atrophy in model mice expressing the human centromeric (SMN2) gene." *J Neurosci* 30(36): 12005-12019.

Passini, M. A., J. Bu, E. M. Roskelley, A. M. Richards, S. P. Sardi, C. R. O'Riordan, K. W. Klinger, L. S. Shihabuddin and S. H. Cheng (2010). "CNS-targeted gene therapy improves survival and motor function in a mouse model of spinal muscular atrophy." *J Clin Invest* 120(4): 1253-1264.

Paushkin, S., A. K. Gubitz, S. Massenet and G. Dreyfuss (2002). "The SMN complex, an assemblyosome of ribonucleoproteins." *Current opinion in cell biology* 14(3): 305-312.

Pellizzoni, L., J. Baccon, J. Rappsilber, M. Mann and G. Dreyfuss (2002). "Purification of native survival of motor neurons complexes and identification of Gemin6 as a novel component." *The Journal of biological chemistry* 277(9): 7540-7545.

Pellizzoni, L., B. Charroux and G. Dreyfuss (1999). "SMN mutants of spinal muscular atrophy patients are defective in binding to snRNP proteins." *Proceedings of the National Academy of Sciences of the United States of America* 96(20): 11167-11172.

Raker, V. A., G. Plessel and R. Luhrmann (1996). "The snRNP core assembly pathway: identification of stable core protein heteromeric complexes and an snRNP subcore particle in vitro." *The EMBO journal* 15(9): 2256-2269.

Riessland, M., B. Ackermann, A. Forster, M. Jakubik, J. Hauke, L. Garbes, I. Fritzsche, Y. Mende, I. Blumcke, E. Hahnen and B. Wirth (2010). "SAHA ameliorates the SMA phenotype in two mouse models for spinal muscular atrophy." *Hum Mol Genet* 19(8): 1492-1506.

Riessland, M., B. Ackermann, A. Forster, M. Jakubik, J. Hauke, L. Garbes, I. Fritzsche, Y. Mende, I. Blumcke, E. Hahnen and B. Wirth (2010). "SAHA ameliorates the SMA phenotype in two mouse models for spinal muscular atrophy." *Human molecular genetics* 19(8): 1492-1506.

Rochette, C. F., N. Gilbert and L. R. Simard (2001). "SMN gene duplication and the emergence of the SMN2 gene occurred in distinct hominids: SMN2 is unique to Homo sapiens." *Human genetics* 108(3): 255-266.

Rose, F. F., Jr., V. B. Mattis, H. Rindt and C. L. Lorson (2009). "Delivery of recombinant follistatin lessens disease severity in a mouse model of spinal muscular atrophy." *Hum Mol Genet* 18(6): 997-1005.

Rudnik-Schoneborn, S., H. H. Goebel, W. Schlote, S. Molaian, H. Omran, U. Ketelsen, R. Korinthenberg, D. Wenzel, H. Lauffer, M. Kreiss-Nachtsheim, B. Wirth and K. Zerres (2003). "Classical infantile spinal muscular atrophy with SMN deficiency causes sensory neuronopathy." *Neurology* 60(6): 983-987.

Rudnik-Schoneborn, S., R. Heller, C. Berg, C. Betzler, T. Grimm, T. Eggermann, K. Eggermann, R. Wirth, B. Wirth and K. Zerres (2008). "Congenital heart disease is a feature of severe infantile spinal muscular atrophy." *Journal of medical genetics* 45(10): 635-638.

Ruiz, R., J. J. Casanas, L. Torres-Benito, R. Cano and L. Tabares (2010). "Altered intracellular Ca2+ homeostasis in nerve terminals of severe spinal muscular atrophy mice." *The Journal of neuroscience : the official journal of the Society for Neuroscience* 30(3): 849-857.

Schrank, B., R. Gotz, J. M. Gunnersen, J. M. Ure, K. V. Toyka, A. G. Smith and M. Sendtner (1997). "Inactivation of the survival motor neuron gene, a candidate gene for human spinal muscular atrophy, leads to massive cell death in early mouse embryos." *Proc Natl Acad Sci U S A* 94(18): 9920-9925.

Shababi, M., J. Habibi, H. T. Yang, S. M. Vale, W. A. Sewell and C. L. Lorson (2010). "Cardiac defects contribute to the pathology of spinal muscular atrophy models." *Human molecular genetics* 19(20): 4059-4071.

Singh, N. K., N. N. Singh, E. J. Androphy and R. N. Singh (2006). "Splicing of a critical exon of human Survival Motor Neuron is regulated by a unique silencer element located in the last intron." *Molecular and cellular biology* 26(4): 1333-1346.

Singh, N. N. and R. N. Singh (2011). "Alternative splicing in spinal muscular atrophy underscores the role of an intron definition model." *RNA biology* 8(4).

Sumner, C. J., C. D. Wee, L. C. Warsing, D. W. Choe, A. S. Ng, C. Lutz and K. R. Wagner (2009). "Inhibition of myostatin does not ameliorate disease features of severe spinal muscular atrophy mice." *Human molecular genetics* 18(17): 3145-3152.

Swoboda, K. J., T. W. Prior, C. B. Scott, T. P. McNaught, M. C. Wride, S. P. Reyna and M. B. Bromberg (2005). "Natural history of denervation in SMA: relation to age, SMN2 copy number, and function." *Annals of neurology* 57(5): 704-712.

Tsai, L. K., M. S. Tsai, C. H. Ting and H. Li (2008). "Multiple therapeutic effects of valproic acid in spinal muscular atrophy model mice." *Journal of molecular medicine* 86(11): 1243-1254.

Valori, C. F., K. Ning, M. Wyles, R. J. Mead, A. J. Grierson, P. J. Shaw and M. Azzouz (2010). "Systemic delivery of scAAV9 expressing SMN prolongs survival in a model of spinal muscular atrophy." *Science translational medicine* 2(35): 35ra42.

Valori, C. F., K. Ning, M. Wyles, R. J. Mead, A. J. Grierson, P. J. Shaw and M. Azzouz (2010). "Systemic delivery of scAAV9 expressing SMN prolongs survival in a model of spinal muscular atrophy." *Sci Transl Med* 2(35): 35ra42.

Vitte, J. M., B. Davoult, N. Roblot, M. Mayer, V. Joshi, S. Courageot, F. Tronche, J. Vadrot, M. H. Moreau, F. Kemeny and J. Melki (2004). "Deletion of murine Smn exon 7 directed to liver leads to severe defect of liver development associated with iron overload." *The American journal of pathology* 165(5): 1731-1741.

Voigt, T., K. Meyer, O. Baum and D. Schumperli (2010). "Ultrastructural changes in diaphragm neuromuscular junctions in a severe mouse model for Spinal Muscular Atrophy and their prevention by bifunctional U7 snRNA correcting SMN2 splicing." *Neuromuscular disorders : NMD* 20(11): 744-752.

Wang, J. and G. Dreyfuss (2001). "Characterization of functional domains of the SMN protein in vivo." *The Journal of biological chemistry* 276(48): 45387-45393.

Williams, J. H., R. C. Schray, C. A. Patterson, S. O. Ayitey, M. K. Tallent and G. J. Lutz (2009). "Oligonucleotide-mediated survival of motor neuron protein expression in CNS improves phenotype in a mouse model of spinal muscular atrophy." *The Journal of neuroscience : the official journal of the Society for Neuroscience* 29(24): 7633-7638.

Wishart, T. M., J. P. Huang, L. M. Murray, D. J. Lamont, C. A. Mutsaers, J. Ross, P. Geldsetzer, O. Ansorge, K. Talbot, S. H. Parson and T. H. Gillingwater (2010). "SMN deficiency disrupts brain development in a mouse model of severe spinal muscular atrophy." *Human molecular genetics* 19(21): 4216-4228.

Workman, E., L. Saieva, T. L. Carrel, T. O. Crawford, D. Liu, C. Lutz, C. E. Beattie, L. Pellizzoni and A. H. Burghes (2009). "A SMN missense mutation complements SMN2 restoring snRNPs and rescuing SMA mice." *Human molecular genetics* 18(12): 2215-2229.

Zerres, K., S. Rudnik-Schoneborn, R. Forkert and B. Wirth (1995). "Genetic basis of adult-onset spinal muscular atrophy." *Lancet* 346(8983): 1162.

Zerres, K., S. Rudnik-Schoneborn, E. Forrest, A. Lusakowska, J. Borkowska and I. Hausmanowa-Petrusewicz (1997). "A collaborative study on the natural history of childhood and juvenile onset proximal spinal muscular atrophy (type II and III SMA): 569 patients." *Journal of the neurological sciences* 146(1): 67-72.

Zerres, K., B. Wirth and S. Rudnik-Schoneborn (1997). "Spinal muscular atrophy--clinical and genetic correlations." *Neuromuscular disorders : NMD* 7(3): 202-207.

Zhang, Z., F. Lotti, K. Dittmar, I. Younis, L. Wan, M. Kasim and G. Dreyfuss (2008). "SMN deficiency causes tissue-specific perturbations in the repertoire of snRNAs and widespread defects in splicing." *Cell* 133(4): 585-600.

6

Mesenchymal Stem Cell Therapy for Apoptosis After Spinal Cord Injury

Venkata Ramesh Dasari[1], Krishna Kumar Veeravalli[1],
Jasti S. Rao[1,2], Dan Fassett[2,3] and Dzung H. Dinh[2,3]
[1]Departments of Cancer Biology and Pharmacology,
[2]Neurosurgery
[3]Illinois Neurological Institute
University of Illinois College of Medicine at Peoria, Peoria, Illinois,
USA

1. Introduction

Spinal cord injury (SCI) is a devastating clinical problem that has irreversible consequences, results in permanent functional loss, and life time disability (Sekhon and Fehlings, 2001). This debilitating condition often affects young and healthy individuals at the prime of their life, creates enormous physical and emotional cost, and places a significant financial burden to society at large (Ackery et al., 2004). Even though years of research have led to a better understanding in the pathophysiology of permanent neural injuries at the cellular level, much of the mechanism and processes of secondary injury at the molecular level remain to be elucidated. With modern molecular strategies and techniques, breakthroughs in the understanding of neuronal injury and neural regeneration provide new promises for reversal of spinal cord injury that once was thought to be permanent and irreversible (Carlson and Gorden, 2002).

Spinal cord injury involves an initial mechanical or primary injury followed by a series of cellular and molecular secondary events that amplify the extent of the initial damage and results in the progressive destruction of spinal cord tissue. After acute contusion, the spinal cord undergoes a sequential progression of pathologic changes, including micro hemorrhage, cytotoxic edema, neuronal necrosis, axonal fragmentation, demyelination, further secondary cellular destruction and eventually cyst formation (Balentine, 1978; Balentine and Greene, 1984; Coutts and Keirstead, 2008). Damage to the spinal cord results in extensive proliferation of microglia and macrophages in and around the injury epicenter. This acute inflammatory response at the injury site is at least partly responsible for secondary spinal cord injury (Popovich et al., 1997; Carlson et al., 1998; Taoka et al., 1998). The inflammatory cells (particularly macrophages/microglia) mediate tissue damage by producing a variety of cytotoxic factors including interleukins (Rice et al., 2007) and tumor necrosis factor-alpha (TNF-α) (Beattie et al., 2002). White matter breakdown begins at the grey-white matter junction with progressive edema (Dohrmann et al., 1972). Axoplasmic stasis and axonal swelling that contains multiple organelles, mitochondria, neurofilament, and smooth endoplasmic reticulum eventually undergo glandular dissolution and myelin disruption (Bresnahan et al., 1976; Balentine, 1978; Bresnahan, 1978; Balentine and Greene, 1984). Within 4h of injury, neuronal and oligodendroglial cell loss is apparent in the lesion epicenter, and extends rostrally and caudally (Grossman et al., 2001). Within days after the injury polymorphonuclear cells and macrophages begin to infiltrate the injured region (Blight, 1985; Means and Anderson, 1983). And within one week, the central necrotic region begins to show cystic changes. By four weeks, chronic changes have occurred, and a cystic cavity remains with astrocytic gliosis and demyelination of the remaining axons (Wagner et al., 1971). Even years after initial trauma, neuronal and oligodendroglial apoptotic cell death processes continues to contribute to demyelination and Wallerian degeneration (Hagg and Oudega, 2006; Taoka and Okajima, 1998). The wave of post-traumatic tissue destruction, as initiated by secondary injury mechanisms, include disruption of spinal cord vasculature and ischemia, glutamatergic excitotoxicity, oxidative cell stress, lipid peroxidation and inflammation (Nashmi and Fehlings, 2001; Tator and Fehlings, 1991) — all of which alone or in concert can trigger apoptosis, contribute to the permanency of functional motor and sensory deficits (Hagg and Oudega, 2006; Taoka and Okajima, 1998).

Apoptotic cell death has been observed to occur for weeks after injury at distance remote from the point of mechanical impact (Crowe et al., 1997; Emery et al., 1998; Springer et al., 1999). Neurons and oligodendrocytes are especially vulnerable to the toxicity of the acute lesion microenvironment after SCI for several reasons (Choi, 1988). Neurons have a high rate of oxidative metabolism that makes them susceptible to injury by reactive oxygen species (ROS) following ischemia (Juurlink and Paterson, 1998). Compared to their supporting astroglial cells, neurons have lower levels of antioxidant levels (e.g., glutathione) and respond differently to molecular mechanisms involving the activation of Phase II enzymes, which are responsible for neutralization of damaging free radicals (Eftekharpour et al., 2000). Oligodendrocytes are also very susceptible to ROS due to their higher iron content and lower levels of glutathione and its related antioxidant enzymes, (Juurlink and Paterson, 1998). The oxidative stress by induction of ROS and pro-inflammatory cytokines initiates a cascade of oxidative events that lead to cell death due to a combination of necrosis and apoptosis (Crowe et al., 1997). Loss of oligodendroglia causes demyelination, impairs axonal function and survival. In the days to weeks after injury, disrupted neuronal axons and extracellular elements of the necrotic core at the site of injury are removed by recruited inflammatory cells and phagocytes (Dusart and Schwab, 1994), leaving in place fluid-filled cystic cavities at the site of injury (Greitz, 2006).

2. Apoptosis after SCI

Apoptosis is a genetically controlled cell death that is characterized by intact membrane integrity, cytoplasmic and nuclear condensation, loss of cellular volume, membrane bleb formation and nuclear disintegration (Yakovlev and Faden, 2001). The cell eventually fragments into apoptotic bodies, which are then engulfed and degraded by neighboring cells. During apoptosis, morphological changes are often accompanied by internucleosomal cleavage of genomic DNA (Wyllie et al., 1980). In the secondary injury process after SCI, apoptosis has been well documented. Emery et al., (1998) analyzed the spinal cords of 15 patients who had died after traumatic SCI and described evidence of apoptotic cells at the edges of the lesion epicenter and in the adjacent white matter. Apoptotic mechanisms of cell death have been implicated in delayed Wallerian degeneration of white matter after spinal cord injury (Crowe et al., 1997). Oligodendrocytes, microglia, and neurons are susceptible to apoptosis. After SCI, some cellular demise was directly related to post-traumatic necrosis, whereas others die due to apoptosis (Crowe et al., 1997; Emery et al., 1998; Shuman et al., 1997; Springer et al., 1999; Keane et al., 2001; Warden et al., 2001; Beattie et al., 2002). Spinal cord trauma activates upregulation of caspases and calpain and the apoptotic machinery, leading to increased expression of death receptors and their ligands (Banik et al., 1997; Casha et al., 2001; Keane et al., 2001; Springer et al., 1999). However, there are conflicting reports as to the role of cell death in SCI— probably a reflection of the known dual capacity of TNF to be both pro- and anti-apoptotic. Fas/CD95, TNFR1 and TNFR2 have been mainly characterized in the immune system and are primarily involved in regulating inflammatory and apoptotic responses. However, these receptors and their ligands are also detectable in CNS tissue (both normal and traumatized), implicating their roles in neuronal maturation as well as in neurological trauma and disease. Apoptotic pathways triggered after SCI are depicted in Figure 1.

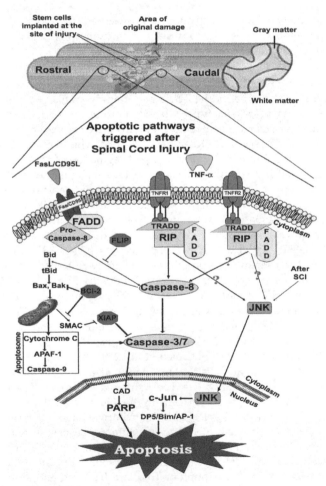

Fig. 1. Apoptotic pathways triggered after SCI

Apoptosis of the cells takes place either rostral or caudal to the area of original damage. These are mainly either Fas-activated or TNF-α or JNK-activated pathways. In Fas-mediated pathway, Fas is activated by Fas ligand, whereby Fas-associated death domain (FADD) and caspase-8 are recruited to Fas to form the death-inducing signaling complex (DISC). Subsequently, caspase-8 can autoactivate and trigger cell death by cleavage of Bid and activation of effector caspases- 3 and -7. The activation and involvement of mitochondria in apoptosis appears to be the main pathway responsible for cell death. In tumor necrosis factor receptor 1 (TNFR1/TNFR2) signaling, early after trauma, increased levels of TNFR1/TNFR2 are activated where they associate with the adaptor protein TRADD, Fas-associated death domain (FADD), TRAF2, TRAF1, and RIP. In later stages after injury, RIP and cIAP-1 appear to dissociate from the TNFR1 complex by an unknown mechanism and this complex signals death by activating caspase-8. In either case, activated caspase-3 translocates to nucleus, and activates CAD resulting in cleavage of PARP leading to apoptotic cell death. In JNK mediated pathway, JNK gets activated after SCI, and translocated to nucleus where it activates c-Jun leading to apoptotic cell death. In mesenchymal stem cell treatment for apoptosis, mesenchymal stem cells are injected at the site of injury or rostral or caudal to the site of injury.

2.1 Apoptosis involving FAS/CD95 and caspases

Fas (CD95 or Apo-1) is a member of the TNFR superfamily and is one of six known death receptors. Fas exists as a 45-kDa, type 1 transmembrane protein with an elongated extracellular domain. This extracellular region contains three cysteine-rich domains (CRDs), which are typical of TNF receptors (Keane et al., 2006). This receptor contains a death domain and plays a central role in the physiological regulation of programmed cell death, and has been implicated in the pathogenesis of various malignancies and diseases of the immune system. The interaction of this receptor with its ligand generates the formation of a death-inducing signaling complex that includes Fas-associated death domain protein (FADD), caspase-8, and caspase-10. The autoproteolytic processing of the caspases in the complex triggers a downstream caspase cascade, and leads to apoptosis. The typical ligand for Fas is FasL (CD95L, Apo-1L, Cd178, TNFSF6), which is a 281–amino acid protein produced as a type 2 transmembrane protein and is highly restricted to immune cells and cells of the CNS. In the nervous system, Fas/CD95 activation can lead to cell death involving neurons and glial cells (D'Souza et al., 1995; Raoul et al., 2002). Activation of Fas/CD95 can also lead to enhanced axonal growth (Desbarats et al., 2003). Fas and FasL are expressed in the normal CNS, and are upregulated in inflamed and degenerated brains (Choi and Benveniste, 2004). Fas and FasL levels have been found to be elevated after SCI (Casha et al., 2001; Dasari et al., 2008; Demjen et al., 2004; Li et al., 2000a). Yoshino *et al.*, (Yoshino et al., 2004) investigated Fas/CD95-mediated apoptosis after SCI using Fas-deficient mutant mice. Mice lacking Fas/FasL showed improved functional recovery, decreased lesion size, and fewer apoptotic cells in the injured cord than control littermates. It appears that Fas-FasL induce apoptosis via both intrinsic and extrinsic pathways. The extrinsic pathway involves Fas-FasL mediated activation of caspase-8, which then directly activates caspase-3 (Salvesen and Dixit, 1999; Stennicke et al., 1998). There was evidence to support the regulation of intrinsic mitochondrial apoptotic pathways by the Bcl-2 family proteins, which consists of both pro-apoptotic (Bid and Bax) and anti-apoptotic (Bcl-2 and Bcl-xL) members (Kim et al., 2000). In addition, the intrinsic pathway can be initiated by the extrinsic pathway, thereby amplifying the apoptotic process. In this scenario, Caspase-8 cleaves Bid into truncated tBid, which translocates from the cytosol into the mitochondria, releasing cytochrome c and activating caspase-3 and -9 (Kuwana et al., 1998; Li et al., 1998; Scaffidi et al., 1998; Stennicke et al., 1998; Verhagen et al., 2000). Also, a mitochondrial apoptotic protein, Apoptosis-inducing factor (AIF), was found capable of inducing neuronal apoptosis when translocated from mitochondria to the nucleus via a caspase-dependent pathway (Tsujimoto, 2003; Tsujimoto and Shimizu, 2000; Yu et al., 2006; Yu et al., 2009).

Strategies to inhibit Fas-FasL cascade may provide effective neuroprotective approaches for mollifying apoptosis after SCI. In one experiment, neutralization of FasL, but not TNF, significantly decreased apoptotic cell death after SCI (Demjen et al., 2004). Mice pretreated with FasL-specific antibodies were capable of initiating active hind-limb movements several weeks after injury with upregulation of growth-associated protein Gap-43 and more abundance in regenerating fibers. Thus, neutralization of FasL appears to diminish apoptotic cell death and promote axonal regeneration and functional improvement in injured adult animals (Demjen et al., 2004). Other experiments have demonstrated that blocking Fas activation using soluble Fas receptors for competitive inhibition or neutralization using anti-FasL antibody diminished brain injury volume and improved outcome in a stroke model of mouse (Gao et al., 2005). The neuroprotective effect of anti-FasL in animal models of SCI, stroke and multiple sclerosis has stimulated considerable interest in elucidation of the role of the Fas/CD95/FasL system in CNS neurons (Demjen et al., 2004; Martin-Villalba et al., 1999; Waldner et al., 1997). However, a true understanding of how FasL antibodies reduce cell death and enhance recovery requires more detailed knowledge. It is not clear if CNS cells exhibit differences in the efficiency of Fas/CD95 signaling and thus can be categorized as type I or type II cells (Keane et al., 2006). The cellular source and target of the ligand in damaged CNS tissue need to be identified, and strategies need to be developed for effective delivering antibodies to the lesion. Recent experimental evidence has provided some knowledge about receptor submembrane localization and the formation of alternative signaling complexes that can alter the fate of cells *in vitro*, but whether these principles hold true *in vivo* remained to be explored. Thus, activation of these signaling pathways might result in promising therapeutic targets for the acute treatment of neurological trauma and disease.

In addition to FasL/CD95 involvement in apoptosis, caspases are also known to be powerful mediators of programmed cell-death in CNS injury and disease processes. All caspases are translated initially as inactive zymogens that are then activated after specific cleavage. They have the following structural features in common: an N-terminal pro-domain of variable length (22 to >200 amino acids), a large subunit (~ 17-20 kDa), a short inter-subunit region (~10 amino acids), and a small subunit (~10−12 kDa). The C-terminal portion of the large subunit contains the catalytic cysteine residue. Flanking this are other conserved residues that, together, form the semiconserved pentapeptide sequence QACXG at the active site (Alnemri et al., 1996; Thornberry and Lazebnik, 1998). Pro-caspases are processed by limited proteolysis into their active form, which consists of a large and small subunit dimer. *In vivo*, however, caspases are more conformationally stable as tetramers consisting of two large/small subunit dimers (Eldadah and Faden, 2000). Once activated by specific cleavage to active forms, caspases can activate other procaspases via extrinsic pathway directly or intrinsic pathway by mitochondrial-dependent mechanisms, thereby amplifying the programmed cell death process (Li et al., 1998; Scaffidi et al., 1998; Slee et al., 1999; Yakovlev and Faden, 2001; Yu et al., 2009). Based on their putative functions and sequence homologies, caspases are often categorized into three groups: apoptotic initiators (caspase-2, 8, -9 and -10), apoptotic executioners (caspase- 3, -6, and -7), and inflammatory mediators (caspase -1, -4,-5, -11, -12, and -13) (Alenzi et al., 2010; Thornberry and Lazebnik, 1998). The apoptotic initiators, act at upstream positions within apoptotic pathways; that is, the cell surface and mitochondria. They have in common long N-terminal pro-domains that contain six anti-parallel α-helices with complementary binding capability. Caspases-8 and -10 have two such domains at their N-termini known as death effector domains (DEDs). Caspases-2 and -9 have only one of these domains, which, in the case of these members, are known as caspase recruitment domains (CARDs). These sequences play an important role in localization and activation of specific procaspases. The apoptotic executioners mediate some of the morphological and biochemical manifestations of apoptosis: plasma membrane blebbing, nuclear membrane dissolution, chromatin condensation and margination, and DNA fragmentation. Executioner caspases have short N-terminal pro-domains whose function remains unclear (Eldadah and Faden, 2000). The third group of caspases is inflammatory mediating proteases that are poor substrates for other caspases and their activation pathways are not well understood.

Numerous studies have demonstrated the presence of multiple caspases and apoptosis following SCI (Beattie et al., 2000; Citron et al., 2000; Crowe et al., 1997; Eldadah and Faden, 2000; Keane et al., 2001; Liu et al., 1997; Lou et al., 1998; Springer et al., 1999; Yong et al., 1998). Emery *et al.*, (1998) have reported substantial labeling of active caspase-3 around the injury site in histological study of injured spinal cords from 15 patients who died after traumatic SCI. The involvement of caspase-3 as a major effector in injury-induced neuronal apoptosis was established by using specific caspase inhibitors in various models of ischemic or traumatic injury (Clark et al., 2000; Gillardon et al., 1997; Gottron et al., 1997; Namura et al., 1998; Yakovlev et al., 1997). Caspase-3 can be activated by caspases-8, -9, -11, and -12 (Kang et al., 2000; Wang et al., 1998). Caspases-11 and -12 in turn can be activated by Calpain and Cathepsin B (Nakagawa and Yuan, 2000; Schotte et al., 1998; Yamashima, 2000). Apoptosis therefore plays an important role in the secondary injury processes following traumatic injury to the CNS (Crowe et al., 1997; Keane et al., 2001; Li et al., 1996; Lu et al., 2000). The permanent neurological deficits after spinal cord injury may be due in part to widespread apoptosis in regions distant from and relatively unaffected by the initial injury (Crowe et al., 1997). Caspases were one of the viable therapeutic targets for modulating apoptosis and remain the viable approach to blocking apoptotic cell death (Nicholson, 2000). A number of caspase inhibitors such as z-VAD fmk (N-benzyloxycarbonyl-Val-Ala-Asp-fluoromethylketones) have been developed to avert apoptotic chain events. X-linked inhibitor of apoptosis proteins (XIAP) has been identified as one of the mammalian homologues in the IAP family, and has been demonstrated to inhibit cell death (Ekert et al., 1999). During apoptosis, XIAP is cleaved to generate fragments with distinct specificity for caspases (Deveraux et al., 1999). However, caspase inhibition has yet to be used in clinical setting despite demonstrated efficacy in treatment of various CNS insults of *in vivo* models (Braun et al., 1999; Hara et al., 1997; Li et al., 2000b; Yakovlev et al., 1997). Several SCI experiments using caspase inhibitors have been reported (Li et al., 2000a; Lou et al., 1998; Springer et al., 1999) to mitigate injury-induced programmed cell death.

2.2 Apoptosis involving TNF-α mediated pathway

Tumor necrosis factor (TNF)-α, also known as cachexin or cachectin, is a pro-inflammatory, pro-apoptotic cytokine that elicits diverse biological actions, including the induction of apoptosis (Tracey, 2011). TNF-α is a trimeric protein primarily produced by the brain resident immune cells such as monocytes and macrophages (the microglia cells) in response to various stimuli (Leung and Cahill, 2010). TNF-α is initially synthesized as a 26-kD cell surface-associated molecule (membrane-bound form) which is then cleaved into a soluble 17-kD form by TNF-converting enzyme (Grewal, 2009). The known roles of TNF-α have extended from the immune system to neuro-inflammatory domain in the nervous system (Leung and Cahill, 2010). TNF-α induces central sensitization and hyperalgesia by increasing excitatory synaptic transmission (Kawasaki et al., 2008). TNF-α initiates the activation of several cytokines and growth factors, as well as the recruitment of some immune cells. Cytokines exist in 'cascades' and interrupting one cytokine can disrupt the cascade. For example, blocking TNF-α reduces the activity of IL-6 and IL-1b (Fong et al., 1989); whereas blocking IL-1b reduces IL-6 (Goldbach-Mansky et al., 2006); and blocking IL-12 and IL-23 reduces IFN-γ. It is this 'master role' in cytokine function that makes TNF-α an attractive target in SCI and other disorders involving inflammation and apoptosis. TNF-α interacts with two distinct receptors – TNFR-55 (TNFR1, p55, CD120a) and TNFR-75 (TNFR2, p75, CD120b). TNF-α can either bind directly to TNFR1 and TNFR2 through cell-to-cell contact or undergo cleavage and binds in its soluble form (Vandenabeele et al., 1995). All nucleated cells express TNF receptors. TNFR1 is expressed constitutively on most cell types, whereas expression of TNFR2 can be induced by TNF-α, interleukin (IL)-1, and interferon (IFN)-α in rat primary astrocytes (Choi et al., 2005). In addition, TNFR2 expression is restricted to hematopoetic cells and can discriminate between murine and human forms of TNF-α (Tartaglia et al., 1991). The receptors also differ significantly in their binding affinity for homotrimeric TNF-α. Although both receptors can be considered high-affinity, the on–off kinetics of the two differs dramatically. Binding of homotrimeric TNF-α to TNFR1 seems to be essentially irreversible, whereas binding to TNFR2 is associated with rapid on–off kinetics (Choi et al., 2005).

Evidence showed that proinflammatory and proapoptotic cytokines, including TNF-α, IL-1γ, and FasL regulate cellular events and contributes to neuronal damage and functional impairment associated with SCI (Harrington et al., 2005; Lee et al., 2000; Martin-Villalba et al., 1999; Streit et al., 1998). TNF-α levels become elevated in human spinal cord after SCI, reaching a peak within 1h after the initial trauma (Dinomais et al., 2009). The expression of TNF-α is upregulated rapidly at the lesion site after SCI (Hayashi et al., 2000; Streit et al., 1998; Wang et al., 1996; Wang et al., 2002; Yan et al., 2001). TNF-α can induce apoptosis of oligodendrocytes and neuronal cell line *in vitro* (D'Souza et al., 1995; Sipe et al., 1996). Rapid accumulation of TNF-α may act as an external signal initiating apoptosis after SCI in neurons and glial cells (Lee et al., 2000; Shuman et al., 1997). Neutralization of TNF-α reduced the number of apoptotic cells after SCI (Lee et al., 2000). Apoptosis induced by TNF-α after SCI could be mediated in part by nitric oxide via upregulation of inducible nitric oxide synthase (iNOS) (Yune et al., 2003). Although, few studies indicate a neuroprotective role of TNF-α and NOS expression in SCI, several investigators support a neurodestructive role of these agents in spinal cord pathology (Bethea et al., 1999; Bethea and Dietrich, 2002; Dolga et al., 2008; Gonz'alez Deniselle et al., 2001; Sharma et al., 1995; Sharma, 2007; Sharma, 2008; Sharma, 2010; Stalberg et al., 1998).

Apoptosis of oligodendrocytes *in vivo* was shown to be induced by the overexpression of TNFR1 (Akassoglou et al., 1998). Following SCI, TNFR1 and TNFR2 expression is elevated in the injured spinal cord and localized on neurons, astrocytes and oligodendrocytes (Yan et al., 2003). TNFR1 and TNFR2 are elevated as soon as 15 min after traumatic SCI in adult rats, reaches the peak at 4h for TNFR2 and 8h for TNFR1, and declines markedly after 1 day and 3 days (Yan et al., 2003). TNFR1 immunoreactivity was demonstrated on cells and afferent fibers of dorsal root and dorsal root ganglia, dorsal root entry zone and within lamina I and II of dorsal horn, whereas TNFR2 expression was absent in these regions (Holmes et al., 2004). These two receptors might work individually or synergistically to mediate the biological activity of TNF-α. It has been suggested that TNF receptors are involved in anti-apoptotic activities through the TNFR1-nuclear factor kappa B (NFκB) signal transduction pathway, which activates a recently identified endogenous caspase inhibitory system that is mediated by cellular inhibitor of apoptosis protein 2 (c-IAP2) (Kim et al., 2001). After TNF binding to TNFR1, a TNFR1 receptor–associated complex (complex-I) forms and contains TRADD, RIP1, TRAF1, TRAF2, and cIAP-1. Complex-I transduce signals that lead to NF-κB activation through recruitment of the IκB kinase 'signalsome' high-molecular-weight complex (Poyet et al., 2000; Zhang et al., 2000). TNFR1$^{-/-}$ mice had greater numbers of apoptotic cells, larger contusion size, and worse functional recovery after SCI. TNFR2$^{-/-}$ mice had similar, although not as pronounced, consequences as the TNFR1$^{-/-}$ mice. However, when new protein synthesis is inhibited prior to TNF stimulation, TNFR1 can initiate apoptosis by activation of apical caspases (Varfolomeev and Ashkenazi, 2004). TNFR1-mediated apoptosis signaling is induced in which TRADD and RIP1 associate with FADD and caspase-8 to form a cytoplasmic complex (complex-II) that dissociates from TNFR1. When complex-I triggers sufficient NF-κB signaling, anti-apoptotic gene expression is induced and the activation of initiator caspases in complex-II is inhibited. If NFκB signaling is deficient, complex-II transduces an apoptotic signal. Thus, early activation of NFκB by complex-I serves as a checkpoint to regulate whether complex-II induces apoptosis at a later time point after TNF binding.

2.3 Apoptosis involving JNK mediated pathway

The mitogen-activated protein kinases (MAPKs) are a family of evolutionarily conserved molecules that play a critical role in cell signaling and gene expression. MAPK family includes three major members: c-Jun N-terminal kinase (JNK), p38 and extracellular signal regulated kinase (ERK), representing three different signaling cascades. The JNK pathway is considered as a key mediator of stress-induced apoptosis (Davis, 2000). Examples include neuronal apoptosis induced by NGF withdrawal (Eilers et al., 1998; Park et al., 1996; Xia et al., 1995), excitotoxic stress (Yang et al., 1997b) and UV radiation (Tournier et al., 2000; Tournier et al., 2001), thymocyte apoptosis induced by anti-CD3 antibody (Rincon et al., 1998; Sabapathy et al., 1999) and endothelial cell apoptosis caused by diabetes-associated hyperglycemia (Ho et al., 2000). JNK pathway activation may also contribute to neuronal death in neurodegenerative diseases including Alzheimer's, Parkinson's, Huntington's Diseases and stroke (Gao et al., 2005; Okuno et al., 2004; Yang et al., 1997b). However, the mechanism by which JNK activation triggers apoptotic processes remains to be fully elucidated. Substrates of JNK, including the Bcl-2 family proteins, regulate cytochrome c release which is an important event in apoptosis secondary to mitochondrial dysfunction. After SCI, JNK3 activity itself is induced by the injury, regulating cytochrome C release by phosphorylating Mcl-1, and thereby facilitating the degradation of Mcl-1, which is necessary for induction of apoptosis of oligodendrocytes (Li et al., 2007). Although JNK3 is also activated in neurons after SCI, it did not induce neuronal apoptosis. A potential role for

JNK3 in neurons is regulation of autophagic death instead of apoptotic death as observed in oligodendrocytes (Li et al., 2007). Several studies demonstrated that the anti-apoptotic proteins Bcl-2, Bcl-xL and Mcl-1 are phosphorylated by JNK *in vitro* and *in vivo* (Inoshita et al., 2002; Maundrell et al., 1997; Yamamoto et al., 1999), there by suppressing the anti-apoptotic activity of these proteins. Another possibility is that JNK phosphorylates the transcription factor c-Jun which might in turn mediate the induction of proteins regulating cytochrome c release in apoptosis (Behrens et al., 1999). Indeed, JNK has been found to regulate some pro-apoptotic BH3-only proteins via transcription-dependent mechanisms (Tournier et al., 2000). Two genes in this subfamily, DP5 and Bim, have AP-1 binding sites on their promoters, and transcription appears to be regulated by JNK activity (Davis, 2000; Harris and Johnson, Jr., 2001; Putcha et al., 2001; Putcha et al., 2003; Whitfield et al., 2001; Yang et al., 1997a; Yin et al., 2005).

Substantial increases in p-JNK expression were noticed after SCI (Esposito et al., 2009; Yin et al., 2005). Activated form of JNK was expressed in the apoptotic cells that were stained by oligodendrocyte antibodies 1–3 days after SCI (Nakahara et al., 1999) and both p-JNK and DP5 colocalization were found in neurons and oligodendrocytes undergoing apoptosis after SCI (Yin et al., 2005). Similarly, the transcription factor, c-Jun (which is an exclusive substrate of JNK), was also phosphorylated shortly after traumatic injury. Furthermore, DP5 is also induced after SCI in a JNK-dependent manner. Suppression of JNK activity by SP600125, a JNK inhibitor, or jnk1 knockdown by an antisense oligodeoxynucleotide (ODN) attenuated SCI-induced DP5 upregulation and caspase-3 activation. Following traumatic SCI, JNK activation contributes to activation of caspase 3, and apoptosis of glia and neurons (Yin et al., 2005). Based on these discoveries, it appears that JNK/c-Jun/DP5/Caspase 3 signaling pathway could represent a potential target for therapeutic interventions in SCI.

3. Stem cell therapy for apoptosis after SCI

During the first few days after injury, there are many microenvironmental features that are detrimental to the survival and integration of transplanted stem cells (Hausmann, 2003). The pathophysiologic processes initiated after acute spinal cord injury are extremely complex, and our limited understanding is reflected in the utilization of i.v. steroid trauma protocol as the only currently available neuroprotective strategy. The limited success of pharmacologic treatment has shifted the focus of medical research away from these traditional treatments to other more promising areas such as cell-based therapy, particularly, the application of stem cell biology (Hipp and Atala, 2004; Stanworth and Newland, 2001). Thus, various cellular transplantation strategies have been utilized in different models of SCI (Eftekharpour et al., 2008). The adult spinal cord harbors endogenous stem/progenitor cells, collectively referred to as NPCs, which might be responsible for normal cell turnover. However, the proliferative activity of endogenous NPCs is too limited to support significant self repair after injury. As such, stem cell transplantation has become a very attractive and viable treatment option for not only CNS injury but also other neurodegenerative disease processes such as Parkinson disease, MS, stroke and ALS (Malgieri et al., 2010). The rationale for cell replacement approach for the treatment of SCI are (1) regeneration, which seeks to replace lost or damaged neurons and induce axonal regeneration or modulate plasticity; and (2) repair, which seeks to replace supportive cells such as oligodendrocytes in order to prevent progressive myelin loss and induce remyelination (Totoiu and Keirstead, 2005). Additionally, stem cell transplantation may promote protection of endogenous cells from further cell loss by attenuation of secondary injury process. Non-embryonic sources of adult stem cells, free from many of the ethical and legal concerns associated with embryonic stem cell research, may offer great promise for the advancement of medicine (Moore et al., 2006). At present, the only non-embryonic stem cells easily available in large numbers are found in the bone marrow, adipose tissue and human umbilical cord blood. These multipotent adult stem cells are ideal vehicles for gene therapy, and genetic engineering for therapeutic treatment of various genetic disorders (Pessina and Gribaldo, 2006). Recent studies have shown that transplanted adult stem cells, including mesenchymal stem cells, human umbilical cord blood stem cells into injured spinal cord promote endogenous myelin repair and modulate immune response, stirring the hope of applying their efficacy to other demyelinating diseases such as MS and stroke.

3.1 Mesenchymal stem cells

Mesenchymal stem cells (MSC) are stromal cells from the bone marrow (BM) and appear as spindle-shaped cells in culture (Friedenstein et al., 1974). Human mesenchymal stem cells are multipotent cells that are present in adult marrow, can replicate as undifferentiated cells and have the potential to differentiate to lineages of mesenchymal tissues, including bone, cartilage, fat, tendon, muscle, and marrow stroma (Pittenger et al., 1999). Even though not immortal, they have the ability to expand many folds in culture while retaining their growth and multilineage potential. MSC are identified by the expression of surface markers including CD105 (SH2) and CD73, and are negative for hematopoietic markers such as CD34, CD45 and CD14. MSC attracted interest for their ability to migrate to the injured site and differentiate into multiple cellular phenotypes *in vivo* (Uccelli et al., 2011). The heterogenity of MSC, and their expression of a large number of regulatory proteins, may explain their wide therapeutic features and capacity to respond differently to injuries depending on the microenvironment, despite their low engraftment *in vivo* (Phinney and Prockop, 2007). MSC produce cytokines and a variety of soluble factors regulating several biological activities as demonstrated by their transcriptome analysis (Phinney et al., 2006). They play a major role in the maintenance of local homeostasis via their supporting activity in the survival of non-proliferating hematopoietic stem cells (HSC) niche in the bone marrow (Mendez-Ferrer et al., 2010). These mesenchymal stem cells are derived from the embryonic mesodermal layer and retain the cardinal abilities of stemcellness for self-renewal and multipotentiality to differentiate into various tissue cell types.

MSCs are attractive candidates for cellular therapies because they are easy to isolate, have a broad differentiation potential, and proliferate *in vitro* (Barry, 2003). Bone Marrow and umbilical cord blood are rich sources of these cells, but MSC have also been isolated from fat (Gronthos et al., 2001), skeletal muscle (Jankowski et al., 2002), human deciduous teeth (Miura et al., 2003), and trabecular bone (Noth et al., 2002). In addition, recent data demonstrated that MSC can give rise to cells of non-mesodermal origin such as hepatocytes, epithelial and neural cells (Chagraoui et al., 2003; Ma et al., 2006; Spees et al., 2003; Woodbury et al., 2000). The choice of the tissue source is governed by availability, as well as by the degree of characterization of the cells and the consistency of the preparations. MSCs from bone marrow and umbilical cord blood have been reasonably well defined in terms of surface markers and differentiation pathways. These donor sites provide a readily available autologous source for cell transplantation, alleviating the need for long-term immunosuppression. Mesenchymal stem cells have been used in experimental models of

SCI and in preliminary clinical trials for SCI (Himes et al., 2006; Sykova et al., 2006) with apparent improvement of behavioral outcome. Stem cells are likely to be therapeutically valuable both in providing permissive substrates for axonal regeneration and as 'cellular minipumps' delivering trophic factors that could enhance white matter sparing and/or axonal regeneration (Enzmann et al., 2006). The functional benefits of MSC transplantation in CNS injuries can be explained by their ability to provide the host tissue with growth factors or modulate the host immune system (Garbuzova-Davis et al., 2006). One of the major goals for the therapeutic use of stem cells is to prevent apoptosis or to replace lost cells, particularly oligodendrocytes, in order to facilitate the remyelination of spared axons. Details showing application of unengineered mesenchymal stem cells from various sources and their applications after SCI are provided in Table 1.

3.1.1 Bone marrow derived mesenchymal stem cells

Human MSCs are isolated from a bone marrow (BM) aspirate, which is often harvested from the superior iliac crest of the pelvis. They represent a very minor fraction of the total nucleated cell population in marrow, but can be plated and enriched using standard cell culture techniques. Frequently, the marrow sample is subjected to fractionation on a density gradient solution, such as Percoll, after which the cells are plated. Primary cultures are usually maintained for 12–16 days, and are then detached by trypsinization and subcultured. Morphologically, the cells resemble adherent fibroblasts (Barry, 2003). Under physiological settings bone marrow derived MSC (BMSC) main function is to regulate hematopoiesis. However, when these cells are grown away from their natural environment, they can be readily and effectively propagated and manipulated genetically into cells of the mesodermal lineage but also, under certain experimental circumstances, into cells of the neuronal and glial lineage (Clark and Keating, 1995). The advantages of using bone marrow as a source for stem cells are numerous: they are relatively easy to isolate, the cells grow and expand well in tissue culture. BMSC may be used in autologous transplantation protocols, and these have already received FDA approval for treatment of hematopoietic diseases (Sykova et al., 2006). BMSC therapeutic value relies on their significant anti-proliferative, anti-inflammatory and anti-apoptotic features. These properties have been demonstrated in the treatment of experimental autoimmune encephalomyelitis (EAE), an animal model of multiple sclerosis where inhibition of the autoimmune response resulted in a significant neuroprotection.

BMSC transplantation results in neuroprotection and increased endogenous neuronal survival in experimental brain ischemia, traumatic brain and spinal cord injury models (Uccelli et al., 2011). There is increasing evidence that MSCs possess immunosuppressive features (Bartholomew et al., 2002; Corcione et al., 2006; Di Nicola et al., 2002; Jiang et al., 2005). These immunosuppressive properties in combination with their restorative functions reduce the acute inflammatory response to SCI, minimize cavity formation, as well as diminish astrocyte and microglia/macrophage reactivity (Abrams et al., 2009; Himes et al., 2006; Neuhuber et al., 2005). BMSC administered 1- week post-SCI had better rates of survival since the microenvironment has become less hostile by then. MSC transplantation in an experimental SCI model has been shown to enhance tissue protection and cellular preservation via reduction in injury-induced sensitivity to mechanical trauma (Abrams et al., 2009). These studies indicated that transplanted MSC attenuates acute inflammation and promote functional recovery following SCI (Hofstetter et al., 2002). Clinically, Park *et al.* (2005)

References	Source of Mesenchymal stem cells	Experimental Animals	Route/site of administration	Treatment timing	Treatment outcome
Cízková et al., 2006	Human bone marrow	Rats	Into right femoral vein	7 days after thoracic SCI	Remyelination of spared white matter tracts, enhancing axonal growth and functional recovery
Dasari et al., 2007a	Rat bone marrow	Rats	Injury epicenter	7 days after thoracic SCI	Downregulation of caspase mediated apoptosis, functional recovery of rats
Dasari et al., 2008	Human umbilical cord blood	Rats	Injury epicenter	7 days after thoracic SCI	Downregulation of Fas mediated apoptosis, functional recovery of rats
Dasari et al., 2009	Human umbilical cord blood	Rats	Injury epicenter	7 days after thoracic SCI	Downregulation of TNF-α mediated neuronal apoptosis
Deng et al., 2006	Rhesus monkey bone marrow	Rhesus monkey	Injury epicenter	7 days after thoracic SCI	*de novo* neurogenesis and functional recovery
Gu et al., 2010	Rat bone marrow	Rats	1mm rostral and caudal from injury epicenter	7 days after thoracic SCI	Reduction in lesion volume; axonal regrowth of injured spinal cord.
Hu et al., 2010	Human umbilical cord blood	Rats	2mm rostral and caudal from injury epicenter	24h after thoracic SCI	Increased length of neurofilament positive fibers and increased numbers of growth cone-like structures around the lesion site, functional recovery
Lee et al., 2007	Human bone marrow	Rats	Injury epicenter	7 days after thoracic SCI	Functional recovery
Lim et al., 2007	Umbilical cord blood of canine fetuses	Dogs	Injury epicenter	7 days after balloon compression at the first lumbar vertebra.	Significant improvement in the nerve conduction velocity based on the somatosensory evoked potentials. Functional recovery.
Osaka et al., 2010	Rat bone marrow	Rats	Intravenous (through the femoral vein)	6h, 1d, 3d, 10d, 14d, 21d, 28d after thoracic SCI	Cavitation in the contused spinal cords was less; functional recovery
Parr et al., 2008	Rat bone marrow	Rats	Injury epicenter	9 days after clip compression injury at the thoracic region	Potential axonal guidance through guiding strands of matrix generated by the bone marrow stromal cells
Satake et al., 2004	Rat bone marrow	Rats	Stem cells injected into the subarachnoid space	3, 5, 7 days after thoracic SCI	MSCs differentiated into Nestin-positive, immature neurons or glial cells
Yang et al., 2008	Wharton's jelly of the human umbilical cord	Rats	2mm rostral and caudal to injury epicenter	After complete transection at the thoracic region.	Functional recovery, regenerated axons in the corticospinal tract and neurofilament-positive fibers around the lesion site.
Zeng et al., 2011	Rat bone marrow derived mesenchymal stem cells grown on 3D gelatin sponge (GS) scaffolds	Rats	Injury epicenter	7 days after thoracic SCI	Attenuating inflammation, promoting angiogenesis and reducing cavity formation.

Table 1. Table showing different authors using mesenchymal stem cells for treatment after SCI

evaluated the therapeutic efficacy of combining autologous BMSC transplantation, administered directly into the spinal cord lesion site, with granulocyte macrophage- colony stimulating factor (GM-CSF), given subcutaneously, in six patients with complete SCI. At the 6-month and 18-month follow-up periods, four of the six patients showed neurological improvements by two ASIA grade (from ASIA A to ASIA C), while another improved from ASIA A to ASIA B. Moreover, BMSC transplantation together with GM-CSF was not associated with increased morbidity or mortality. In another clinical trial, safety of autologous bone marrow cell implantation was tested in 20 patients (Sykova et al., 2006). Motor evoked potential, somatosensory evoked potential, magnetic resonance imaging, and ASIA scores were measured in patient follow-up. This study demonstrated that BMSC transplantation is a relatively safe procedure and BMSC-mediated repair can lead to modest improvements in some injured patients. Thus, it is anticipated that a Phase II clinical trial designed to test the efficacy will be initiated in the near future. In another study using human mesenchymal stem cells (hMSCs) derived from adult bone marrow, the transplanted cells were found to infiltrate mainly into the ventrolateral white matter tracts, spreading to adjacent segments rostro-caudal to the injury epicenter, and facilitate recovery from SCI by remyelinating spared white matter tracts and/or by enhancing axonal growth (Cizkova et al., 2006). In our laboratory, we used mesenchymal stem cells from rat bone marrow to evaluate the therapeutic potential after SCI (Dasari et al., 2007a). Immunohistochemistry confirmed a large number of apoptotic neurons and oligodendrocytes in caudal segments 2 mm away from the lesion site. Expression of caspase-3 on both neurons and oligodendrocytes after SCI was significantly downregulated by BMSC. Treatment with BMSC had a positive effect on behavioral outcome and better structural integrity preservation as seen on histopathological analysis. BMSC secrete protective factors that prevent neuronal apoptosis through stimulation of endogenous survival signaling pathways, namely the PI3-K/Akt and the MAPK/Erk1, 2-cascade (Isele et al., 2007). The potential of bone marrow cell transplantation as a method of repair in the injured CNS may serve a number of different purposes that span various therapeutic targets. Animal studies have demonstrated that transplanted MSCs mollify the inflammatory response in the acute setting and reduce the inhibitory effects of scar tissue in the subacute/chronic setting to provide a permissive environment for axonal extension. In addition, grafted cells may provide a source of growth factors to enhance axonal elongation across spinal cord lesions (Wright et al., 2011). Moreover, SCI initiates an innate immune response that participates not only in secondary pathogenesis but also in wound healing (Trivedi et al., 2006). Even though the present data are promising, further research is needed to establish whether bone marrow cell treatments can serve as a safe and efficacious autologous source for the treatment of the injured SCI (Wright et al., 2011). Downregulation of TNF-α expression in macrophages/microglia was observed at an early stage after SCI in rats transplanted with a gelatin sponge scaffold impregnated with rat bone marrow-derived mesenchymal stem cells at the site of injury (Zeng et al., 2011).

3.1.2 Human umbilical cord blood derived mesenchymal stem cells

Human umbilical cord blood collected from umbilical vein following birth is a valuable source of mesenchymal stem cells (hUCB or hUCBSC) and has been used as an alternative source of allogenic donor cells to treat a variety of hematologic, immunologic and oncologic disorders (Broxmeyer et al., 1989; Gluckman et al., 1997; Han et al., 2003; Kim et al., 2002).

Human umbilical cord blood contains a heterogeneous population of cells enriched in hematopoietic stem cells and display a high proliferative capacity (Mayani and Lansdorp, 1998). These mesenchymal multipotent progenitor cells possess the capability of differentiating into diverse functional progenitors, including hematopoietic cell lineages, dendritic cells, cardiomyocytes, mesenchymal stem cell (MSC) progenitors, neural stem cell (NSC) progenitors, keratinocytes, hepatocytes, pancreatic β-cells, and endothelial cells in specific culture conditions *in vitro* and *in vivo* (Brunstein et al., 2007; Hemmoranta et al., 2006; Mimeault and Batra, 2006; Weiss and Troyer, 2006). Complex interactions between adult stem cells, host cells and the specialized microenvironment may influence their behavior (Arai and Suda, 2007; Barrilleaux et al., 2006; Bryder et al., 2006; Moore et al., 2006; Wilson and Stice, 2006). More specifically, the reciprocal interactions of adult stem cells with neighboring cells *via* the formation of adherens junctions and the secretion of diverse soluble factors might contribute to their restricted mobility and the adoption of a quiescent or activated state within niches (Mimeault and Batra, 2006). There are many advantages of human umbilical cord blood as a source of MSC as compared to bone marrow or adipose tissue. First, the collection of cord blood is easy and painless. The cord blood can be stored for later use. Second, hUCBSC are more primitive than MSCs isolated from other tissue sources (Can and Karahuseyinoglu, 2007; Lu et al., 2006; Sarugaser et al., 2005; Wu et al., 2007). Third, hUCBSC have a higher proliferative capacity and a faster population doubling time that remains unaltered after 30 passages. In contrast, BMSC showed significantly slower doubling time which became even longer after 6 passages (Malgieri et al., 2010). Finally, hUCBSC has lower immunogenicity and graft-versus-host reactivity when compared to BMSC (Malgieri et al., 2010). There are four different methods for isolation and purification of hUCBSC: density gradient centrifugation, flow cytometry isolation, attachment screening and two-step enzymatic digestion (Zhang et al., 2006). In our laboratory, the cord blood is subjected to fractionation on a density gradient solution, such as Ficoll, after which the cells are plated. Primary cultures are usually maintained for 12–16 days, and are then detached by trypsinization and subcultured. As such, umbilical cord blood bank represents a rich source of multipotent stem cells that are readily available for transplantation or for generating diverse tissue-specific adult stem/progenitor cells and their further differentiated progeny for cellular therapies of various disorders in humans (Barrilleaux et al., 2006; Brunstein et al., 2007; Mimeault and Batra, 2006).

Human umbilical cord blood stem cells offer great potential for novel therapeutic approaches targeted against many CNS diseases. The therapeutic potential of hUCBSC may either be attributed to the inherent ability of stem cell populations to replace damaged tissues outright, or alternatively, to their ability to repair damaged tissues through neural protection and secretion of neurotrophic factors by various cell types within the graft (Park et al., 2011; Sanberg et al., 2005). Previous studies have reported that hUCBSC are beneficial in reversing the deleterious behavioral effects of spinal cord injury, even when infused 5 days after injury (Saporta et al., 2003). Transplanted hUCBSC differentiate into various neural cells and induce motor function improvement in SCI rat models (Kuh et al., 2005). However, to date, very few reports have utilized hUCBSC in SCI. More thorough experiments are needed to evaluate how hUCBSC modulates improvement after SCI and whether it possesses the potential of tissue plasticity (Enzmann et al., 2006). In our laboratory, using SCI injury model in rats, we transplanted hUCBSC one week after SCI to evaluate neural cell differentiation and functional improvement. We have shown that hUCBSC transdifferentiated into neurons and oligodendrocytes, and downregulated Fas-mediated apoptosis (Dasari et al., 2007b; Dasari et al., 2008). The hUCBSC-transdifferentiated oligodendrocytes facilitate the secretion of neurotrophic hormones NT3 and BDNF and synthesize MBP and PLP, promoting the remyelination of demyelinated axons in the injured spinal cord (Dasari et al., 2007b). Furthermore, apoptotic pathways mediated by both Fas and TNF-α were downregulated by hUCBSC (Dasari et al., 2008). Our findings confirmed that mesenchymal stem cells were able to downregulate apoptotic pathways mediated by Fas and Caspase-3 (Figure 2) (Dasari et al., 2007b; Dasari et al., 2008). In hUCBSC-treated rats, the PI3K/Akt pathway was also involved in anti-apoptotic actions. Further, the structural integrity of the cytoskeletal proteins α-tubulin, MAP-2A and -2B and NF-200 has been maintained with hUCBSC treatments. The locomotor scale scores in hUCBSC-treated rats were significantly improved compared to those of the injured group. Taken together, hUCBSC-mediated down-regulation of Fas and caspases may lead to functional recovery of the hind limbs of rats after SCI. With extension of this study, using RT-PCR microarray and analyzing 84 apoptotic genes, we identified the genes that render the injured spinal cord harmful and the hUCBSC-treated spinal cord conducive to regeneration and repair at 3 weeks (Dasari et al., 2009). We observed that the genes involved in inflammation and apoptosis were up-regulated (phospho-p53 and Bax) in the injured spinal cords of rats (Kotipatruni et al., 2011), whereas the genes involved in neuroprotection were up-regulated in the hUCBSC-treated rats (Dasari et al., 2008). Changes in the expressions of TNF-α, TNFR1 and TNFR2 were detected over 3 weeks after SCI and after transplantation with hUCBSC cells. The expression of P50 and P65 on neurons after SCI was efficiently inhibited by application of hUCBSC. Both the *in vivo* and *in vitro* studies support our hypothesis that the therapeutic mechanism of hUCBSC is inhibition of the neuronal apoptosis during the repair of injured spinal cord. Veeravalli *et al.* (2009a) reported the involvement of tissue plasminogen activator (tPA) after SCI in rats and the role of hUCB stem cells. The tPA expression and activity were studied *in vivo* after SCI in rats and *in vitro* in rat embryonic spinal neurons in response to injury with staurosporine, hydrogen peroxide and glutamate. The expression of tPA increased after SCI and reached peak levels at 3 weeks post-SCI. The MBP expression was minimal at the time of the peak tPA activity and *vice versa*. By contrast, infusion of hUCBSC stem cells down-regulated the elevated tPA activity *in vivo* in rats as well as *in vitro* in the spinal neurons. Further, MMP-2 is upregulated after hUCBSC treatment in spinal cord injured rats and in spinal neurons injured either with staurosporine or hydrogen peroxide. Also, hUCBSC-induced upregulation of MMP-2 diminished formation of the glial scar at the site of injury along with reduced immunoreactivity to chondroitin sulfate proteoglycans. This upregulation of MMP-2 levels and reduction of glial scar formation by hUCBSC treatment after SCI created an environment more favorable for endogenous repair mechanisms (Veeravalli et al., 2009b). There have been an increasing number of studies suggesting that these hUCB derived-CD34+ cells can induce angiogenesis and endo/exogenous neurogenesis in stroke (Taguchi et al., 2004) and SCI (Kao et al., 2008). In addition, Chen *et al.* (2008) recently showed that hUCB cells have the ability to secrete multiple neurotrophic factors. Their study demonstrated elevation of neuroprotective cytokine serum IL-10 levels and depression of TNF-α levels after hUCB cell infusion. Moreover, both GDNF and VEGF could be detected in the injured spinal cord after the transplantation of hUCB cells, promoting angiogenesis and neuronal regeneration.

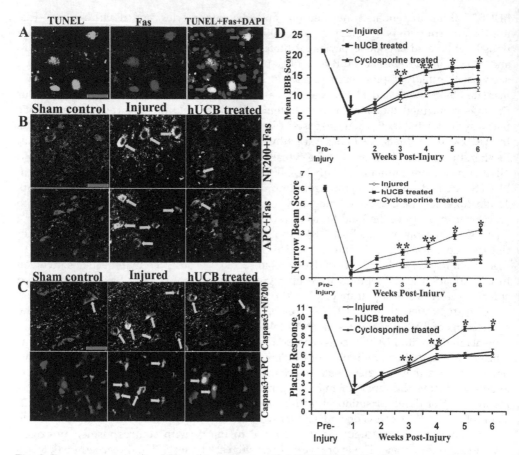

Fig. 2. Fas expression after SCI and treatment with hUCBSC: (A) Fas immunoreactivity on
TUNEL positive cells. Expression of Fas (Texas-red conjugated) on TUNEL positive cells
(green) from injured sections. (B) Cryo-sections showing co-localization of Fas and NF-200
(specific for neurons) and Fas and APC (mature marker for oligodendrocytes) showing
expression of Fas on neurons and oligodendrocytes (↑) undergoing apoptosis. Fas is FITC-
conjugated and NF-200 and APC are Texas-red conjugated. Results are from 3 sections
between 1 and 2mm caudal to the injury epicenter after 3 weeks SCI (n≥3). (C) Confocal
images of cryo-sections illustrate co-localization (yellow) of activated caspase-3 (FITC-
conjugated) with NF-200 (Texas-red conjugated) and APC (Texas-red conjugated) within the
dorsal region(↑), following spinal cord contusion. For panels A, B and C Bar = 100μm.
(D) Top panel shows BBB scores of rats with SCI before and after hUCB transplantation.
Repeated-measures of ANOVA followed by Bonferroni's post hoc tests showed that BBB
scores in hUCB-grafted animals were significantly higher than those in injured-untreated
animals. Each point represents the highest locomotor score achieved each day. Middle panel
shows Narrow beam scores of injured and treated rats over a period of 6 weeks and bottom
panel shows number of placing responses of injured and treated animals. Arrow (↓) indicates
hUCB transplantation point. Error bars indicate ±SEM (n≥5/group) (*p<0.01 and **p<0.05)

4. Conclusions

Transplantation of mesenchymal stem cells into the injured spinal cord and therapeutic applications of mesenchymal stem cells represent exciting new approaches to managing spinal cord injury. Improvements in molecular techniques and strategies along with the availability of modified stem cell lines have fostered our understanding in the mechanism of SCI and advanced the application of stem cell transplantation for treatment of other neurological disorders beyond traumatic brain and spinal cord injury. However, cell-based therapy for SCI is still at an early stage and faces numerous challenges: among them safety problem, patient's genetic diversity and variability, differences in the extent of injury, translational clinical issues, regulatory and ethical concerns. There are numerous ongoing clinical trials utilizing MSC transplantation for treatment of various genetic and neurological disorders. However, the ultimate value of cell-based therapy will need continued expansion of basic scientific knowledge of disease processes and proven therapeutic efficacy via rigorous controlled, randomized, double blind clinical trials.

5. Acknowledgements

This research was supported by a grant from Illinois Neurological Institute to DHD. We also thank Shellee Abraham for manuscript preparation and Diana Meister and Sushma Jasti for manuscript review.

6. References

Abrams M.B., Dominguez C., Pernold K., Reger R., Wiesenfeld-Hallin Z., Olson L. et al. (2009). Multipotent mesenchymal stromal cells attenuate chronic inflammation and injury-induced sensitivity to mechanical stimuli in experimental spinal cord injury. *Restor Neurol Neurosci* 27: 307-321.

Ackery A., Tator C., & Krassioukov A. (2004). A global perspective on spinal cord injury epidemiology. *J Neurotrauma* 21: 1355-1370.

Akassoglou K., Bauer J., Kassiotis G., Pasparakis M., Lassmann H., Kollias G. et al. (1998). Oligodendrocyte apoptosis and primary demyelination induced by local TNF/p55TNF receptor signaling in the central nervous system of transgenic mice: models for multiple sclerosis with primary oligodendrogliopathy. *Am J Pathol* 153: 801-813.

Alenzi F.Q., Lotfy M., & Wyse R. (2010). Swords of cell death: caspase activation and regulation. *Asian Pac J Cancer Prev* 11: 271-280.

Alnemri E.S., Livingston D.J., Nicholson D.W., Salvesen G., Thornberry N.A., Wong W.W. et al. (1996). Human ICE/CED-3 protease nomenclature. *Cell* 87: 171.

Arai F. & Suda T. (2007). Regulation of hematopoietic stem cells in the osteoblastic niche. *Adv Exp Med Biol* 602: 61-67.

Balentine J.D. (1978). Pathology of experimental spinal cord trauma. II. Ultrastructure of axons and myelin. *Lab Invest* 39: 254-266.

Balentine J.D. & Greene W.B. (1984). Ultrastructural pathology of nerve fibers in calcium-induced myelopathy. *J Neuropathol Exp Neurol* 43: 500-510.

Banik N.L., Matzelle D., Gantt-Wilford G., & Hogan E.L. (1997). Role of calpain and its inhibitors in tissue degeneration and neuroprotection in spinal cord injury. *Ann NY Acad Sci* 825: 120-127.

Barrilleaux B., Phinney D.G., Prockop D.J., & O'Connor K.C. (2006). Review: ex vivo engineering of living tissues with adult stem cells. *Tissue Eng* 12: 3007-3019.

Barry F.P. (2003). Biology and clinical applications of mesenchymal stem cells. *Birth Defects Res C Embryo Today* 69: 250-256.

Bartholomew A., Sturgeon C., Siatskas M., Ferrer K., McIntosh K., Patil S. et al. (2002). Mesenchymal stem cells suppress lymphocyte proliferation *in vitro* and prolong skin graft survival *in vivo*. *Exp Hematol* 30: 42-48.

Beattie M.S., Hermann G.E., Rogers R.C., & Bresnahan J.C. (2002). Cell death in models of spinal cord injury. *Prog Brain Res* 137: 37-47.

Beattie M.S., Li Q., & Bresnahan J.C. (2000). Cell death and plasticity after experimental spinal cord injury. *Prog Brain Res* 128: 9-21.

Behrens A., Sibilia M., & Wagner E.F. (1999). Amino-terminal phosphorylation of c-Jun regulates stress-induced apoptosis and cellular proliferation. *Nat Genet* 21: 326-329.

Bethea J.R. & Dietrich W.D. (2002). Targeting the host inflammatory response in traumatic spinal cord injury. *Curr Opin Neurol* 15: 355-360.

Bethea J.R., Nagashima H., Acosta M.C., Briceno C., Gomez F., Marcillo A.E. et al. (1999). Systemically administered interleukin-10 reduces tumor necrosis factor-alpha production and significantly improves functional recovery following traumatic spinal cord injury in rats. *J Neurotrauma* 16: 851-863.

Blight A.R. (1985). Delayed demyelination and macrophage invasion: a candidate for secondary cell damage in spinal cord injury. *Cent Nerv Syst Trauma* 2: 299-315.

Braun J.S., Novak R., Herzog K.H., Bodner S.M., Cleveland J.L., & Tuomanen E.I. (1999). Neuroprotection by a caspase inhibitor in acute bacterial meningitis. *Nat Med* 5: 298-302.

Bresnahan J.C. (1978). An electron-microscopic analysis of axonal alterations following blunt contusion of the spinal cord of the rhesus monkey (*Macaca mulatta*). *J Neurol Sci* 37: 59-82.

Bresnahan J.C., King J.S., Martin G.F., & Yashon D. (1976). A neuroanatomical analysis of spinal cord injury in the rhesus monkey (*Macaca mulatta*). *J Neurol Sci* 28: 521-542.

Broxmeyer H.E., Douglas G.W., Hangoc G., Cooper S., Bard J., English D. et al. (1989). Human umbilical cord blood as a potential source of transplantable hematopoietic stem/progenitor cells. *Proc Natl Acad Sci USA* 86: 3828-3832.

Brunstein C.G., Setubal D.C., & Wagner J.E. (2007). Expanding the role of umbilical cord blood transplantation. *Br J Haematol* 137: 20-35.

Bryder D., Rossi D.J., & Weissman I.L. (2006). Hematopoietic stem cells: the paradigmatic tissue-specific stem cell. *Am J Pathol* 169: 338-346.

Can A. & Karahuseyinoglu S. (2007). Concise review: human umbilical cord stroma with regard to the source of fetus-derived stem cells. *Stem Cells* 25: 2886-2895.

Carlson G.D. & Gorden C. (2002). Current developments in spinal cord injury research. *Spine J* 2: 116-128.

Carlson S.L., Parrish M.E., Springer J.E., Doty K., & Dossett L. (1998). Acute inflammatory response in spinal cord following impact injury. *Exp Neurol* 151: 77-88.

Casha S., Yu W.R., & Fehlings M.G. (2001). Oligodendroglial apoptosis occurs along degenerating axons and is associated with FAS and p75 expression following spinal cord injury in the rat. *Neuroscience* 103: 203-218.

Chagraoui J., Lepage-Noll A., Anjo A., Uzan G., & Charbord P. (2003). Fetal liver stroma consists of cells in epithelial-to-mesenchymal transition. *Blood* 101: 2973-2982.

Chen C.T., Foo N.H., Liu W.S., & Chen S.H. (2008). Infusion of human umbilical cord blood cells ameliorates hind limb dysfunction in experimental spinal cord injury through anti-inflammatory, vasculogenic and neurotrophic mechanisms. *Pediatr Neonatol* 49: 77-83.

Choi C. & Benveniste E.N. (2004). Fas ligand/Fas system in the brain: regulator of immune and apoptotic responses. *Brain Res Brain Res Rev* 44: 65-81.

Choi D.W. (1988). Glutamate neurotoxicity and diseases of the nervous system. *Neuron* 1: 623-634.

Choi S.J., Lee K.H., Park H.S., Kim S.K., Koh C.M., & Park J.Y. (2005). Differential expression, shedding, cytokine regulation and function of TNFR1 and TNFR2 in human fetal astrocytes. *Yonsei Med J* 46: 818-826.

Citron B.A., Arnold P.M., Sebastian C., Qin F., Malladi S., Ameenuddin S. et al. (2000). Rapid upregulation of caspase-3 in rat spinal cord after injury: mRNA, protein, and cellular localization correlates with apoptotic cell death. *Exp Neurol* 166: 213-226.

Cizkova D., Rosocha J., Vanicky I., Jergova S., & Cizek M. (2006). Transplants of human mesenchymal stem cells improve functional recovery after spinal cord injury in the rat. *Cell Mol Neurobiol* 26: 1167-1180.

Clark B.R. & Keating A. (1995). Biology of bone marrow stroma. *Ann N Y Acad Sci* 770: 70-78.

Clark R.S., Kochanek P.M., Watkins S.C., Chen M., Dixon C.E., Seidberg N.A. et al. (2000). Caspase-3 mediated neuronal death after traumatic brain injury in rats. *J Neurochem* 74: 740-753.

Corcione A., Benvenuto F., Ferretti E., Giunti D., Cappiello V., Cazzanti F. et al. (2006). Human mesenchymal stem cells modulate B-cell functions. *Blood* 107: 367-372.

Coutts M. & Keirstead H.S. (2008). Stem cells for the treatment of spinal cord injury. *Exp Neurol* 209: 368-377.

Crowe M.J., Bresnahan J.C., Shuman S.L., Masters J.N., & Beattie M.S. (1997). Apoptosis and delayed degeneration after spinal cord injury in rats and monkeys. *Nat Med* 3: 73-76.

D'Souza S., Alinauskas K., McCrea E., Goodyer C., & Antel J.P. (1995). Differential susceptibility of human CNS-derived cell populations to TNF-dependent and independent immune-mediated injury. *J Neurosci* 15: 7293-7300.

Dasari V.R., Spomar D.G., Cady C., Gujrati M., Rao J.S., & Dinh D.H. (2007a). Mesenchymal stem cells from rat bone marrow downregulate caspase-3-mediated apoptotic pathway after spinal cord injury in rats. *Neurochem Res* 32: 2080-2093.

Dasari V.R., Spomar D.G., Gondi C.S., Sloffer C.A., Saving K.L., Gujrati M. et al. (2007b). Axonal remyelination by cord blood stem cells after spinal cord injury. *J Neurotrauma* 24: 391-410.

Dasari V.R., Spomar D.G., Li L., Gujrati M., Rao J.S., & Dinh D.H. (2008). Umbilical cord blood stem cell mediated downregulation of Fas improves functional recovery of rats after spinal cord injury. *Neurochem Res* 33: 134-149.

Dasari V.R., Veeravalli K.K., Tsung A.J., Gondi C.S., Gujrati M., Dinh D.H. et al. (2009). Neuronal apoptosis is inhibited by cord blood stem cells after spinal cord injury. *J Neurotrauma* 26: 2057-2069.

Davis R.J. (2000). Signal transduction by the JNK group of MAP kinases. *Cell* 103: 239-252.

Demjen D., Klussmann S., Kleber S., Zuliani C., Stieltjes B., Metzger C. et al. (2004). Neutralization of CD95 ligand promotes regeneration and functional recovery after spinal cord injury. *Nat Med* 10: 389-395.

Deng Y.B., Liu X.G., Liu Z.G., Liu X.L., Liu Y., Zhou G.Q. (2006). Implantation of BM mesenchymal stem cells into injured spinal cord elicits de novo neurogenesis and functional recovery: evidence from a study in rhesus monkeys. *Cytotherapy* 8:210-214.

Desbarats J., Birge R.B., Mimouni-Rongy M., Weinstein D.E., Palerme J.S., & Newell M.K. (2003). Fas engagement induces neurite growth through ERK activation and p35 upregulation. *Nat Cell Biol* 5: 118-125.

Deveraux Q.L., Leo E., Stennicke H.R., Welsh K., Salvesen G.S., & Reed J.C. (1999). Cleavage of human inhibitor of apoptosis protein XIAP results in fragments with distinct specificities for caspases. *EMBO J* 18: 5242-5251.

Di Nicola M., Carlo-Stella C., Magni M., Milanesi M., Longoni P.D., Matteucci P. et al. (2002). Human bone marrow stromal cells suppress T-lymphocyte proliferation induced by cellular or nonspecific mitogenic stimuli. *Blood* 99: 3838-3843.

Dinomais M., Stana L., Egon G., Richard I., & Menei P. (2009). Significant recovery of motor function in a patient with complete T7 paraplegia receiving etanercept. *J Rehabil Med* 41: 286-288.

Dohrmann G.J., Wagner F.C., Jr., & Bucy P.C. (1972). Transitory traumatic paraplegia: electron microscopy of early alterations in myelinated nerve fibers. *J Neurosurg* 36: 407-415.

Dolga A.M., Granic I., Blank T., Knaus H.G., Spiess J., Luiten P.G. et al. (2008). TNF-alpha-mediates neuroprotection against glutamate-induced excitotoxicity via NF-kappaB-dependent up-regulation of K2.2 channels. *J Neurochem* 107: 1158-1167.

Dusart I. & Schwab M.E. (1994). Secondary cell death and the inflammatory reaction after dorsal hemisection of the rat spinal cord. *Eur J Neurosci* 6: 712-724.

Eftekharpour E., Holmgren A., & Juurlink B.H. (2000). Thioredoxin reductase and glutathione synthesis is upregulated by t-butylhydroquinone in cortical astrocytes but not in cortical neurons. *Glia* 31: 241-248.

Eftekharpour E., Karimi-Abdolrezaee S., & Fehlings M.G. (2008). Current status of experimental cell replacement approaches to spinal cord injury. *Neurosurg Focus* 24: E19.

Eilers A., Whitfield J., Babij C., Rubin L.L., & Ham J. (1998). Role of the Jun kinase pathway in the regulation of c-Jun expression and apoptosis in sympathetic neurons. *J Neurosci* 18: 1713-1724.

Ekert P.G., Silke J., & Vaux D.L. (1999). Caspase inhibitors. *Cell Death Differ* 6: 1081-1086.

Eldadah B.A. & Faden A.I. (2000). Caspase pathways, neuronal apoptosis, and CNS injury. *J Neurotrauma* 17: 811-829.

Emery E., Aldana P., Bunge M.B., Puckett W., Srinivasan A., Keane R.W. et al. (1998). Apoptosis after traumatic human spinal cord injury. *J Neurosurg* 89: 911-920.

Enzmann G.U., Benton R.L., Talbott J.F., Cao Q., & Whittemore S.R. (2006). Functional considerations of stem cell transplantation therapy for spinal cord repair. *J Neurotrauma* 23: 479-495.

Esposito E., Genovese T., Caminiti R., Bramanti P., Meli R., & Cuzzocrea S. (2009). Melatonin reduces stress-activated/mitogen-activated protein kinases in spinal cord injury. *J Pineal Res* 46: 79-86.

Fong Y., Moldawer L.L., Marano M., Wei H., Barber A., Manogue K. et al. (1989). Cachectin/TNF or IL-1 alpha induces cachexia with redistribution of body proteins. *Am J Physiol* 256: R659-R665.

Friedenstein A.J., Chailakhyan R.K., Latsinik N.V., Panasyuk A.F., & Keiliss-Borok I.V. (1974). Stromal cells responsible for transferring the microenvironment of the hemopoietic tissues. Cloning *in vitro* and retransplantation *in vivo*. *Transplantation* 17: 331-340.

Gao Y., Signore A.P., Yin W., Cao G., Yin X.M., Sun F. et al. (2005). Neuroprotection against focal ischemic brain injury by inhibition of c-Jun N-terminal kinase and attenuation of the mitochondrial apoptosis-signaling pathway. *J Cereb Blood Flow Metab* 25: 694-712.

Garbuzova-Davis S., Willing A.E., Saporta S., Bickford P.C., Gemma C., Chen N. et al. (2006). Novel cell therapy approaches for brain repair. *Prog Brain Res* 157: 207-222.

Gillardon F., Bottiger B., Schmitz B., Zimmermann M., & Hossmann K.A. (1997). Activation of CPP-32 protease in hippocampal neurons following ischemia and epilepsy. *Brain Res Mol Brain Res* 50: 16-22.

Gluckman E., Rocha V., Boyer-Chammard A., Locatelli F., Arcese W., Pasquini R. et al. (1997). Outcome of cord-blood transplantation from related and unrelated donors. Eurocord Transplant Group and the European Blood and Marrow Transplantation Group. *N Engl J Med* 337: 373-381.

Goldbach-Mansky R., Dailey N.J., Canna S.W., Gelabert A., Jones J., Rubin B.I. et al. (2006). Neonatal-onset multisystem inflammatory disease responsive to interleukin-1beta inhibition. *N Engl J Med* 355: 581-592.

Gonz'alez Deniselle M.C., Gonz'alez S.L., & De Nicola A.F. (2001). Cellular basis of steroid neuroprotection in the wobbler mouse, a genetic model of motoneuron disease. *Cell Mol Neurobiol* 21: 237-254.

Gottron F.J., Ying H.S., & Choi D.W. (1997). Caspase inhibition selectively reduces the apoptotic component of oxygen-glucose deprivation-induced cortical neuronal cell death. *Mol Cell Neurosci* 9: 159-169.

Greitz D. (2006). Unraveling the riddle of syringomyelia. *Neurosurg Rev* 29: 251-263.

Grewal I.S. (2009). Overview of TNF superfamily: a chest full of potential therapeutic targets. *Adv Exp Med Biol* 647: 1-7.

Gronthos S., Franklin D.M., Leddy H.A., Robey P.G., Storms R.W., & Gimble J.M. (2001). Surface protein characterization of human adipose tissue-derived stromal cells. *J Cell Physiol* 189: 54-63.

Grossman S.D., Rosenberg L.J., & Wrathall J.R. (2001). Temporal-spatial pattern of acute neuronal and glial loss after spinal cord contusion. *Exp Neurol* 168: 273-282.

Gu W, Zhang F, Xue Q, Ma Z, Lu P, Yu B. (2010). Transplantation of bone marrow mesenchymal stem cells reduces lesion volume and induces axonal regrowth of injured spinal cord. *Neuropathology* 30:205-217.

Hagg T. & Oudega M. (2006). Degenerative and spontaneous regenerative processes after spinal cord injury. *J Neurotrauma* 23: 264-280.

Han I.S., Ra J.S., Kim M.W., Lee E.A., Jun H.Y., Park S.K. et al. (2003). Differentiation of CD34+ cells from human cord blood and murine bone marrow is suppressed by C6 beta-chemokines. *Mol Cells* 15: 176-180.

Hara H., Friedlander R.M., Gagliardini V., Ayata C., Fink K., Huang Z. et al. (1997). Inhibition of interleukin 1beta converting enzyme family proteases reduces ischemic and excitotoxic neuronal damage. *Proc Natl Acad Sci USA* 94: 2007-2012.

Harrington J.F., Messier A.A., Levine A., Szmydynger-Chodobska J., & Chodobski A. (2005). Shedding of tumor necrosis factor type 1 receptor after experimental spinal cord injury. *J Neurotrauma* 22: 919-928.

Harris C.A. & Johnson E.M., Jr. (2001). BH3-only Bcl-2 family members are coordinately regulated by the JNK pathway and require Bax to induce apoptosis in neurons. *J Biol Chem* 276: 37754-37760.

Hausmann O.N. (2003). Post-traumatic inflammation following spinal cord injury. *Spinal Cord* 41: 369-378.

Hayashi M., Ueyama T., Nemoto K., Tamaki T., & Senba E. (2000). Sequential mRNA expression for immediate early genes, cytokines, and neurotrophins in spinal cord injury. *J Neurotrauma* 17: 203-218.

Hemmoranta H., Hautaniemi S., Niemi J., Nicorici D., Laine J., Yli-Harja O. et al. (2006). Transcriptional profiling reflects shared and unique characters for CD34+ and CD133+ cells. *Stem Cells Dev* 15: 839-851.

Himes B.T., Neuhuber B., Coleman C., Kushner R., Swanger S.A., Kopen G.C. et al. (2006). Recovery of function following grafting of human bone marrow-derived stromal cells into the injured spinal cord. *Neurorehabil Neural Repair* 20: 278-296.

Hipp J. & Atala A. (2004). Tissue engineering, stem cells, cloning, and parthenogenesis: new paradigms for therapy. *J Exp Clin Assist Reprod* 1: 3.

Ho F.M., Liu S.H., Liau C.S., Huang P.J., & Lin-Shiau S.Y. (2000). High glucose-induced apoptosis in human endothelial cells is mediated by sequential activations of c-Jun NH(2)-terminal kinase and caspase-3. *Circulation* 101: 2618-2624.

Hofstetter C.P., Schwarz E.J., Hess D., Widenfalk J., El M.A., Prockop D.J. et al. (2002). Marrow stromal cells form guiding strands in the injured spinal cord and promote recovery. *Proc Natl Acad Sci USA* 99: 2199-2204.

Holmes G.M., Hebert S.L., Rogers R.C., & Hermann G.E. (2004). Immunocytochemical localization of TNF type 1 and type 2 receptors in the rat spinal cord. *Brain Res* 1025: 210-219.

Hu S.L., Luo H.S., Li J.T., Xia Y.Z., Li L., Zhang L.J., Meng H., Cui G.Y., Chen Z., Wu N., Lin J.K., Zhu G., Feng H. (2010) Functional recovery in acute traumatic spinal cord injury after transplantation of human umbilical cord mesenchymal stem cells. *Crit Care Med.* 38:2181-2189.

Inoshita S., Takeda K., Hatai T., Terada Y., Sano M., Hata J. et al. (2002). Phosphorylation and inactivation of myeloid cell leukemia 1 by JNK in response to oxidative stress. *J Biol Chem* 277: 43730-43734.

Isele N.B., Lee H.S., Landshamer S., Straube A., Padovan C.S., Plesnila N. et al. (2007). Bone marrow stromal cells mediate protection through stimulation of PI3-K/Akt and MAPK signaling in neurons. *Neurochem Int* 50: 243-250.

Jankowski R.J., Deasy B.M., & Huard J. (2002). Muscle-derived stem cells. *Gene Ther* 9: 642-647.

Jiang X.X., Zhang Y., Liu B., Zhang S.X., Wu Y., Yu X.D. et al. (2005). Human mesenchymal stem cells inhibit differentiation and function of monocyte-derived dendritic cells. *Blood* 105: 4120-4126.

Juurlink B.H. & Paterson P.G. (1998). Review of oxidative stress in brain and spinal cord injury: suggestions for pharmacological and nutritional management strategies. *J Spinal Cord Med* 21: 309-334.

Kang S.J., Wang S., Hara H., Peterson E.P., Namura S., min-Hanjani S. et al. (2000). Dual role of caspase-11 in mediating activation of caspase-1 and caspase-3 under pathological conditions. *J Cell Biol* 149: 613-622.

Kao C.H., Chen S.H., Chio C.C., & Lin M.T. (2008). Human umbilical cord blood-derived CD34+ cells may attenuate spinal cord injury by stimulating vascular endothelial and neurotrophic factors. *Shock* 29: 49-55.

Kawasaki Y., Zhang L., Cheng J.K., & Ji R.R. (2008). Cytokine mechanisms of central sensitization: distinct and overlapping role of interleukin-1beta, interleukin-6, and tumor necrosis factor-alpha in regulating synaptic and neuronal activity in the superficial spinal cord. *J Neurosci* 28: 5189-5194.

Keane R.W., Davis A.R., & Dietrich W.D. (2006). Inflammatory and apoptotic signaling after spinal cord injury. *J Neurotrauma* 23: 335-344.

Keane R.W., Kraydieh S., Lotocki G., Alonso O.F., Aldana P., & Dietrich W.D. (2001). Apoptotic and antiapoptotic mechanisms after traumatic brain injury. *J Cereb Blood Flow Metab* 21: 1189-1198.

Kim G.M., Xu J., Xu J., Song S.K., Yan P., Ku G. et al. (2001). Tumor necrosis factor receptor deletion reduces nuclear factor-kappaB activation, cellular inhibitor of apoptosis protein 2 expression, and functional recovery after traumatic spinal cord injury. *J Neurosci* 21: 6617-6625.

Kim S.K., Koh S.K., Song S.U., Shin S.H., Choi G.S., Kim W.C. et al. (2002). Ex vivo expansion and clonality of CD34+ selected cells from bone marrow and cord blood in a serum-free media. *Mol Cells* 14: 367-373.

Kim T.H., Zhao Y., Barber M.J., Kuharsky D.K., & Yin X.M. (2000). Bid-induced cytochrome c release is mediated by a pathway independent of mitochondrial permeability transition pore and Bax. *J Biol Chem* 275: 39474-39481.

Kotipatruni R.R., Dasari V.R., Veeravalli K.K., Dinh D.H., Fassett D., & Rao J.S. (2011). p53- and Bax-Mediated Apoptosis in Injured Rat Spinal Cord. *Neurochem Res* e-pub ahead of print.

Kuh S.U., Cho Y.E., Yoon D.H., Kim K.N., & Ha Y. (2005). Functional recovery after human umbilical cord blood cells transplantation with brain-derived neutrophic factor into the spinal cord injured rat. *Acta Neurochir (Wien)* 147: 985-992.

Kuwana T., Smith J.J., Muzio M., Dixit V., Newmeyer D.D., & Kornbluth S. (1998). Apoptosis induction by caspase-8 is amplified through the mitochondrial release of cytochrome c. *J Biol Chem* 273: 16589-16594.

Lee K.H., Suh-Kim H., Choi J.S., Jeun S.S., Kim E.J., Kim S.S., Yoon do H., Lee B.H. (2007) Human mesenchymal stem cell transplantation promotes functional recovery following acute spinal cord injury in rats. *Acta Neurobiol Exp (Wars)*. 67:13-22.

Lee Y.B., Yune T.Y., Baik S.Y., Shin Y.H., Du S., Rhim H. et al. (2000). Role of tumor necrosis factor-alpha in neuronal and glial apoptosis after spinal cord injury. *Exp Neurol* 166: 190-195.

Leung L. & Cahill C.M. (2010). TNF-alpha and neuropathic pain--a review. *J Neuroinflammation* 7: 27-38.

Li G.L., Brodin G., Farooque M., Funa K., Holtz A., Wang W.L. et al. (1996). Apoptosis and expression of Bcl-2 after compression trauma to rat spinal cord. *J Neuropathol Exp Neurol* 55: 280-289.

Li H., Zhu H., Xu C.J., & Yuan J. (1998). Cleavage of BID by caspase 8 mediates the mitochondrial damage in the Fas pathway of apoptosis. *Cell* 94: 491-501.

Li M., Ona V.O., Chen M., Kaul M., Tenneti L., Zhang X. et al. (2000a). Functional role and therapeutic implications of neuronal caspase-1 and -3 in a mouse model of traumatic spinal cord injury. *Neuroscience* 99: 333-342.

Li M., Ona V.O., Guegan C., Chen M., Jackson-Lewis V., Andrews L.J. et al. (2000b). Functional role of caspase-1 and caspase-3 in an ALS transgenic mouse model. *Science* 288: 335-339.

Li Q.M., Tep C., Yune T.Y., Zhou X.Z., Uchida T., Lu K.P. et al. (2007). Opposite regulation of oligodendrocyte apoptosis by JNK3 and Pin1 after spinal cord injury. *J Neurosci* 27: 8395-8404.

Lim J.H., Byeon Y.E., Ryu H.H., Jeong Y.H., Lee Y.W., Kim W.H., Kang K. S., Kweon O.K. (2007) Transplantation of canine umbilical cord blood-derived mesenchymal stem cells in experimentally induced spinal cord injured dogs. *J Vet Sci.* 8:275-282.

Liu X.Z., Xu X.M., Hu R., Du C., Zhang S.X., McDonald J.W. et al. (1997). Neuronal and glial apoptosis after traumatic spinal cord injury. *J Neurosci* 17: 5395-5406.

Lou J., Lenke L.G., Ludwig F.J., & O'Brien M.F. (1998). Apoptosis as a mechanism of neuronal cell death following acute experimental spinal cord injury. *Spinal Cord* 36: 683-690.

Lu J., Ashwell K.W., & Waite P. (2000). Advances in secondary spinal cord injury: role of apoptosis. *Spine* 25: 1859-1866.

Lu L.L., Liu Y.J., Yang S.G., Zhao Q.J., Wang X., Gong W. et al. (2006). Isolation and characterization of human umbilical cord mesenchymal stem cells with hematopoiesis-supportive function and other potentials. *Haematologica* 91: 1017-1026.

Ma Y., Xu Y., Xiao Z., Yang W., Zhang C., Song E. et al. (2006). Reconstruction of chemically burned rat corneal surface by bone marrow-derived human mesenchymal stem cells. *Stem Cells* 24: 315-321.

Malgieri A., Kantzari E., Patrizi M.P., & Gambardella S. (2010). Bone marrow and umbilical cord blood human mesenchymal stem cells: state of the art. *Int J Clin Exp Med* 3: 248-269.

Martin-Villalba A., Herr I., Jeremias I., Hahne M., Brandt R., Vogel J. et al. (1999). CD95 ligand (Fas-L/APO-1L) and tumor necrosis factor-related apoptosis-inducing ligand mediate ischemia-induced apoptosis in neurons. *J Neurosci* 19: 3809-3817.

Maundrell K., Antonsson B., Magnenat E., Camps M., Muda M., Chabert C. et al. (1997). Bcl-2 undergoes phosphorylation by c-Jun N-terminal kinase/stress-activated protein kinases in the presence of the constitutively active GTP-binding protein Rac1. *J Biol Chem* 272: 25238-25242.

Mayani H. & Lansdorp P.M. (1998). Biology of human umbilical cord blood-derived hematopoietic stem/progenitor cells. *Stem Cells* 16: 153-165.

Means E.D. & Anderson D.K. (1983). Neuronophagia by leukocytes in experimental spinal cord injury. *J Neuropathol Exp Neurol* 42: 707-719.

Mendez-Ferrer S., Michurina T.V., Ferraro F., Mazloom A.R., Macarthur B.D., Lira S.A. et al. (2010). Mesenchymal and haematopoietic stem cells form a unique bone marrow niche. *Nature* 466: 829-834.

Mimeault M. & Batra S.K. (2006). Concise review: recent advances on the significance of stem cells in tissue regeneration and cancer therapies. *Stem Cells* 24: 2319-2345.

Miura M., Gronthos S., Zhao M., Lu B., Fisher L.W., Robey P.G. et al. (2003). SHED: stem cells from human exfoliated deciduous teeth. *Proc Natl Acad Sci U S A* 100: 5807-5812.

Moore K.E., Mills J.F., & Thornton M.M. (2006). Alternative sources of adult stem cells: a possible solution to the embryonic stem cell debate. *Gend Med* 3: 161-168.

Nakagawa T. & Yuan J. (2000). Cross-talk between two cysteine protease families. Activation of caspase-12 by calpain in apoptosis. *J Cell Biol* 150: 887-894.

Nakahara S., Yone K., Sakou T., Wada S., Nagamine T., Niiyama T. et al. (1999). Induction of apoptosis signal regulating kinase 1 (ASK1) after spinal cord injury in rats: possible involvement of ASK1-JNK and -p38 pathways in neuronal apoptosis. *J Neuropathol Exp Neurol* 58: 442-450.

Namura S., Zhu J., Fink K., Endres M., Srinivasan A., Tomaselli K.J. et al. (1998). Activation and cleavage of caspase-3 in apoptosis induced by experimental cerebral ischemia. *J Neurosci* 18: 3659-3668.

Nashmi R. & Fehlings M.G. (2001). Mechanisms of axonal dysfunction after spinal cord injury: with an emphasis on the role of voltage-gated potassium channels. *Brain Res Brain Res Rev* 38: 165-191.

Neuhuber B., Timothy H.B., Shumsky J.S., Gallo G., & Fischer I. (2005). Axon growth and recovery of function supported by human bone marrow stromal cells in the injured spinal cord exhibit donor variations. *Brain Res* 1035: 73-85.

Nicholson D.W. (2000). From bench to clinic with apoptosis-based therapeutic agents. *Nature* 407: 810-816.

Noth U., Osyczka A.M., Tuli R., Hickok N.J., Danielson K.G., & Tuan R.S. (2002). Multilineage mesenchymal differentiation potential of human trabecular bone-derived cells. *J Orthop Res* 20: 1060-1069.

Okuno S., Saito A., Hayashi T., & Chan P.H. (2004). The c-Jun N-terminal protein kinase signaling pathway mediates Bax activation and subsequent neuronal apoptosis through interaction with Bim after transient focal cerebral ischemia. *J Neurosci* 24: 7879-7887.

Osaka M., Honmou O., Murakami T., Nonaka T., Houkin K., Hamada H., Kocsis J. D. (2010) Intravenous administration of mesenchymal stem cells derived from bone marrow after contusive spinal cord injury improves functional outcome. *Brain Res.* 1343:226-235.

Park D.H., Lee J.H., Borlongan C.V., Sanberg P.R., Chung Y.G., & Cho T.H. (2011). Transplantation of umbilical cord blood stem cells for treating spinal cord injury. *Stem Cell Rev* 7: 181-194.

Park D.S., Stefanis L., Yan C.Y., Farinelli S.E., & Greene L.A. (1996). Ordering the cell death pathway. Differential effects of BCL2, an interleukin-1-converting enzyme family protease inhibitor, and other survival agents on JNK activation in serum/nerve growth factor-deprived PC12 cells. *J Biol Chem* 271: 21898-21905.

Park H.C., Shim Y.S., Ha Y., Yoon S.H., Park S.R., Choi B.H. et al. (2005). Treatment of complete spinal cord injury patients by autologous bone marrow cell transplantation and administration of granulocyte-macrophage colony stimulating factor. *Tissue Eng* 11: 913-922.

Parr A.M., Kulbatski I., Wang X.H., Keating A., Tator C.H. (2008) Fate of transplanted adult neural stem/progenitor cells and bone marrow-derived mesenchymal stromal cells in the injured adult rat spinal cord and impact on functional recovery. *Surg Neurol.* 70:600-607; discussion 607.

Pessina A. & Gribaldo L. (2006). The key role of adult stem cells: therapeutic perspectives. *Curr Med Res Opin* 22: 2287-2300.

Phinney D.G., Baddoo M., Dutreil M., Gaupp D., Lai W.T., & Isakova I.A. (2006). Murine mesenchymal stem cells transplanted to the central nervous system of neonatal versus adult mice exhibit distinct engraftment kinetics and express receptors that guide neuronal cell migration. *Stem Cells Dev* 15: 437-447.

Phinney D.G. & Prockop D.J. (2007). Concise review: mesenchymal stem/multipotent stromal cells: the state of transdifferentiation and modes of tissue repair--current views. *Stem Cells* 25: 2896-2902.

Pittenger M.F., Mackay A.M., Beck S.C., Jaiswal R.K., Douglas R., Mosca J.D. et al. (1999). Multilineage potential of adult human mesenchymal stem cells. *Science* 284: 143-147.

Popovich P.G., Wei P., & Stokes B.T. (1997). Cellular inflammatory response after spinal cord injury in Sprague-Dawley and Lewis rats. *J Comp Neurol* 377: 443-464.

Poyet J.L., Srinivasula S.M., Lin J.H., Fernandes-Alnemri T., Yamaoka S., Tsichlis P.N. et al. (2000). Activation of the Ikappa B kinases by RIP via IKKgamma /NEMO-mediated oligomerization. *J Biol Chem* 275: 37966-37977.

Putcha G.V., Le S., Frank S., Besirli C.G., Clark K., Chu B. et al. (2003). JNK-mediated BIM phosphorylation potentiates BAX-dependent apoptosis. *Neuron* 38:899-914.

Putcha G.V., Moulder K.L., Golden J.P., Bouillet P., Adams J.A., Strasser A. et al. (2001). Induction of BIM, a proapoptotic BH3-only BCL-2 family member, is critical for neuronal apoptosis. *Neuron* 29: 615-628.

Raoul C., Estevez A.G., Nishimune H., Cleveland D.W., deLapeyriere O., Henderson C.E. et al. (2002). Motoneuron death triggered by a specific pathway downstream of Fas. potentiation by ALS-linked SOD1 mutations. *Neuron* 35: 1067-1083.

Rice T., Larsen J., Rivest S., & Yong V.W. (2007). Characterization of the early neuroinflammation after spinal cord injury in mice. *J Neuropathol Exp Neurol* 66: 184-195.

Rincon M., Whitmarsh A., Yang D.D., Weiss L., Derijard B., Jayaraj P. et al. (1998). The JNK pathway regulates the In vivo deletion of immature CD4(+)CD8(+) thymocytes. *J Exp Med* 188: 1817-1830.

Sabapathy K., Hu Y., Kallunki T., Schreiber M., David J.P., Jochum W. et al. (1999). JNK2 is required for efficient T-cell activation and apoptosis but not for normal lymphocyte development. *Curr Biol* 9: 116-125.

Salvesen G.S. & Dixit V.M. (1999). Caspase activation: the induced-proximity model. *Proc Natl Acad Sci USA* 96: 10964-10967.

Sanberg P.R., Willing A.E., Garbuzova-Davis S., Saporta S., Liu G., Sanberg C.D. et al. (2005). Umbilical cord blood-derived stem cells and brain repair. *Ann NY Acad Sci* 1049: 67-83.

Saporta S., Kim J.J., Willing A.E., Fu E.S., Davis C.D., & Sanberg P.R. (2003). Human umbilical cord blood stem cells infusion in spinal cord injury: engraftment and beneficial influence on behavior. *J Hematother Stem Cell Res* 12: 271-278.

Sarugaser R., Lickorish D., Baksh D., Hosseini M.M., & Davies J.E. (2005). Human umbilical cord perivascular (HUCPV) cells: a source of mesenchymal progenitors. *Stem Cells* 23: 220-229.

Satake K., Lou J., Lenke L.G. (2004) Migration of mesenchymal stem cells through cerebrospinal fluid into injured spinal cord tissue. *Spine (Phila Pa 1976).* 29:1971-1979.

Scaffidi C., Fulda S., Srinivasan A., Friesen C., Li F., Tomaselli K.J. et al. (1998). Two CD95 (APO-1/Fas) signaling pathways. *EMBO J* 17: 1675-1687.

Schotte P., Van C.W., Van de C.M., Van L.G., Desmedt M., Grooten J. et al. (1998). Cathepsin B-mediated activation of the proinflammatory caspase-11. *Biochem Biophys Res Commun* 251: 379-387.

Sekhon L.H. & Fehlings M.G. (2001). Epidemiology, demographics, and pathophysiology of acute spinal cord injury. *Spine (Phila Pa)* 26: S2-12.

Sharma H.S. (2007). A select combination of neurotrophins enhances neuroprotection and functional recovery following spinal cord injury. *Ann N Y Acad Sci* 1122: 95-111.

Sharma H.S. (2008). New perspectives for the treatment options in spinal cord injury. *Expert Opin Pharmacother* 9: 2773-2800.

Sharma H.S. (2010). A combination of tumor necrosis factor-alpha and neuronal nitric oxide synthase antibodies applied topically over the traumatized spinal cord enhances neuroprotection and functional recovery in the rat. *Ann N Y Acad Sci* 1199: 175-185.

Sharma H.S., Olsson Y., & Nyberg F. (1995). Influence of dynorphin A antibodies on the formation of edema and cell changes in spinal cord trauma. *Prog Brain Res* 104: 401-416.

Shuman S.L., Bresnahan J.C., & Beattie M.S. (1997). Apoptosis of microglia and oligodendrocytes after spinal cord contusion in rats. *J Neurosci Res* 50: 798-808.

Sipe K.J., Srisawasdi D., Dantzer R., Kelley K.W., & Weyhenmeyer J.A. (1996). An endogenous 55 kDa TNF receptor mediates cell death in a neural cell line. *Brain Res Mol Brain Res* 38: 222-232.

Slee E.A., Harte M.T., Kluck R.M., Wolf B.B., Casiano C.A., Newmeyer D.D. et al. (1999). Ordering the cytochrome c-initiated caspase cascade: hierarchical activation of caspases-2, -3, -6, -7, -8, and -10 in a caspase-9-dependent manner. *J Cell Biol* 144: 281-292.

Spees J.L., Olson S.D., Ylostalo J., Lynch P.J., Smith J., Perry A. et al. (2003). Differentiation, cell fusion, and nuclear fusion during *ex vivo* repair of epithelium by human adult stem cells from bone marrow stroma. *Proc Natl Acad Sci U S A* 100: 2397-2402.

Springer J.E., Azbill R.D., & Knapp P.E. (1999). Activation of the caspase-3 apoptotic cascade in traumatic spinal cord injury. *Nat Med* 5: 943-946.

Stalberg E., Sharma H.S., & Olsson Y. (1998). *Spinal Cord Monitoring. Basic principles, regeneration, pathophysiology and clinical aspects.*, Springer, Wien., New York.

Stanworth S.J. & Newland A.C. (2001). Stem cells: progress in research and edging towards the clinical setting. *Clin Med* 1: 378-382.

Stennicke H.R., Jurgensmeier J.M., Shin H., Deveraux Q., Wolf B.B., Yang X. et al. (1998). Pro-caspase-3 is a major physiologic target of caspase-8. *J Biol Chem* 273: 27084-27090.

Streit W.J., Semple-Rowland S.L., Hurley S.D., Miller R.C., Popovich P.G., & Stokes B.T. (1998). Cytokine mRNA profiles in contused spinal cord and axotomized facial nucleus suggest a beneficial role for inflammation and gliosis. *Exp Neurol* 152: 74-87.

Sykova E., Jendelova P., Urdzikova L., Lesny P., & Hejcl A. (2006). Bone marrow stem cells and polymer hydrogels--two strategies for spinal cord injury repair. *Cell Mol Neurobiol* 26: 1113-1129.

Taguchi A., Soma T., Tanaka H., Kanda T., Nishimura H., Yoshikawa H. et al. (2004). Administration of CD34+ cells after stroke enhances neurogenesis via angiogenesis in a mouse model. *J Clin Invest* 114: 330-338.

Taoka Y. & Okajima K. (1998). Spinal cord injury in the rat. *Prog Neurobiol* 56: 341-358.

Taoka Y., Okajima K., Murakami K., Johno M., & Naruo M. (1998). Role of neutrophil elastase in compression-induced spinal cord injury in rats. *Brain Res* 799: 264-269.

Tartaglia L.A., Weber R.F., Figari I.S., Reynolds C., Palladino M.A., Jr., & Goeddel D.V. (1991). The two different receptors for tumor necrosis factor mediate distinct cellular responses. *Proc Natl Acad Sci USA* 88: 9292-9296.

Tator C.H. & Fehlings M.G. (1991). Review of the secondary injury theory of acute spinal cord trauma with emphasis on vascular mechanisms. *J Neurosurg* 75: 15-26.

Thornberry N.A. & Lazebnik Y. (1998). Caspases: enemies within. *Science* 281: 1312-1316.

Totoiu M.O. & Keirstead H.S. (2005). Spinal cord injury is accompanied by chronic progressive demyelination. *J Comp Neurol* 486: 373-383.

Tournier C., Dong C., Turner T.K., Jones S.N., Flavell R.A., & Davis R.J. (2001). MKK7 is an essential component of the JNK signal transduction pathway activated by proinflammatory cytokines. *Genes Dev* 15: 1419-1426.

Tournier C., Hess P., Yang D.D., Xu J., Turner T.K., Nimnual A. et al. (2000). Requirement of JNK for stress-induced activation of the cytochrome c-mediated death pathway. *Science* 288: 870-874.

Tracey K.J. (2011). Tumor necrosis factor. In: *The Cytokine Handbook*. Thompson A.W. (ed.), pp. 289-304, Academic Press: New York.

Trivedi A., Olivas A.D., & Noble-Haeusslein L.J. (2006). Inflammation and Spinal Cord Injury: Infiltrating Leukocytes as Determinants of Injury and Repair Processes. *Clin Neurosci Res* 6: 283-292.

Tsujimoto Y. (2003). Cell death regulation by the Bcl-2 protein family in the mitochondria. *J Cell Physiol* 195: 158-167.

Tsujimoto Y. & Shimizu S. (2000). Bcl-2 family: life-or-death switch. *FEBS Lett* 466: 6-10.

Uccelli A., Benvenuto F., Laroni A., & Giunti D. (2011). Neuroprotective features of mesenchymal stem cells. *Best Pract Res Clin Haematol* 24: 59-64.

Vandenabeele P., Declercq W., Beyaert R., & Fiers W. (1995). Two tumour necrosis factor receptors: structure and function. *Trends Cell Biol* 5: 392-399.

Varfolomeev E.E. & Ashkenazi A. (2004). Tumor necrosis factor: an apoptosis JuNKie? *Cell* 116: 491-497.

Veeravalli K.K., Dasari V.R., Tsung A.J., Dinh D.H., Gujrati M., Fassett D. et al. (2009a). Human umbilical cord blood stem cells upregulate matrix metalloproteinase-2 in rats after spinal cord injury. *Neurobiol Dis* 36: 200-212.

Veeravalli K.K., Dasari V.R., Tsung A.J., Dinh D.H., Gujrati M., Fassett D. et al. (2009b). Stem Cells Downregulate the Elevated Levels of Tissue Plasminogen Activator in Rats After Spinal Cord Injury. *Neurochem Res* 34: 1183-1194.

Verhagen A.M., Ekert P.G., Pakusch M., Silke J., Connolly L.M., Reid G.E. et al. (2000). Identification of DIABLO, a mammalian protein that promotes apoptosis by binding to and antagonizing IAP proteins. *Cell* 102: 43-53.

Wagner F., Dhormann G., & Bucy P. (1971). Histopathology of transitory traumatic paraplegia in the monkey. *J Neurosurg* 35: 272-276.

Waldner H., Sobel R.A., Howard E., & Kuchroo V.K. (1997). Fas- and FasL-deficient mice are resistant to induction of autoimmune encephalomyelitis. *J Immunol* 159: 3100-3103.

Wang C.X., Nuttin B., Heremans H., Dom R., & Gybels J. (1996). Production of tumor necrosis factor in spinal cord following traumatic injury in rats. *J Neuroimmunol* 69: 151-156.

Wang C.X., Reece C., Wrathall J.R., Shuaib A., Olschowka J.A., & Hao C. (2002). Expression of tumor necrosis factor alpha and its mRNA in the spinal cord following a weight-drop injury. *Neuroreport* 13: 1391-1393.

Wang S., Miura M., Jung Y.K., Zhu H., Li E., & Yuan J. (1998). Murine caspase-11, an ICE-interacting protease, is essential for the activation of ICE. *Cell* 92: 501-509.

Warden P., Bamber N.I., Li H., Esposito A., Ahmad K.A., Hsu C.Y. et al. (2001). Delayed glial cell death following wallerian degeneration in white matter tracts after spinal cord dorsal column cordotomy in adult rats. *Exp Neurol* 168: 213-224.

Weiss M.L. & Troyer D.L. (2006). Stem cells in the umbilical cord. *Stem Cell Rev* 2: 155-162.

Whitfield J., Neame S.J., Paquet L., Bernard O., & Ham J. (2001). Dominant-negative c-Jun promotes neuronal survival by reducing BIM expression and inhibiting mitochondrial cytochrome c release. *Neuron* 29: 629-643.

Wilson P.G. & Stice S.S. (2006). Development and differentiation of neural rosettes derived from human embryonic stem cells. *Stem Cell Rev* 2: 67-77.

Woodbury D., Schwarz E.J., Prockop D.J., & Black I.B. (2000). Adult rat and human bone marrow stromal cells differentiate into neurons. *J Neurosci Res* 61: 364-370.

Wright K.T., Masri W.E., Osman A., Chowdhury J., & Johnson W.E. (2011). Concise review: bone marrow for the treatment of spinal cord injury: mechanisms and clinical applications. *Stem Cells* 29: 169-178.

Wu K.H., Zhou B., Lu S.H., Feng B., Yang S.G., Du W.T. et al. (2007). *In vitro* and *in vivo* differentiation of human umbilical cord derived stem cells into endothelial cells. *J Cell Biochem* 100: 608-616.

Wyllie A.H., Kerr J.F., & Currie A.R. (1980). Cell death: the significance of apoptosis. *Int Rev Cytol* 68: 251-306.

Xia Z., Dickens M., Raingeaud J., Davis R.J., & Greenberg M.E. (1995). Opposing effects of ERK and JNK-p38 MAP kinases on apoptosis. *Science* 270: 1326-1331.

Yakovlev A.G. & Faden A.I. (2001). Caspase-dependent apoptotic pathways in CNS injury. *Mol Neurobiol* 24: 131-144.

Yakovlev A.G., Knoblach S.M., Fan L., Fox G.B., Goodnight R., & Faden A.I. (1997). Activation of CPP32-like caspases contributes to neuronal apoptosis and neurological dysfunction after traumatic brain injury. *J Neurosci* 17: 7415-7424.

Yamamoto K., Ichijo H., & Korsmeyer S.J. (1999). BCL-2 is phosphorylated and inactivated by an ASK1/Jun N-terminal protein kinase pathway normally activated at G(2)/M. *Mol Cell Biol* 19: 8469-8478.

Yamashima T. (2000). Implication of cysteine proteases calpain, cathepsin and caspase in ischemic neuronal death of primates. *Prog Neurobiol* 62: 273-295.

Yan P., Li Q., Kim G.M., Xu J., Hsu C.Y., & Xu X.M. (2001). Cellular localization of tumor necrosis factor-alpha following acute spinal cord injury in adult rats. *J Neurotrauma* 18: 563-568.

Yan P., Liu N., Kim G.M., Xu J., Xu J., Li Q. et al. (2003). Expression of the type 1 and type 2 receptors for tumor necrosis factor after traumatic spinal cord injury in adult rats. *Exp Neurol* 183: 286-297.

Yang C.C., Shih Y.H., Ko M.H., Hsu S.Y., Cheng H, Fu Y.S. (2008) Transplantation of human umbilical mesenchymal stem cells from Wharton's jelly after complete transection of the rat spinal cord. *PLoS One*. 3(10):e3336.

Yang D., Tournier C., Wysk M., Lu H.T., Xu J., Davis R.J. et al. (1997a). Targeted disruption of the MKK4 gene causes embryonic death, inhibition of c-Jun NH2-terminal kinase activation, and defects in AP-1 transcriptional activity. *Proc Natl Acad Sci USA* 94: 3004-3009.

Yang D.D., Kuan C.Y., Whitmarsh A.J., Rincon M., Zheng T.S., Davis R.J. et al. (1997b). Absence of excitotoxicity-induced apoptosis in the hippocampus of mice lacking the Jnk3 gene. *Nature* 389: 865-870.

Yin K.J., Kim G.M., Lee J.M., He Y.Y., Xu J., & Hsu C.Y. (2005). JNK activation contributes to DP5 induction and apoptosis following traumatic spinal cord injury. *Neurobiol Dis* 20: 881-889.

Yong C., Arnold P.M., Zoubine M.N., Citron B.A., Watanabe I., Berman N.E. et al. (1998). Apoptosis in cellular compartments of rat spinal cord after severe contusion injury. *J Neurotrauma* 15: 459-472.

Yoshino O., Matsuno H., Nakamura H., Yudoh K., Abe Y., Sawai T. et al. (2004). The role of Fas-mediated apoptosis after traumatic spinal cord injury. *Spine* 29: 1394-1404.

Yu S.W., Andrabi S.A., Wang H., Kim N.S., Poirier G.G., Dawson T.M. et al. (2006). Apoptosis-inducing factor mediates poly(ADP-ribose) (PAR) polymer-induced cell death. *Proc Natl Acad Sci USA* 103: 18314-18319.

Yu W.R., Liu T., Fehlings T.K., & Fehlings M.G. (2009). Involvement of mitochondrial signaling pathways in the mechanism of Fas-mediated apoptosis after spinal cord injury. *Eur J Neurosci* 29: 114-131.

Yune T.Y., Chang M.J., Kim S.J., Lee Y.B., Shin S.W., Rhim H. et al. (2003). Increased production of tumor necrosis factor-alpha induces apoptosis after traumatic spinal cord injury in rats. *J Neurotrauma* 20: 207-219.

Zeng X., Zeng Y.S., Ma Y.H., Lu L.Y., Du B.L., Zhang W. et al. (2011). Bone Marrow Mesenchymal Stem Cells in a Three Dimensional Gelatin Sponge Scaffold Attenuate Inflammation, Promote Angiogenesis and Reduce Cavity Formation in Experimental Spinal Cord Injury. *Cell Transplant*.

Zhang L., Liu Y., Lu L., Wang A., Xu Z., & Zhu X. (2006). Mesenchymal stem cells derived from human umbilical cord inhibit activation and proliferation of allogenic umbilical cord blood. *Chin J Cancer Biother* 13: 191-195.

Zhang S.Q., Kovalenko A., Cantarella G., & Wallach D. (2000). Recruitment of the IKK signalosome to the p55 TNF receptor: RIP and A20 bind to NEMO (IKKgamma) upon receptor stimulation. *Immunity* 12: 301-311.

7

Wallerian Degeneration in Injury and Diseases: Concepts and Prevention

Bruno S. Mietto[1], Rodrigo M. Costa[1],
Silmara V. de Lima[1], Sérgio T. Ferreira[1,2] and Ana M. B. Martinez[1]
[1]*Program of Basic and Clinical Neuroscience,*
[2]*Institute of Medical Biochemistry, Federal University of Rio de Janeiro,*
Brazil

1. Introduction

The axon is a highly specialized compartment of neurons. Besides their basic function connecting neurons to their targets, axons play key roles in the nervous system. They are involved in the transport of several molecules indispensable to neuronal activity, act as sensors to guidance cues during development and regeneration, and are essential to maintain normal glial cell functions and myelin sheath assembly (Nave & Trap 2008). Recent evidence indicates that mRNA and Schwann cells-delivered ribosomes can be found within the axoplasm, suggesting that axons may be capable of synthesizing specific proteins (Court et al., 2008). However, most axonal structural proteins are synthesized in the neuronal cell body and transported along the length of the axon. Interruption of this supply leads to a degenerative process known as Wallerian degeneration (WD) in the distal portion of the axon (Coleman, 2005). WD is triggered by intrinsic degenerative pathways that are not correlated to cellular apoptosis (Finn et al., 2000). Axon degeneration is a final common pathway observed not only after a traumatic nerve injury, but also in many neurodegenerative disorders (e.g., Parkinson`s and Alzheimer`s diseases) and in demyelinating diseases such as multiple sclerosis (Coleman, 2005; Coleman & Freeman, 2010). Uncovering the mechanisms that trigger and control axon degeneration is extremely relevant, as such knowledge may offer novel tools to treat severed or damaged axons as well as several neurodegenerative disorders in which WD takes place. In this chapter, we will review the basic concepts of WD, with emphasis on the mechanisms that control axon degeneration following trauma. Next, we will address the issue whether or not current anti-degenerative strategies are efficient and can be envisioned to be applied to humans in the near future.

2. Overview of Wallerian degeneration

WD is classically referred to as a series of degenerative processes triggered in the distal portion of axons after a traumatic injury. WD was originally described by Augustus Waller in 1850 based on his observations in transected glossopharyngeal and hypoglossal nerves (Waller, 1850). Waller observed that, upon transection, the distal nerve stump underwent typical morphological alterations which resulted in total nerve fiber fragmentation followed by disintegration. Although Waller`s description of WD was based on studies with transected peripheral nerves, the main features of WD are observed after many types of insults (crush, transection, chemical and/or toxic) both in the central nervous system (CNS) and in the peripheral nervous system (PNS), and are also present in the course of neurodegenerative and demyelinating diseases, suggesting a common triggering mechanism (Coleman & Perry, 2002).

Axons respond rapidly to an injury. Just a few hours after lesion, ultra-structural analysis reveals swollen axons with their axoplasms filled with an amorphous matrix (Figure 1) resulting from the fact that the major cytoskeleton proteins (microtubules and neurofilaments) are being degraded by activation of ubiquitin-proteasome system (UPS) and calcium-dependent proteases, respectively (to review, see Vargas & Barres, 2007). This event is called granular disintegration of the axonal cytoskeleton resulting in complete degradation of axonal organelles and proteins and is the main ultra-structural characteristic of axons undergoing WD in the PNS. In central nerve fibers, axon disruption may present in two distinct patterns of axoplasm degeneration, as based on the ultra-structural aspect of the axoplasm (Figure 1) (Narciso et al., 2001).

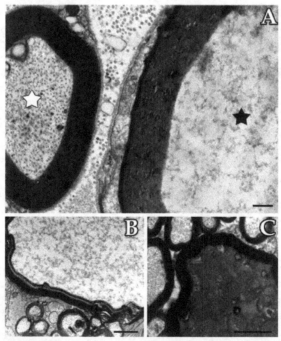

Fig. 1. Ultra-structural images showing different aspects of axon degeneration. Image A represents a sciatic nerve transverse ultra-thin section 48 hours after crush injury in C57BL/6 mice. Note a normal nerve fiber (white star) next to a fiber showing aspects of degeneration with the dissolution of its axoplasmic elements (black star). Images B and C show ultra-thin sections of rat optic nerve, 96 hours after crush injury. Note in B one fiber undergoing watery degeneration, whereas panel C shows a fiber undergoing dark degeneration. Scale bar = 0.3 μm (A) and 1 μm (B and C)

With the onset of WD, the axon will progressively deteriorate and the myelin lamellae will be disrupted into small fragments known as myelin ovoids (Lubińska, 1977) (Figure 2). To date, this criterion is widely used by several groups to study WD in different models (Farah et al., 2011; Narciso et al., 2009).

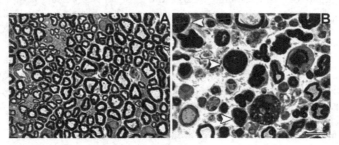

Fig. 2. Wallerian degeneration in C57BL/6 sciatic nerve after crush injury. A. Semi-thin transverse section (toluidine blue staining) from a normal mouse sciatic nerve. B. Semi-thin transverse section from an injured mouse sciatic nerve 96 hours after crush. Note the presence of myelin ovoids (arrowheads). Scale bar = 20 μm

At a later stage of degeneration, myelin and axonal debris will be removed by resident and newly-recruited inflammatory cells (monocytes/macrophages) and microglia (in the CNS) and by Schwann cells (in PNS). The clearance of debris is crucial to create a favorable microenvironment for axon regrowth, since myelin-proteins block axon regeneration by inducing growth-cone collapse (Yiu & He, 2006). During WD, there is an important inflammatory reaction which is highly regulated by immune cells (monocytes/macrophages, T and B lymphocytes, dendritic cells, neutrophils) and by resident non-neuronal cells (microglia and astrocytes in the CNS and Schwann cells in the PNS) (Hawthorne & Popovich, 2011; Sanders & Jones, 2006). Activation of these cells is temporally-orchestrated and triggers the release of several inflammatory molecules that may favor axon degeneration or regeneration. Whether an exacerbated or attenuated inflammatory reaction would be beneficial or harmful to lesioned nerves is still a matter of investigation. Several reports indicate that, in the damaged PNS, inflammation enhances axons regeneration by augmenting macrophages recruitment and myelin debris clearance (Barrete et al., 2008; Narciso et al., 2009). On the other hand, in the damaged CNS, the scenario is not simple: some reports show that recruited macrophages favor axon regeneration (Leon et al., 2000; Yin et al., 2006), while other studies show that it can also be toxic to neurons (Gensel et al., 2009; Popovich & Longbrake, 2008). These conflicting results are currently subject of an intense debate among neuro-immunological researchers and represent an important challenge in the field of neurotrauma (for a review, see Crutcher et al., 2006).

Since Waller`s seminal observations, much has been done in the field of WD. Much of this knowledge was produced with the development of the electron microscope, which allowed researchers to explore in detail the ultra-structural alterations of damaged axons. For a long time, much attention was given to the main mechanisms that control neuronal cell body death; however, to this date, there are several unsolved questions, many of them related to the molecular and cellular pathways that regulate axon destruction, that make this a challenging field for neuroscientists.

3. Molecular and cellular basis of WD

The cascade of events that takes place during axonal degeneration follows a very coordinated sequence determined by the type of nerve fiber affected (motor or sensory neurons, myelinated or unmyelinated fibers), the type and severity of injury, which may vary from a slight crush to complete transection, and by consequences such as deficits in axonal transport (Coleman, 2005) or demyelination (De Vos et al., 2008; Nave & Trapp, 2008). All these factors can affect limb function and recovery in different ways and with different timeframes. But, independently of how severe was the injury, axonal degeneration will occur in a defined fashion. The sequence of steps in axonal degeneration will be discussed in this section. In order to understand the process of axonal degeneration in more detail, however, we first need to cover some basic concepts on axon structure and function.

Each neuron has a highly specialized cylinder-like process that ensures the conduction of information from the cell body to the nerve terminals (Debanne et al., 2011). This process is called "axon" and differs from the other protrusions named "dendrites" in terms of its particular structure and function. The axon emerges from the cell body and varies in length and thickness depending on the function and region of the body it innervates (Wang et al., 2008). Another important feature of axon morphology is the presence or not of a myelin sheath, made by oligodendrocytes in the CNS and by Schwann cells in the PNS. The axonal cylindrical shape is due to the highly organized cytoskeleton components, mainly microtubules and neurofilaments, which are longitudinally aligned along axons. These cytoskeletal components are also responsible for maintenance of axon thickness and are directly implicated in axonal transport of cargoes in association with motor proteins such as dynein and kinesins (De Vos et al., 2008; Perrot et al., 2008).

As previously mentioned, WD is described as the degeneration of axons distal to the point of injury (Waller, 1850). Axonal degeneration is triggered by a large Ca^{2+} influx (George et al., 1995; Martinez & Ribeiro, 1998; Schlaepfer, 1971, 1974), attributed to reversal of the function of the plasma membrane Na^+/Ca^{2+} exchanger as a consequence of dysfunction of the Na^+-K^+ ATPase (reviewed in LoPachin & Lehning, 1997). This intracellular Ca^{2+} overload is presumed to cause disruption of mitochondrial oxidative phosphorylation, excessive formation of free radicals (Anderson et al., 1995; Young et al., 1982) and activation of calpains, calcium-activated neutral cysteine proteases that are responsible for cytoskeleton breakdown and myelin protein degradation (Martinez & Canavarro, 2000; Stokes et al., 1983) (Figure 1). Cytoskeleton disruption leads to failure of axon structural integrity and of important intracellular mechanisms such as axonal trafficking of cargoes and energy supply (De Vos et al., 2008). Intracellular calcium stores are also involved in important cellular changes that boost secondary degeneration (Staal et al., 2010). Another intra-axonal degradation mechanism is the activation of the UPS, which has been implicated as a common mechanism for selective protein degradation in a variety of biological processes including axonal degradation during WD (Zhai et al., 2003). Axon swelling and myelin sheath degradation are the next steps in WD. At this stage, it is possible to observe a bead-like pattern formation along the degenerating axon, classically known as myelin ovoids; this is followed by disconnection and complete degradation of the distal stump (Vargas & Barres, 2007) (Figure 2).

One of the key events in WD is the clearance of axon and myelin debris. Immediately after axonal fragmentation and degradation, Schwann cells in the PNS enter continuous cell division, degrade their own membrane and phagocyte myelin and axonal debris (Liu et al.,

1995; Murinson et al., 2005). Besides, macrophage recruitment and infiltration is initiated via cytokine and chemokine signalling, enhancing myelin debris clearance and creating an appropriated environment for axonal regeneration in the PNS. A different scenario is observed in the CNS, where oligodendrocytes undergo apoptosis and are not involved in myelin debris phagocytosis and signaling for macrophage help. This results in delayed macrophage recruitment, exposure of myelin inhibitory proteins, formation of an astroglial scar and secretion of inhibitory molecules such as chondroitin-sulphate proteoglycans which result in a hostile microenvironment for axon regeneration (George & Griffin, 1994) and establish irreversible loss of function of the target organs. In contrast, microglia, which are considered the resident macrophages of the CNS, are activated after an injury by pro-inflammatory cytokines, among other signals, and undergo several rounds of cell division and morphological changes in order to help phagocytosis of dead cells and myelin debris (Ferrer et al., 1990; Kreutzberg, 1995).

An important tool to better understand the steps and mechanisms involved in WD was the discovery of the slow Wallerian degeneration mouse (Wld^s) (Lunn et al., 1989). In these mutant mice, the active process of neurodegeneration and synapse breakdown after an experimental injury presents a ten-fold delay (Lunn et al., 1989). The chimeric Wld^s gene resulted from a spontaneous mutation in the C57BL/6 mouse strain, causing a tandem triplication in the distal region of chromosome 4 (Conforti et al., 2000), and is known to protect axons in both CNS and PNS from degeneration induced by injury, neurotoxins and neurodegenerative diseases (Wang et al., 2001). The mutation on chromosome 4 comprises a stable 85-kb tandem triplication encoding the N-terminal 70 amino acids of the multiubiquitination factor Ube4b fused in frame to the nuclear nicotinamide adenine dinucleotide (NAD) producing enzyme nicotinamide mononucleotide adenylyltransferase (Nmnat1) (Coleman et al., 1998; Mi et al., 2003). Interestingly, some research groups have described a significant therapeutic potential for this mutation. The Wld^s gene can be used to confer neuroprotection using delivery methods such as gene therapy (Wang et al., 2001), with the advantage of no side or detrimental effects on other non-neuronal cell types (Wishart et al., 2009).

The differences between CNS and PNS, as pointed out here, include important features regarding molecular mechanisms in nervous system degeneration. Therapeutic approaches such as anti-degenerative strategies must thus be designed and tested according to the target region of the nervous system, type of injury and severity.

4. Anti-degenerative strategies

The main goal of an anti-degenerative strategy is to halt the progress of neurodegeneration in order to rescue neural and non-neural cells from death. Delaying degeneration can also represent a useful approach to open a time-window in which to introduce combinations treatments, e.g., administration of trophic factors. To achieve its goal, such approach should down-regulate genes related to cellular degeneration and up-regulate those related to regeneration. However, this scenario is not simple. During WD, innumerous signaling pathways are triggered within the neuron's cell body, axon, synaptic terminals and also in glial cells. To make things worse, we still do not know with certainty the identities of the main proteins that control WD. Nonetheless, based on results from animal model experiments, promising strategies have been proven to be effective in modulating WD progression, raising hopes that they may, in the near future, be applied to humans.

Importantly, several studies have shown that the mechanisms that activate neuronal cell death pathways and axonal degeneration are different from each other. Blocking neuronal death does not prevent axonal degeneration, and inhibiting axonal degeneration does not necessarily block neuronal death (Beirowsky et al., 2008; Vohra et al., 2010). In an attempt to block or decrease tissue damage after neuronal injury, one should simultaneously take into consideration the need to inhibit neuronal death, prevent axonal degeneration and, finally, stimulate neuronal regeneration.

4.1 Neuronal survival

Following a lesion to peripheral nerves, there are molecular and cellular events that occur within the axons acutely after injury and that are followed by other alterations in non-neuronal and neuronal cells. These changes culminate in the activation of signals responsible for initiating the regeneration program but also activate neuronal death pathways (Chen et al., 2007; Makwana & Raivich, 2005). The interruption of axonal transport is one of the first events that take place after injury and its impact on the flow of trophic factors, specially the retrograde transport of ciliary neurotrophic factor (CNTF), brain-derived neurotrophic factor (BDNF) and nerve growth factor (NGF) from target areas, promotes neuronal death (Koliatsos et al., 1993; Sendtner et al., 1997). On the other hand, activation of the signal transducer and activator of transcription 3 (STAT3) and its retrograde transport activates genes important for axonal regeneration (Cafferty et al., 2004). The main components of the axoplasm, the microtubules and neurofilaments, are degraded through the UPS and calpain, respectively (Ehlers, 2004; Zhai et al., 2003), leading to disconnection of the neuronal cell bodies to their targets (Makwana & Raivich, 2005).

Numerous studies have shown the effects of neutrophic factor and neurotrophins (NT) on neuronal survival after injury (Arenas & Persson, 1994; Koliatsos et al., 1993; Yan et al., 1992). Administration of NGF after sciatic nerve transection completely prevented cell loss of dorsal root ganglia neurons (Otto et al., 1987). CNTF and BDNF also prevent death of motor neurons after axotomy (Koliatsos et al., 1993; Yan et al., 1992). This role in preventing neuronal death is important to preserve a certain amount of neuronal cells that can potentially regenerate, resulting in better functional recovery (Chen et al., 2007). The importance of NT in neuronal survival after injury was first appreciated when researchers found that the levels of some NT and neurotrophic factors, and also their receptors, change after lesion and this could account for the roles of different NT on neuronal survival and regeneration (Funakoshi et al., 1993). Funakoshi and collaborators (1993) demonstrated changes in the profile of NT and their receptors at different times after lesion to the sciatic nerve. They showed that levels of BDNF mRNA in the neuronal cell body did not change after sciatic nerve transection but, in contrast, there was a marked increase in the proximal stump. They also found an increase in BDNF mRNA levels at the target, the gastrocnemius muscle, two weeks after lesion. In the case of NT-3, mRNA levels decreased in the cell body after injury but returned to baseline levels 3 days after, while levels in the sciatic nerve dropped within hours after lesion and came back to baseline levels by 2 weeks after the injury. For NT-4, there was no change in the levels of mRNA in the cell body, but there was a 5-fold increase in the proximal stump and a strong decrease in the neuronal target; this latter event suggests that expression of NT-4 by target organs depends upon neuronal stimulation. Concomitant with changes in the expression of NT, the levels of their receptors also changed and this occurred specially in the nerve's proximal stump. All these changes are important to support neuronal survival after damage and they imply that these factors are produced by glial cells and targets organs in an attempt to promote neuronal survival, regeneration and re-myelination of the growing axons (Chan et al., 2001; Cosgaya et al., 2002).

Another strategy that has been used to prevent cell death is the use of apoptotic and necrotic blockers with the aim of inhibiting activation of cell death pathways. However, the outcomes from these strategies have only impacted on neuronal survival, and not on axonal neuroprotection and regeneration. For example, overexpression of Bcl-2, a mitochondrial protein that inhibits the intrinsic pathway of caspase activation, enhances retinal ganglion cell (RGC) survival after injury, but its effect is only temporary (for a review, see Isenmann et al., 2003). Moreover, BCL-2 overexpression results only in histological improvement after traumatic brain injury without better behavior outcomes (Tehranian et al., 2006). Calpains are also involved in cell death after injury and are implicated in necrotic and apoptotic pathways (McKernan et al., 2007; Paquet-Durand et al., 2007). *In vitro* studies have shown that by inhibiting calpain activation it is possible to attenuate apoptosis in RGC after injury to the optic nerve (Smith et al., 2011). Although calpain inhibition can affect neuronal survival and provide axonal neuroprotection, there is no evidence that its inhibition can promote axonal neuroprotection and neuronal survival at the same time, which is another indicative that neuronal death and axonal degeneration are triggered and controlled by distinct pathways.

4.2 Axonal neuroprotection

As mentioned above, one of the first events triggered upon injury is the degradation of cytoskeleton proteins by calpains. Several studies have shown positive effects of calpain inhibition in different types of lesion and animal models of CNS and PNS disorders, but the precise relationship between calpain activation and neuronal death is not fully understood (Couto et al., 2004; Kieran & Greensmith, 2004; McKernan et al., 2007). It has been shown that use of calpain inhibitors improves the outcomes of muscle function and cell survival after PNS injury (Kieran & Greensmith, 2004). Application of a calpain inhibitor in the distal target organ improved the rate of cell survival and muscular function 12 weeks after a crush lesion of the sciatic nerve (Harding et al., 1996). To test whether calpain inhibition in neuronal cell bodies would have an impact on neuronal survival and muscle function, Kieran & Greensmith (2004) delivered a calpain inhibitor to the spinal cord after injuring the sciatic nerve. Twelve weeks later they observed an improvement in neuronal survival and muscle function, suggesting that calpain inhibition plays an important role on both neuronal survival and axonal neuroprotection. Couto and collaborators (2004) showed that a calpain inhibitor applied to the site of a crush injury had a neuroprotective effect on optic nerve fibers 4 days after injury (Figure 3), while Silmara de Lima and collaborators (unpublished dada) observed that the delay in axonal degeneration promoted by calpain inhibition had no effect on RGC survival 14 days after optic nerve lesion. These results are important since the delay in the onset of WD can create a time-window to add other strategies and investigate whether different types of combinational treatments can lead to better results.

Sodium or calcium channel blockers have also been used in anti-degenerative strategies to prevent axonal disintegration. Lo and colleagues (2003) demonstrated that neuroprotection to spinal cord axons was achieved using a sodium channel blocker in a model of experimental allergic encephalomyelitis. Those authors reported that, besides preventing axonal degeneration, nerve fibers from animals treated with the sodium channel blocker maintained the ability to conduct action potentials. Calcium channel blockers also proved effective in protecting axons from degeneration and improving neuronal survival in models of spinal cord and optic nerve injury, with loss of myelin basic protein and alterations in spinal cord evoked potentials attenuated in the former case (Winkler et al., 2003), and RGC survival increased in the latter (Karim et al., 2006).

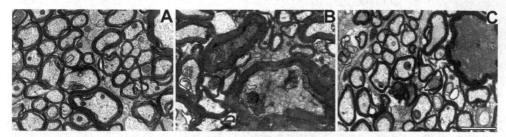

Fig. 3. Transverse ultrathin section from rat optic nerve. A represents a normal optic nerve. B shows a 4 day-injured optic nerve with numerous axons undergoing WD. C shows a 4 day post-injury optic nerve treated with calpain inhibitor prior to the lesion and during the survival time. Note that there are more intact fibers with preserved axoplasm when compared to the image in B. Scale bar = 2 μm

Another important system involved in WD is the UPS, which has been implicated in many biological processes including protein degradation and axonal pathfinding (Campbell & Holt, 2001). The involvement of UPS in the early stages of WD was demonstrated in explanted superior cervical ganglion neurons by Zhai and collaborators (2003), who showed that they could delay axonal degeneration by using a UPS inhibitor. In the same study, they showed that by combining UPS and calpain inhibitors there was also a delay in axonal degeneration. However, better results were obtained when the UPS inhibitor was used prior to the lesion, suggesting that the UPS is involved in the early phase of WD. According to Walker and collaborators (2001), microtubule degradation is sufficient to trigger axonal degeneration, whereas neurofilament disruption *per se* does not affect the distribution of microtubules and other elements of the axon cytoskeleton. For these reasons, maintaining the integrity of axons and improving neuronal survival may be a way to promote a better outcome after nerve fiber injury and to accelerate functional recovery. Therefore, the combined use of calpain and UPS inhibitors may be a promising approach for testing in clinical trials, as inhibitors can be applied peripherally onto neuronal targets.

Another promising strategy is to prevent or slow down axonal degeneration using pharmacological agents. For example, Da Costa et al. (2010) recently showed that intra-peritoneal injections of 2,4-dinitrophenol (DNP) every 24 hours following injury significantly reduced axonal degeneration in a mouse model of sciatic nerve crush injury.

Besides, expression of amyloid precursor protein (APP) and neuregulin-1 (NRG1) were increased in sciatic nerve longitudinal sections after DNP treatment. APP is related to neuronal development, growth and survival (reviewed in Gralle & Ferreira, 2007) and NRG1 plays important roles in development and neurodegeneration (Falls, 2003) and is involved in myelin thickness control (Michailov et al., 2004). DNP is a well-known uncoupler of mitochondrial oxidative phosphorylation (Parascandola, 1974). However, at low concentrations, insufficient to produce mitochondrial uncoupling, DNP has been shown to be a powerful neuroprotective agent against a variety of insults (reviewed in De Felice & Ferreira, 2006; De Felice et al., 2007).

5. Conclusions and perspectives

Since Waller's first experiments and important observations, huge advances have been made in terms of imaging technology, molecular biology tools, genomics and chemical compound synthesis and screening. All this progress has allowed a detailed view of the mechanisms and molecular intimacy of degenerating axons. From accurate freehand drawings to live 3D multiphoton microscopy, researchers have unveiled some of the mysteries behind the dynamics of morphological changes of injured nerves. However, we still face some basic questions regarding axon degeneration: What are the main molecular pathways that trigger axon breakdown after injury? Can we manipulate these key molecules in order to prevent axon degeneration? Furthermore, although it is possible to precisely monitor specific events during degeneration, there are still many open questions about how efficient and which is the best anti-degenerative strategy depending on the type of injury, lesioned region (PNS or CNS) and how far from the cell bodies were the axons damaged. The time between the injury and the beginning of treatment is also a big issue in terms of WD progression and is an important factor regarding limb function recovery. The crosstalk between basic and clinical research is one of the key points in developing new strategies and testing therapeutic hypothesis. Longitudinal screenings on different types of injuries and evaluations of therapies that were applied to each single subject may help to create a blueprint for a personalized nervous system injury treatment.

6. Acknowledgements

Work in the author's laboratories is funded by grants from the Brazilian agencies Conselho Nacional de Desenvolvimento Científico e Tecnológico, Fundação de Amparo à Pesquisa do Estado do Rio de Janeiro and Instituto de Neurociência Translacional.

7. References

Anderson, D.K.; Means, E.D.; Waters, T.R. & Spears, C. J. (1995). Spinal cord energy metabolism following compression trauma to the feline spinal cord. *J. Neurosurg.* 53:375–380.

Arenas, E. & Persson, H. (1994). Neurotrophin-3 prevents the death of adult central noradrenergic neurons in vivo. *Nature.* 6461:368-71.

Barrete, B.; Hébert, M.A.; Filadi, M.; Lafortune, K.; Vallières, N.; Gowing, G.; Julien, J.P. & Lacroix, S. (2008). Requirement of myeloid cells for axon regeneration. *J. Neurosci.* 38:9363-9376.

Beirowski, B.; Babetto, E.; Coleman, M.P. & Martin, K.R. (2008). The WldS gene delays axonal but not somatic degeneration in a rat glaucoma model. *Eur. J. Neurosci.* 6:1166-79.

Cafferty, W.B.; Gardiner, N.J.; Das P, Q.J.; McMahon, S.B. & Thompson S.W. (2004). Conditioning injury-induced spinal axon regeneration fails in interleukin-6 knock-out mice. *J. Neurosci.* 18:4432-43.

Campbell, D.S. & Holt, C.E. (2001). Chemotropic responses of retinal growth cones mediated by rapid local protein synthesis and degradation. *Neuron.* 6:1013-26.

Chan, J.R.; Cosgava, J.M.; Wu, Y.J. & Shooter, E.M. (2001). Neurotrophins are key mediators of the myelination program in the peripheral nervous system. *Proc. Natl. Acad. Sci.* 25:14661-8. 2001.

Chen, Z.L.; Yu, W.M. & Strickland, S. (2007). Peripheral regeneration. *Annu. Rev. Neurosci.* 30:209-33.

Coleman, M. (2005). Axon degeneration mechanisms: commonality amid diversity. *Nat. Rev. Neurosci.* 6:889-898.

Coleman, M.P. & Freeman, M.R. (2010). Wallerian degeneration, Wlds and Nmnat. *Annu. Rev. Neurosci.* 33:245-267.

Coleman, M. P.; Conforti, L.; Buckmaster, E.A.; Tarlton, A.; Ewing, R.M.; Brown, M.C.; Lyon, M.F. & Perry, V.H. (1998). An 85-kb tandem triplication in the slow Wallerian degeneration (Wlds) mouse. *Proc. Natl. Acad. Sci. USA.* 95:9985-9990

Coleman, M.P. & Perry, V.H. (2002). Axon pathology in neurological diseases: a neglected therapeutic target. *Trends Neurosci.* 25:532-537.

Conforti, L.; Tarlton, A.; Mack, T.G.; Mi, W. & Buckmaster, E. A. (2000). A Ufd2/D4Cole1e chimeric protein and overexpression of Rbp7 in the slow Wallerian degeneration (WldS) mouse. *Proc. Natl. Acad. Sci. USA.* 97: 11377-11382.

Cosgaya, J.M.; Chan, J.R. & Shooter, E.M. (2002). The neurotrophin receptor p75NTR as a positive modulator of myelination. *Science.* 5596:1245-8.

Court, F.A.; Hendriks, W.T.J.; MacGillavry, H.D.; Alvarez, J. & Van Minnen, J. (2008). Schwann cell to axon transfer of ribosomes: toward a novel understanding of the role of glia in the nervous system. *J. Neurosci.* 43:11024-11029.

Couto, L.A.; Narciso, M.S.; Hokoç, J. N. & Blanco Martinez, A. M. (2004). Calpain inhibitor 2 prevents axonal degeneration of opossum optic nerve fibers. *J Neurosci Res.* 77: 410-419.

Crutcher, K.A.; Gendelman, H.E.; Kipnis, J.; Perez-Polo, J.R.; Perry, V.H.; Popovich, P.G. & Weaver, L.C. (2006). Debate: "is increasing neuroinflammation beneficial for neural repair?". *J Neuroimmune Pharmacol.* 1:165-211.

Da Costa, R.M.; Martinez, A.M.B. & Ferreira, S.T. (2010). 2,4-Dinitrophenol blocks neurodegeneration and preserves sciatic nerve function after trauma. *J. Neurotauma.* 5:829-841.

De Felice, F.G. & Ferreira, S.T. (2006). Novel neuroprotective, neuritogenic and anti-amyloidogenic properties of 2,4-dinitrophenol: The gentle face of Janus. *IUBMB Life* 58:185-191.

De Felice, F.G.; Wasilewska-sampaio, A.P.; Gomes, F.A.; Klein, W.L. & Ferreira, S.T. (2007). Cyclic AMP enhances Abeta oligomerization blockers as potential theraqpeutics agents in Alzheimers diseases. *Curr. Alzheimer Res.* 3:263-271.

De Vos, K.J.; Grierson, A.J.; Ackerley, S. & Miller, C.C. (2008). Role of axonal transport in neurodegenerative diseases. *Annu. Rev. Neurosci.* 31:151-73.

Debanne, D.; Campanac, E.; Bialowas, A.; Carlier, E. & Alcaraz, G. (2011). Axon physiology. *Physiol. Rev.* 91(2):555-602.

Ehlers, M.D. (2004). Deconstructing the axon: Wallerian degeneration and the ubiquitin-proteasome system. *Trends. Neurosci.* 1:3-6.

Falls, D.L. (2003). Neuregulins: Functions, forms, and signaling strategies. *Exp. Cell. Res.* 284:14-30.

Farah, M.H.; Pan, B.H.; Hoffman, P.N.; Ferraris, D.; Tsukamoto, T.; Nguyen, T.; Wong, P.C.; Price, D.L.; Slusher, B.S. & Griffin, J.W. (2011). Reduced BACE1 activity enhances clearance of myelin debris and regeneration of axons in the injured peripheral nervous system. *J. Neurosci.* 15:5744-5754.

Ferrer, I.; Bernet, E.; Soriano, E.; Del Rio, T. & Fonseca, M. (1990). Naturally occurring cell death in the cerebral cortex of the rat and removal of dead cells by transitory phagocytes. *Neuroscience.* 39:451–458.

Finn, J.T.; Weil, M.; Archer, F.; Siman, R.; Srinivasan, A. & Raff, M.C. (2000). Evidence that wallerian degeneration and localized axon degeneration induced by local neurotrophin deprivation do not involve caspases. *J. Neurosci.* 20:1333-1341.

Funakoshi, H.; Frisén, J.; Barbany, G.; Timmusk, T.; Zachrisson, O.; Verge, V.M. & Persson, H. (1993). Differential expression of mRNAs for neurotrophins and their receptors after axotomy of the sciatic nerve. *J. Cell. Biol.* 2:455-65.

Gensel, J.C.; Nakamura, S.; Guan, Z.; Rooijen, N.V.; Ankeny, D.P. & Popovich, P.G. (2009). Macrophages promote axon regeneration with concurrent neurotoxicity. *J. Neurosci.* 12:3956-3968.

George, R. & Griffin, J.W. (1994). Delayed macrophage responses and myelin clearance during Wallerian degeneration in the central nervous system: the dorsal radiculotomy model. *Exp. Neurol.* 129:225–36.

George, E.B.; Glass, J.D. & Griffin, J.W. (1995). Axotomy-induced axonal degeneration is mediated by calcium influx through ion-specific channels. *J. Neurosci.* 15:6445–6452.

Gralle, M. & Ferreira, S.T. (2007). Structure and functions of the human amyloid precursor protein: The whole is more than the sum of its parts. *Prog. Neurobiol.* 82:11–32.

Harding, D.I.; Greensmith, L.; Connold, A.L. & Vrbová, G. (1996). Stabilizing neuromuscular contacts increases motoneuron survival after neonatal nerve injury in rats. *Neuroscience.* 3:799-805.

Hawthorne, A.L. & Popovich, P.G. (2011). Emerging concepts in myeloid cell biology after spinal cord injury. *Neurotherapeutics.* 2:252-261.

Isenmann, S.; Kretz, A. & Cellerino, A. (2003). Molecular determinants of retinal ganglion cell development, survival, and regeneration. *Prog. Retin Eye Res.* 4:483-543.

Karim, Z.; Sawada, A.; Kawakami, H.; Yamamoto, T. & Taniguchi, T. (2006). A new calcium channel antagonist, lomerizine, alleviates secondary retinal ganglion cell death after optic nerve injury in the rat. *Curr. Eye Res.* 3:273-283.

Kieran, D. & Greensmith, L. (2004). Inhibition of calpains, by treatment with leupeptin, improves motoneuron survival and muscle function in models of motoneuron degeneration. *Neuroscience.* 2:427-39.

Koliatsos, V.E.; Clatterbuck, R.E.; Winslow, J.W.; Cayouette, M.H. & Price, D.L. (1993). Evidence that brain-derived neurotrophic factor is a trophic factor for motor neurons in vivo. *Neuron.* 3:359-67.

Kreutzberg, G.W. (1995) The First Line of Defense in Brain Pathologies. *Drug Research.* 45: 357–360

Leon, S.; Yin, Y.; Nguyen, J.; Irwin, N. & Benowitz, L.I. (2000). Lens injury stimulates axon regeneration in the mature rat optic nerve. *J. Neurosci.* 12:4615-4626.

Liu, H.M.; Yang, L.H. & Yang, Y.J. (1995). Schwann cell properties: 3. C-fos expression, bFGF production, phagocytosis and proliferation during Wallerian degeneration. *J. Neuropathol. Exp. Neurol.* 54:487–96.

Lo, A.C.; Saab, C.Y.; Black, J.A. & Waxman, S.G. (2003). Phenytoin protects spinal cord axons and preserves axonal conduction and neurological function in a model of neuroinflammation in vivo. *.J Neurophysiol.* 5:3566-71.

LoPachin, R.M. & Lehning, E.J. (1997) Mechanism of calcium entry during axon injury and degeneration. *Toxicol. Appl. Pharmacol.* 143:233–244

Lubińska, L. (1977). Early course of wallerian degeneration in myelinated fibers of the rat phrenic nerve. *Brain Res.* 1:47-63.

Lunn, E.R.; Perry, V.H.; Brown, M.C.; Rosen, H. & Gordon, S. (1989). Absence of Wallerian degeneration does not hinder regeneration in peripheral nerve. *Eur. J. Neurosci.* 1:27–33.

Makwana, M. & Raivich, G. (2005). Molecular mechanisms in successful peripheral regeneration. *FEBS. J.* 11:2628-38.

Martinez, A.M.B. & Canavarro, S. (2000). Early myelin breakdown following sural nerve crush: a freeze-fracture study. *Braz. J. Med. Biol. Res.* 12:1477-1482.

Martinez, A.M.B. & Ribeiro, L.C.V. (1998). Ultrastructural localization of calcium in peripheral nerve fibers undergoing Wallerian degeneration: an oxalate-pyroantimonate and x-ray microanalysis Study. *J. Submicrosc Cytol Pathol.* 3:451-458.

McKernan, D.P.; Guerin, M.B.; O'Brien, C.J. & Cotter, T.G. (2007). A key role for calpains in retinal ganglion cell death. *Invest. Ophthalmol. Vis. Sci.* 12:5420-5430.

Mi, W.; Glass, J. D. & Coleman, M. P. (2003). Stable inheritance of an 85-kb triplication in C57BL/WldS mice. *Mutat. Res.* 526:33-37.

Michailov, G.V.; Sereda, M.W.; Brinkmann, B.G.; Fischer, T.M.; Haug, B.; Birchmeier, C.; Role, L.; Lai, C.; Schwab, M.H. & Nave, K.A. (2004). Axonal neuregulin-1 regulates myelin sheath thickness. *Science* 304:700–703.

Murinson, B.B.; Archer, D.R.; Li, Y. & Griffin, J.W. (2005). Degeneration of efferent myelinated fibers prompts mitosis in Remak Schwann cells of uninjured C-fibers afferents. *J. Neurosci.* 25:1179-1187.

Narciso, M.S.; Hokoç, J.N. & Martinez, A.M.B. (2001). Watery and dark axons in Wallerian degeneration of the opossum`s optic nerve: different patterns of cytoskeletal breakdown?. *An. Acad. Bras. Cienc.* 2:231-243.

Narciso, M.S.; Mietto, B.S.; Marques, S.A.; Soares, C.P.; Mermelstein, C.S.; El-Cheikh, M.C. & Martinez, A.M.B. (2009). Sciatic nerve regeneration is accelerated in galectin-3 knockout mice. *Exp. Neurol.* 217:7-15.

Nave, K.A. & Trapp, B.D. (2008). Axon-glial signaling and the glial support of axon function. *Annu. Rev. Neurosci.* 31: 535–561.

Otto, D.; Unsicker, K. & Grothe, C. (1987). Pharmacological effects of nerve growth factor and fibroblast growth factor applied to the transectioned sciatic nerve on neuron death in adult rat dorsal root ganglia. *Neurosci. Lett.* 1-2:156-60.

Paquet-Durand, F.; Johnson, L. & Ekström, P. (2007). Calpain activity in retinal degeneration. *J. Neurosci. Res.* 4:693-702.

Parascandola, J. (1974). Dinitrophenol and bioenergetics: A historical perspective. *Mol. Cell Biochem.* 5:69–77.

Perrot, R.; Berges, R.; Bocquet, A. & Eyer, J. (2008). Review of the multiple aspects of neurofilament functions, and their possible contribution to neurodegeneration. *Mol. Neurobiol.* 38:27–65.

Popovich, P.G. & Longbrake, E.E. (2008). Can the immune system be harnessed to repair the CNS?. *Nat. Rev. Neurosci.* 6:481-493.

Sanders, V.M. & Jones, K.J. (2006). Role of immunity in recovery from a peripheral nerve. *J. Neuroimmune. Pharmacol.* 1:11-19.

Schlaepfer, W.W. (1971). Experimental alterations of neurofilaments and neurotubules by calcium and other ions. *Exp. Cell Res.* 67:73–80.

Schlaepfer, W.W. (1974). Calcium-induced degeneration of axoplasm in isolated segments of rat peripheral nerve. *Brain Res.* 69:203–215.

Sendtner, M.; Götz, R.; Holtmann, B. & Thoenen, H. (1997). Endogenous ciliary neurotrophic factor is a lesion factor for axotomized motoneurons I adult mice. *J. Neurosci.* 18:6999-7006.

Smith, A.W.; Das, A.; Guyton, M.K.; Ray, S.K.; Rohrer, B. & Banik N.L. (2011). Calpain inhibition attenuates apoptosis of retinal ganglion cells in acute optic neuritis. *Invest. Ophthalmol. Vis. Sci.* 7:4935-41.

Staal, J.A., Dickson, T.C., Gasperini, R., Liu, Y., Foa, L. & Vickers, J.C. (2010) Initial calcium release from intracellular stores followed by calcium dysregulation is linked to secondary axotomy following transient axonal stretch injury. *J. Neurochem.* 112:1147-1155.

Stokes, B.T.; Fox, P. & Hollinden, G. (1983). Extracellular calcium activity in the injured spinal cord. *Exp. Neurol.* 80:561–572.

Tehranian, R.; Rose, M.E.; Vagni, V.; Griffith, R.P.; Wu, S.; Maits, S.; Zhang, X.; Clark, R.S.; Dixon, C.E.; Kochanek, P.M.; Bernard, O. & Graham, S.H. (2006). Transgenic mice that overexpress the anti-apoptotic Bcl-2 protein have improved histological outcome but unchanged behavioral outcome after traumatic brain injury. Brain Res. 1:126-35.

Vargas, M.E. & Barres, B.A. (2007). Why is Wallerian Degeneration in the CNS so slow? *Ann. Rev. Neurosci.* 30:157-179.

Vohra, B.P.; Sasaki, Y.; Miller, B.R.; Chang, J.; DiAntonio, A. & Milbrandt J. (2010). Amyloid precursor protein cleavage-dependent and -independent axonal degeneration programs share a common nicotinamide mononucleotide adenylyltransferase 1-sensitive pathway. *J. Neurosci.* 41:13729-13738.

Walker, K.L.; Yoo, H.K.; Undamatla, J. & Szaro, B.G. (2001). Loss of neurofilaments alters axonal growth dynamics. *J Neurosci.* 24:9655-66

Waller, A. (1850). Experiments on the section of glossopharyngeal and hypoglossal nerves of the frog and observations of the alternatives produced thereby in the structure of their primitive fibers. *Philos. Trans. R. Soc. Lond. B Biol. Sci.* 140:423–29.

Wang, M.S.; Fang, G.; Culver, D.G.; Davis, A.A.; Rich, M.M. & Glass, J.D. (2001). The WldS protein protects against axonal degeneration: a model of gene therapy for peripheral neuropathy. *Ann. Neurol.* 50:773-9.

Wang, S.S.; Shultz, J.R.; Burish, M.J.; Harrison, K.H.; Hof, P.R.; Towns, L.C.; Wagers, M.W. & Wyatt, K.D. (2008). Functional trade-offs in white matter axonal scaling. *J. Neurosci.* 28:4047–4056.

Winkler, T.; Sharma, H.S.; Stålberg, E.; Badgaiyan, R.D.; Gordh, T. & Westman, J. (2003). An L-type calcium channel blocker, nimodipine influences trauma induced spinal cord conduction and axonal injury in the rat. *Acta Neurochir. Suppl.* 86:425-32.

Wishart, T.M.; Brownstein, D.G.; Thomson, D.; Tabakova, A.M.; Boothe, K.M.; Tsao, J.W. & Gillingwater, T.H. (2009) Expression of the neuroprotective slow Wallerian degeneration (WldS) gene in non-neuronal tissues. *BMC Neurosci.* 10:148.

Yan, Q.; Elliott, J. & Snider, W.D. (1992). Brain-derived neurotrophic factor rescues spinal motor neurons from axotomy-induced cell death. *Nature.* 6406:753-755.

Yin, Y.; Henzl, M.T.; Lorber, B.; Nakazawa, T.; Thomas, T.T.; Jiang, F.; Langer, R.; Benowitz, L.I. (2006). Oncomodulin is a macrophage-derived signal for axon regeneration in retinal ganglion cells. *Nat. Neurosci.* 6:843-852.

Yiu, G. & He, Z. (2006). Glial inhibition of CNS axon regeneration. *Nat Rev Neurosci.* 8:617-627.

Young, W.; Yen, V. & Blight, A. (1982) Extracellular calcium ionic activity in experimental spinal cord contusion. *Brain Res.* 253:105–113.

Zhai, Q.; Wang, J.; Kim, A.; Liu, Q.; Watts, R.; Hoopfer, E.; Mitchison, T.; Luo, L. & He, Z. (2003). Involvement of the ubiquitin-proteasome system in the early stages of wallerian degeneration. *Neuron.* 2:217-25.

8

Modelling Multiple Sclerosis *In Vitro* and the Influence of Activated Macrophages

E.J.F. Vereyken, C.D. Dijkstra and C.E. Teunissen
VU University Medical Center
Amsterdam,
The Netherlands

1. Introduction

Multiple sclerosis (MS) is a chronic inflammatory disease of the central nervous system (CNS). The prevalence of MS is approximately 2 million people worldwide, with an incidence of about 1:1000 in Europe and Northern America, and women are affected more often compared to men, at a ratio of approximately 2:1. It is the most common cause of neurological disability among young adults with an onset generally between 20 and 40 years of age [Pugliatti et al., 2002]. The major neuropathological hallmarks of MS are demyelinating lesions associated with perivascular infiltrates, consisting of macrophages/microglia and lymphocytes. The lesions are characterized by destruction of myelin sheaths, oligodendrocyte death, axonal damage and glial scar formation, called astrogliosis. Demyelination is a central event in MS pathology. Although some remyelination occurs, it ultimately fails [Franklin, 2002]. The cause of the remyelination failure is not clear, although several processes have been suggested to play a role [Franklin and Ffrench-Constant, 2008; Wolswijk, 2002; John et al., 2002]. Not only processes behind remyelination failure remain elusive, also the cellular mechanisms behind the demyelination and axonal damage are largely unknown. Modelling MS both in animals and *in vitro* could help with understanding this.

This chapter will focus on MS pathology and the models that exist for investigating this disease, especially zooming in on *in vitro* models.

2. Multiple sclerosis

2.1 Clinical symptoms and diagnosis

MS is characterized by multiple sclerotic lesions affecting areas such as the cerebellum, cerebrum (periventricular white matter), optic nerve, brainstem and spinal cord [Compston and Coles, 2008]. The clinical symptoms of MS are very heterogeneous depending on the location, size and number of lesions. Symptoms include motor function disturbances, such as muscle weakness, tremor and paralysis, and progressive sensory malfunction, for instance impaired vision. The main criterion for diagnosis of MS is the occurrence of two (or more) independent episodes of clinical symptoms consistent with focal demyelination separated in space (part of the CNS) and time (more than one occasion) [Polman et al., 2011; McDonald et al., 2001]. Magnetic resonance imaging (MRI) techniques have become very important for verification of diagnosis [Barkhof et al., 1997; Nielsen et al., 2005; Polman et al., 2005], for detection of the number and size of the lesions and to differentiate between ongoing inflammation and blood-brain-barrier leakage [Bruck et al., 1997; Miller et al., 1998; Nesbit et al., 1991; Katz et al., 1993]. The presence of oligoclonal bands in cerebrospinal fluid (CSF) of MS patients and elevated immunoglobulin G (IgG) levels are supportive of MS diagnosis [Polman et al., 2011]. Furthermore, they corroborate the inflammatory demyelinating nature of the underlying condition, are used to evaluate alternative diagnoses and to predict clinical definite MS [Correale and de los Milagros Bassani Molinas, 2002]. In approximately 90% of MS patients oligoclonal immunoglobulin bands are detected [Bourahoui et al., 2004]. These oligoclonal bands are also detected in other neurological diseases, although not as consistently and persistently as in MS. In patients with clinically isolated syndrome the presence of oligoclonal bands is predictive for the progression to clinically definite MS [Paolino et al., 1996]. In MS patients the absence of oligoclonal bands is associated with a benign disease course, while high levels of oligoclonal bands are correlated with a severe disease, suggesting that oligoclonal bands may be clinically relevant [Correale and de los Milagros Bassani Molinas, 2002]. The identification of biomarkers for diagnosis and prognosis of MS is the subject of intense ongoing research [Teunissen et al., 2011; Ziemann et al., 2011; Junker et al., 2011; Teunissen et al., 2009]. One example is neurofilament light, which was found to be increased in clinically isolated syndrome patients, especially in those that converted to MS, and was observed to correlate with relapses and the number of gadolinium enhancing lesions [Teunissen et al., 2009].

Four major subtypes of MS with different progression and relapse characteristics have been recognized: the relapsing-remitting (RR-MS), the secondary-progressive (SP-MS), primary progressive (PP-MS) and progressive-relapsing (PR-MS) subtype [Lublin and Reingold, 1996]. Approximately 70% of the cases start with the RR subtype, which is characterized by clinical attacks that are followed by a clinically silent period with almost complete recovery. After a period of 15 to 20 years most cases of the RR-MS subtype develop progressive neurological deterioration without apparent remission, the SP-MS subtype. About 15-20% of MS patients show a progressive disease course without relapses and remissions from the beginning, the PP-MS subtype. Finally, less than 5% suffer from PR-MS, characterized by progressive neurological impairment with occasional relapses.

2.2 Pathology

The major neuropathological hallmarks of MS are multiple focal inflammatory demyelinating lesions spread throughout the CNS. These lesions are associated with perivascular infiltrates containing macrophages and lymphocytes. Other features of MS plaques are axonal damage and loss, oligodendrocyte death and astrogliosis [Charcot, 1868], which is hypertrophy and an abnormal increase in the number of astrocytes. Lesions are classified based on the degree of myelin loss, the presence of inflammatory cells and HLA-DR expression on leukocytes and microglial cells. Four different stages in MS lesions have been identified: (p)reactive, active, chronic active and chronic inactive lesions [van der Valk and De Groot, 2000; de Groot et al., 2001].

In (p)reactive lesions no demyelination is apparent. Clusters of activated microglia can be observed with increased expression of HLA-DR expression and occasionally perivascular leukocyte infiltrations can be seen.

Active lesions are characterized by areas of demyelination containing macrophages, activated microglia and activated hypertrophic astrocytes. Activated astrocytes fill up the lesion area and form a gliotic scar. T-cells and some B-cells can be found, mostly in the perivascular space. The macrophages and microglia in the lesions contain myelin degradation products, such as myelin proteins and lipids, giving them a foamy appearance. The presence of myelin proteins in these macrophages reflect ongoing demyelination, since these myelin proteins are degraded in a known time frame [Bruck et al., 1995; van der Goes A. et al., 2005]. Oligodendrocyte death occurs in these lesions, often via apoptotic mechanisms [Wolswijk, 2000; Rodriguez and Lucchinetti, 1999]. This apoptosis of oligodendrocytes may be a disease initiating event, since it precedes leukocyte infiltration [Barnett and Prineas, 2004; Henderson et al., 2009].

Chronic active lesions are defined by a hypocellular demyelinated centre surrounded by a hypercellular rim with high numbers of foamy macrophages and reactive astrocytes. In these lesions oligodendrocyte numbers are reduced and lymphocytes are present in perivascular spaces.

In chronic inactive lesions almost no cellular infiltrates are present. They are hypocellular, demyelinated and contain widened extracellular spaces and gliotic scar tissue. In the CNS parenchyma and perivascular spaces relatively small numbers of macrophages and lymphocytes still remain. No myelin proteins can be detected in the macrophages.

Next to demyelination, remyelination also occurs [Franklin, 2002]. Remyelination can be restricted to the lesion edge, but can also extend throughout the lesions which are then called shadow-plaques [Bruck et al., 2003; Prineas et al., 1993; Prineas and Connell, 1979; Raine and Wu, 1993; Lassmann et al., 1997]. Oligodendrocyte precursor cells, after maturation into mature oligodendrocytes, generate thin myelin sheaths and could therefore contribute to recovery in MS patients. Remyelination in MS is limited. The cause of remyelination failure in MS is unknown, but several mechanisms have been proposed, such as restricted oligodendrocyte precursor cell migration, maturation and a growth inhibitory environment [Franklin, 2002; Wolswijk, 2002; John et al., 2002; Charles et al., 2002]. Macrophages could play an important role in remyelination as well [Doring and Yong, 2011].

It is clear from the above that macrophages are an important characteristic defining lesion stage. They likely play a central role in lesion formation in MS. In the next sections, we will describe the role of these immune cells in disease and particularly in MS in more detail.

3. Macrophages in MS

3.1 Macrophages and innate immunity

Macrophages (meaning "big eaters") are phagocytic cells that play a vital role in innate immunity, the first line of defense against pathogens. Cells of the innate immune system such as macrophages are able, to some extent, to discriminate between "self" and "non-self" antigens (reviewed by Janeway [Janeway, Jr. and Medzhitov, 2002]). Via a limited number of germline-encoded pattern recognition receptors, macrophages recognize highly conserved structures from bacteria, viruses and fungi. Several different families of pattern recognition receptors have been identified, for example macrophage scavenger receptors and the family of Toll-like receptors [Takeda and Akira, 2005; Akira et al., 2006]. After recognition, the binding of the receptor with its ligand on the pathogen, macrophages usually engulf the pathogen, a process called phagocytosis. This process results in the containment of microbes in the phagosome, which fuses with lysosomal vesicles containing a multitude of microbicidal products. Both oxygen-dependent, called the respiratory burst, and oxygen-independent microbicidal mechanisms exist. The respiratory burst uses an enzymatic complex called nicotinamide adenine dinucleotide phosphate reduced (NADPH) oxidase. Upon stimulation active NADPH oxidase forms. This active complex transfers two electrons from NADPH to two molecules of oxygen to form superoxide anion [DeLeo et al., 1999; Babior, 1999]. From this superoxide anion other ROS, such as hydrogen peroxide, are formed [Babior, 1999]. Oxygen-independent microbicidal mechanisms include acidification of the phagolysosome, nutrient depletion and antimicrobial proteins or peptides.

Macrophages differentiate from circulating monocytes. Once a monocyte migrates into a specific tissue, during steady-state or inflammation, it develops into a macrophage. Macrophages are present in virtually all tissues and usually specialize according to the tissue they are in, for instance osteoclasts (in bone), Kupffer cells (in liver) and microglia (in the CNS) [Gordon and Taylor, 2005].

Next to their role in innate immunity they have an important function in tissue homeostasis, since they are crucial for the clearance of apoptotic cells and the remodeling and repair of tissues after inflammation [Gordon, 1986; Gordon, 1998]. Phagocytosis of apoptotic cells does not induce the expression of inflammatory mediators in unstimulated macrophages [Kono and Rock, 2008].

During an infection macrophages also clear cellular debris of necrotic cells that contain endogenous danger signals, such as heat-shock proteins and nuclear proteins [Zhang and Mosser, 2008]. The detection of these danger signals alters the physiology of the macrophages, including expression of cell surface proteins, cytokines and pro-inflammatory mediators, increasing immune function of macrophages. However, macrophages can respond to many signals in the microenvironment of tissues and not all increase immune function.

3.2 Macrophage activation results in different subtypes

Macrophages are highly plastic cells and are able to respond to a variety of environmental cues changing their phenotype and physiology, resulting in different subtypes of macrophages. These different subtypes of macrophages have different functions in immune response, homeostasis and tissue repair [Gordon, 2003; Mosser, 2003; Mosser and Edwards, 2008].

Based on activation pathways several subtypes of macrophages have been described [Edwards et al., 2006b; Martinez et al., 2008]. The two most studied subtypes are: 1) the classically activated macrophages (CA, also called M1), induced by interferon-gamma (IFN-γ) and lipopolysaccharide (LPS); 2) the alternatively activated macrophages (AA, also called M2), stimulated by IL-4/13 and/or glucocorticoids. In 1992 Stein et al. introduced the concept of alternatively activated macrophages [Stein et al., 1992]. In contrast to the classically activated macrophages, macrophages stimulated with interleukin-4 (IL-4) increased the expression of mannose receptor (MR). Another study showed that Th1 cytokines (e.g. IFN-γ) and Th2 cytokines (e.g. IL-4) induced two distinct functional states in macrophages. Exposure of macrophages to Th2 cytokines led to an upregulation of certain phagocytic receptors and arginase, which reduced ability to kill intracellular pathogens, while Th1 cytokines led to induction of inducible nitric oxide synthase (iNOS) in macrophages [Modolell et al., 1995].

CA macrophages are cytotoxic and secrete high amounts of oxygen and nitrogen radicals in order to kill pathogens [Nathan and Shiloh, 2000]. CA macrophages also produce pro-inflammatory cytokines [O'Shea and Murray, 2008]. In mice, CA macrophages are

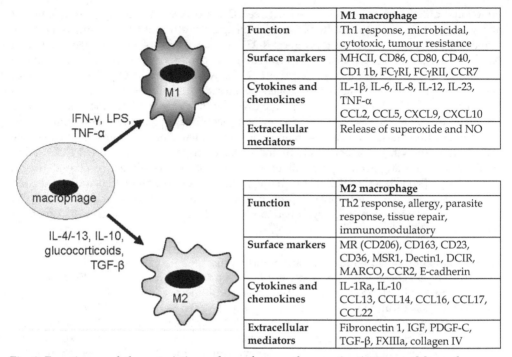

	M1 macrophage
Function	Th1 response, microbicidal, cytotoxic, tumour resistance
Surface markers	MHCII, CD86, CD80, CD40, CD1 1b, FCγRI, FCγRII, CCR7
Cytokines and chemokines	IL-1β, IL-6, IL-8, IL-12, IL-23, TNF-α CCL2, CCL5, CXCL9, CXCL10
Extracellular mediators	Release of superoxide and NO

	M2 macrophage
Function	Th2 response, allergy, parasite response, tissue repair, immunomodulatory
Surface markers	MR (CD206), CD163, CD23, CD36, MSR1, Dectin1, DCIR, MARCO, CCR2, E-cadherin
Cytokines and chemokines	IL-1Ra, IL-10 CCL13, CCL14, CCL16, CCL17, CCL22
Extracellular mediators	Fibronectin 1, IGF, PDGF-C, TGF-β, FXIIIa, collagen IV

Fig. 1. Functions and characteristic markers of macrophage activation types. Macrophages can change their phenotype and function in response to signals from the environment. The most studied phenotypes are M1 and M2 macrophages. M1 macrophages are induced in vitro by IFN-γ, LPS and/or TNF-α, while the induction of the M2 phenotype requires IL-4/13, IL-10, glucocorticoids or TGF-β

characterized by their production of nitric oxide (NO) [Edwards et al., 2006b; MacMicking et al., 1997; Hibbs, Jr., 2002]. Human macrophages derived from circulating monocytes do not generally produce NO [Mosser, 2003], therefore other markers should be used to discriminate between CA and AA macrophages, such as MR, E-cadherin [Van den Bossche J. et al., 2009], CD40 [Zeyda et al., 2007] and Fc-gamma receptor I (FcγRI). CA macrophages are essential for host defence [Gordon and Taylor, 2005; Nathan, 2008] and tumor killing. The pro-inflammatory mediators produced by CA macrophages can cause extensive damage to the host.

AA macrophages seem to play a role in immune suppression and tissue repair, due to production of anti-inflammatory cytokines and extracellular matrix components and lack of production of NO [Edwards et al., 2006b]. The most commonly used distinctive marker for AA macrophages, in mice, is the high expression and activity of arginase [Edwards et al., 2006b]. Due to the activation of arginase, arginine is converted to ornithine, a precursor for polyamines and collagen, which contributes to the production of extracellular matrix [Kreider et al., 2007; Albina et al., 1990; Gratchev et al., 2001; Hesse et al., 2001]. Furtermore, the polyamines produced can influence production of cytokines and suppress clonal expansion of lymphocytes, thereby regulating the immune response [Cordeiro-da-Silva et al., 2004].

Functional differences can be observed between CA and AA macrophages. As mentioned above, due to the production of ROS, CA macrophages are efficient in the killing of bacteria, while AA macrophages do not produce ROS and are therefore less efficient in killing bacteria [Gordon and Taylor, 2005]. Furthermore, CA macrophages are efficient antigen presenting cells, while AA macrophages are not [Edwards et al., 2006b]. CA macrophages are also more efficient in activating T-cell proliferation compared to AA macrophages [Edwards et al., 2006b]. AA macrophages are involved in scar formation, since they enhance fibrogenesis, while CA macrophages do not. AA macrophages stimulate proliferation and activation of fibroblasts, by expression and release of potent fibrogenic growth factors, like transforming growth factor-beta (TGF-β) and platelet derived growth factor (PDGF) [Song et al., 2000]. The angiogenic potential of AA macrophages is higher compared to CA macrophages [Kodelja et al., 1997]. Due to the production of growth factors and stimulation of angiogenesis, AA macrophages are considered tumor promoting. In vitro CA macrophages were shown to be cytotoxic to tumor cells but not to normal cells [Romieu-Mourez et al., 2006].

3.3 Macrophages in MS lesion formation and repair

It is widely accepted that macrophages play an important role in MS pathology. Macrophages are implicated in mechanisms that lead to demyelination and axonal damage [Bitsch et al., 2000; Kuhlmann et al., 2002; Trapp et al., 1998; Koning et al., 2007; Huitinga et al., 1990; Heppner et al., 2005; Hendriks et al., 2005; Newman et al., 2001]. Inflammatory infiltrates in MS lesions contain large amounts of macrophages. In experimental autoimmune encephalomyelitis (EAE), an animal model for MS, it has been shown that elimination of infiltrating macrophages reduced both clinical signs and axonal damage [Heppner et al., 2005]. Furthermore, during spinal cord injury (SCI), elimination of infiltrating macrophages increased axonal repair and functional outcome [Popovich et al., 1999; Stirling et al., 2004]. Clinical signs of EAE were significantly enhanced when the macrophage inhibitory signal of CD200/CD200R between neurons and macrophages was blocked [Koning et al., 2007]. This suggests a direct link between increased macrophage activity and aggravated disease course in EAE. Finally, macrophages are able to secrete a plethora of neurotoxic substances, such as matrix metalloproteinases [Newman et al., 2001], reactive oxygen species (ROS) [Nathan and Shiloh, 2000] and nitric oxide (NO) [Smith et al., 2001]. These studies all indicate that macrophages are detrimental.

However the role of macrophages is more complex. Several studies have shown that activated macrophages can actually be beneficial during CNS repair. During SCI macrophages can create a growth-permissive environment in which axonal regeneration can take place [Rapalino et al., 1998; Barrette et al., 2008]. In MS lesions, activated macrophages can be observed in areas with increased growth-associated protein-43 (GAP-43) expression [Teunissen et al., 2006]. In vitro AA macrophage conditioned medium has been found to promote axonal outgrowth [Kigerl et al., 2009]. Furthermore, macrophages are beneficial because they remove myelin debris, which is growth inhibiting for axons [Baer et al., 2009; Kotter et al., 2006], they release growth factors [Song et al., 2000; Kodelja et al., 1997] and they support axonal repair [Shechter et al., 2009; Bouhy et al., 2006; Batchelor et al., 2002]. These different roles ascribed to macrophages could be due to polarization in macrophage activation [Edwards et al., 2006a; Mosser and Edwards, 2008; Mantovani et al., 2004a] (Figure 1).

4. Models for MS

4.1 In vivo models

Research on the mechanisms of demyelinating diseases is highly dependent on experimental animal models, due to the inaccessibility of the human brain for experimental research. Most frequently allergic autoimmune encephalitis (EAE) models are used as a model for MS. In EAE, an autoimmune reaction is induced by injection of myelin proteins or myelin-specific inflammatory T-cells into rats or mice. Disability starts with loss of tail tonus, leading to complete paralysis, which can be recovered. Demyelination occurs after a chronic induction paradigm. The model poses very serious discomfort to the many animals involved. Other animal models use viruses or chemical agents such as cuprizone or lysophosphatidylcholine (LPC) to induce demyelination [Ercolini and Miller, 2006; Matsushima and Morell, 2001; Woodruff and Franklin, 1999]. Another model that is currently increasingly used is the mutant shiverer mouse that carries a deletion in the myelin basic protein (MBP) gene [Nave, 1994]. Several drawbacks of using animal models are: i) per animal only one condition can be tested, making the use of many animals unavoidable, ii) investigating the mechanism behind demyelination at a cellular level is difficult, due to the complex interactions of the CNS with the immune system, iii) *in vivo* it is very difficult to control all experimental conditions.

4.2 *In vitro* models

Only few alternative *in-vitro* models for de- and remyelination are available. This is due to the complex interactions between axons, oligodendrocytes and astrocytes needed for the development of multilayered myelin around axons, which cannot be accomplished by cell lines or monolayer cultures. A demyelination model in slice cultures has been described using LPC [Birgbauer et al., 2004; Miron et al., 2010]. Slice cultures contain intact myelin of specific brain areas, and are therefore very suitable for experiments. A drawback, but also advantage, of the use of slice cultures is the fact that the cellular composition of the slice can not be altered. Furthermore, the top and bottom layer of the slice consists of damaged cells, which might influence the behavior of the layers underneath.

Another good and flexible *in vitro* model for the CNS is the culture of 3-dimensional brain spheroids. Spheroids are formed by continuous rotation of a single cell suspension of primary brain cells. These cells aggregate within 24 hours and start to differentiate. The result after 4 weeks of maturation is a spheroid containing all different brain cell types that make 3-dimensional contacts [Figure 2: 3-dimensional aspect of spheroid cultures]. The high level of differentiation is exemplified by the presence of myelinated axons and spontaneous synaptic activity. The model has been used for studying brain development, neurotoxicity, and neurodegenerative diseases [Berglund et al., 2004; Diemel et al., 2004; Honegger and Richelson, 1976].

In previous studies, immune-mediated demyelination has been induced in this model, using anti-myelin antibodies and complement [Diemel et al., 2004; Loughlin et al., 1994]. The major drawback of that model is that only modest and variable effects of antibodies were observed (personal observations C. Teunissen). We were able to induce non-inflammatory demyelination using LPC as well as subsequent recovery after LPC-withdrawal, in rodent brain spheroids. The effect of LPC was specific for myelin, since other CNS cell types present in the cultures were only slightly or not affected [Vereyken et al., 2009]. After cessation of LPC treatment, remyelination was observed in these culture (Figure 3) . These data demonstrate the potential of this model to study several fundamental aspects of de- and remyelination.

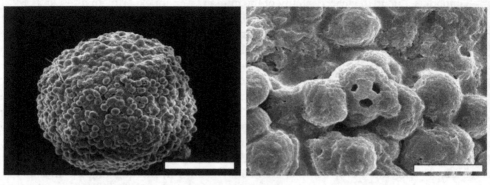

Copyright permission has been obtained from Brain Research.

(A)   (B)

Fig. 2. Scanning electron microscopy photograph of a cultured spheroid. (A) Example of 3-week-old whole brain spheroids showing a typical three-dimensional appearance. Bar represents 50 mm. (B) Higher magnification than (A), bar represents 5 mm. Teunissen et al 2000 [Teunissen et al., 2000]

5. Macrophage-CNS interaction in an in vitro model for MS

Microglia are present in spheroids, and these can be activated to study the effects of macrophages on myelin formation and demyelination. Alternatively, activated macrophages can be supplemented to the cultures. We set out to study whether the spheroid culture model is suitable for studying effects of supplemented macrophages. An important first question was whether macrophages are able to migrate into the spheroids, which would be a benefit of this model over *in vivo* models as there is no blood brain barrier (BBB) and the influence of BBB interruption can be circumvented. Next, we were especially interested to determine the effects of macrophages on CNS cell types inside the spheroids. Our hypothesis was that CA macrophages would have toxic effects and AA macrophages positive effects on myelin, glia and axonal integrity. No studies so far have addressed the question if these differential macrophage phenotypes have differential effects on intact CNS tissue. Therefore, we also set out to compare the effects of CA and AA macrophages on cellular structures within whole brain spheroid cultures.

5.1 Number of macrophages in spheroids
First, we established whether macrophages could migrate into the spheroids, and whether the numbers were similar for the CA and AA macrophage phenotypes. For this, we cultured rat whole brain spheroids during 4 weeks, to reach optimal myelin development, and exposed them to differently activated macrophages, that were fluorescently labeled, [method of macrophage activation: Vereyken et al., 2011] during maximal 1 week. At several time points, cryostat sections were cut of the spheroids and the number of spheroids containing macrophages were counted.

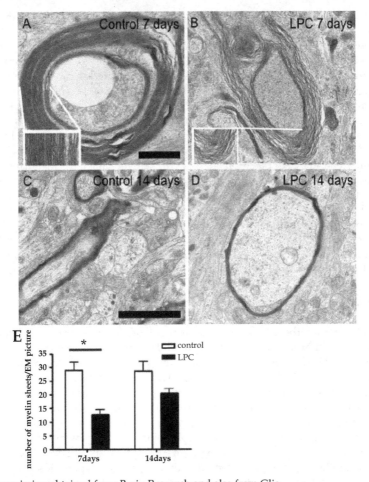

Fig. 3. EM picture of demyelinated rat whole brain spheroid cultures. A: After 4 weeks of culturing the experiment was started at day 0. After 7 days (5 weeks of culturing) multilayered compact myelin was present. See insert for more detail. B: After a week of exposure to LPC (three times addition of 0.12 mM LPC), at day 7 (= week 5 of culturing), the myelin layers were loosely packed. See insert for more detail. C: Control cultures at day 14 (6 week old cultures), show compact myelin. D: At day 14, after 1 week of exposure to LPC and 1 week of recovery, LPC-exposed cultures show compact myelin. Bar is 500 nm. E: Quantification of the number of myelin sheets present in EM pictures from two separate experiments (four pictures from three spheroids). After LPC treatment at 7 days 12.5 myelin sheets per picture were counted. When compared with control spheroids, 29 myelin sheets per picture, a significant decrease of 56% was, therefore, visible. At 14 days, the number of myelin sheets was not significantly different between control, 28 myelin sheets per picture, and LPC treated, 20 myelin sheets per picture, cultures. Results are presented as mean ± SEM. Open bars: control; closed bars: LPC treated; asterisks indicate
P < 0.05. [Vereyken et al.. 2009]

We observed a temporal pattern. After 1 day no macrophages were visible in the spheroids (data not shown). At 2 days after macrophage addition, low numbers of macrophages were present in spheroids exposed to AA and unstimulated (US) macrophages (data not shown). At 3 days macrophages were observed in 40-70% of the spheroid sections (Figure 4A and D). After 8 days the macrophage numbers were decreased compared to day 3 (data not shown).

Most macrophages were associated with spheroids on the outside rim of the spheroid, but several also migrated into the center of the spheroids (Figure 4A, B, C). A larger number of spheroids contained one or more macrophages when exposed to either AA or US macrophages compared to CA macrophages (Figure 4D). These results were in agreement with our previous observations showing that AA macrophages have a higher intrinsic motility compared to CA macrophages [Vereyken et al., 2011]. Furthermore, CA macrophages had been observed to express higher levels of adhesion receptors compared to both AA and US macrophages [Vereyken et al., 2011]. Thus, the lower motility and higher adhesion could contribute to the lower migration of CA macrophages into spheroids.

After induction of demyelination, a similar pattern was observed for the differentially activated macrophages, i.e. a higher percentage of spheroids contained AA and US macrophages (Figure 4E). Taken together, all different macrophage phenotypes could migrate into the spheroids, while the extend of migration differed between phenotypes.

5.2 Effect of differentially activated macrophages on CNS cells in spheroid cultures

Next, we tested whether CA and AA macrophages had and effect on CNS cells in the spheroids and whether the effects were dependent on the macrophage phenotype. We quantified the total immunoreactivity per spheroid section using image analysis software [Vereyken et al., 2009]. Figure 5A-D. show the results of the quantification of the immunereactivity (IR). MBP immunereactivity was 50% increased in spheroid cultures exposed to CA and AA macrophages, compared to control spheroid cultures (spheroids exposed to unstimulated macrophages and spheroid cultures without macrophages). Figure 6A-D shows representative images of MBP staining after exposure of intact spheroids to differently activated macrophages. In control spheroids, MBP IR was present in structures in the center and at the borders (Figure 6A). In the spheroids exposed to unstimulated macrophages a similar picture was observed, although, in some spheroids a higher number of MBP-positive structures near the border was observed (Figure 6B). Note that in this specific section, no intact macrophages are visible, which is likely due to the relatively low numbers of macrophages inside the spheroids in combination with the low thickness of the sections. After exposure to CA macrophages, a higher mean IR was observed at the spheroid border (Figure 6C). The mean IR was also increased in spheroids exposed to AA macrophages (Figure 6D). This increase was mainly observed in the area just below the border.

GFAP IR was not affected by addition of the macrophages. GFAP IR was slightly lower in spheroids exposed to AA macrophages compared to spheroids exposed to CA macrophages (Fig 5B). β-tubulin IR was decreased by 50% in CA macrophage-exposed spheroids compared to control spheroids, not exposed to any macrophages. Tubulin staining was present in center of the control spheroids, as described before [Vereyken et al., 2009]. After exposure of the spheroids to CA macrophages especially the β-tubulin IR in the center of the spheroids was decreased (Figure 5C). A slight increase in GAP-43 IR was observed in spheroids exposed to CA macrophages compared to control spheroids not exposed to macrophages (Figure 5D).

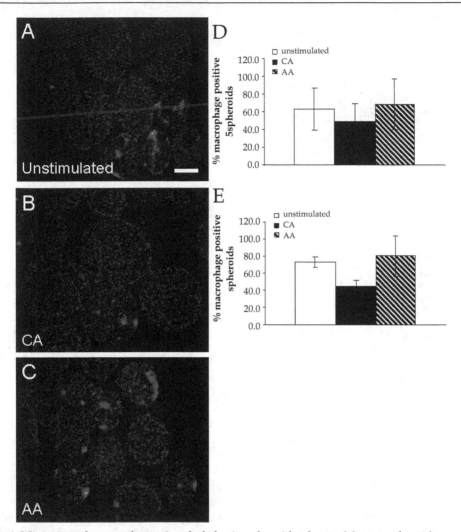

Fig. 4. Migration of macrophages in whole brain spheroid cultures. Mature spheroids were exposed to unstimulated (A); classically activated (CA); of alternatively activated (AA) macrophages during three days. Macrophages were labelled with DiI before addition to the cultures. Sections were prepared and nuclei stained with Hoechst. Bar in A is 200 µm. Figure 4D and E: Quantification of migration of differently activated macrophages in whole brain spheroids. D: The number of positive spheroids was determined as the number of spheroids containing one or more macrophages/total number of control spheroids. A trend could be seen of a lower migration of CA macrophages into spheroids compared to unstimulated and AA macrophages. E: Quantification of migration of macrophages is higher in demyelinated spheroids. Unstimulated macrophages were present in 73% (± 6) of the LPC-demyelineated spheroids. Spheroids exposed to CA macrophages. Only 45% (± 6) of the LPC-demyelineated spheroids were positive for CA macrophages. With AA macrophages the percentage of spheroids positive was 80 % (± 24)

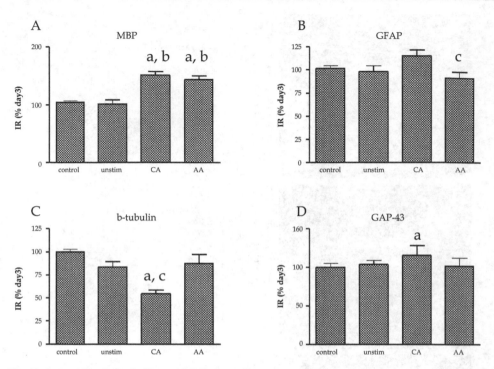

Fig. 5. Quantification of effects of differentially activated macrophages on immunereactivity of specific CNS cell proteins in spheroid cultures. Unstim=unstimulated macrophages; CA: classically activated macrophages; AA: Alternatively activated macrophages. Four-weeks old whole brain spheroid cultures exposed to unstim, CA or AA macrophages during 3 days. a: P< 0.05 compared to control; b: P<0.05 compared to unstimulated macrophages; c: P<0.05 for differences between CA and AA macrophages

5.3 Discussion of the experimental results in spheroid cultures

The first aim of the experiments described above was to study whether macrophages can migrate into the spheroid cultures. This was indeed the case. Externally supplemented macrophages can be labeled to trace them within the spheroid and we observed that they can migrate into the center of the spheroid.

The second aim was to study effects of classically and alternatively activated macrophages on cellular structures of whole brain spheroid cultures. Our hypothesis was that CA macrophages would have toxic effects and that AA macrophages have positive effects on myelin and axonal integrity. Our results were in part supportive for this hypothesis: CA macrophages had a slight negative effect on tubulin immune reactivity in intact spheroids, while AA macrophages had no effect on tubulin immune reactivity. This indicates that CA macrophages were toxic to neurons, while AA macrophages were not. These data are in agreement with our observations in monolayers (EJFV Unpublished observation). The GFAP immunereactivity was slightly higher in CA exposed macrophages compared to AA exposed macrophages. However, for many of our read-outs there were no substantial differences between the differently activated macrophages. A similar positive effect of both

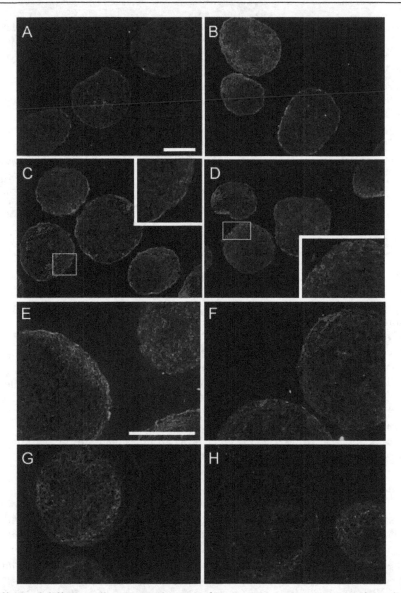

Fig. 6. Effects of differentially activated macrophages on immunereactivity of myelin basic protein (MBP) in spheroid cultures. Four-weeks old whole brain spheroid cultures were exposed to unstim, CA or AA macrophages during 3 days. A: MBP immune reactivity in control spheroids without exposure to macrophages.; B-D: MBP immune reactivity in spheroids exposed to (B) unstimulated macrophages, (C) classically activated (CA) macrophages, and (D) Alternatively activated macrophages (AA). E: GFAP IR in spheroids exposed to CA macrophages; F: GFAP IR in spheroids exposed to AA macrophages. G: β-tubulin IR in control spheroids. H: β-tubulin IR in spheroids exposed to CA macrophages. Bar in A and G= 200 μm

CA and AA macrophages on MBP immunereactivity in spheroids was observed. The lack of large differences between the different macrophage phenotypes could be related to the length of the experiments and the flexibility of the macrophage phenotypes, as a fundamental characteristic of macrophages is their ability to change their phenotype and they could all have a similar phenotype after a few days of contact with the CNS tissue. However, the duration of the experiments was three days, and we observed differences in migration between the phenotypes after 3 days. The different phenotypes do contain similar receptors, and it is possible that MBP expression is influenced by growth factors that may be differently, but at least sufficient on both phenotypes for induction of the observed.

Taken together, our results have shown that CA and AA macrophages can both affect myelin formation in spheroid cultures. Future studies must show whether macrophages can enhance myelin formation after demyelination and the conditions under which they can have regenerative effects.

6. Future perspectives

There are various in vivo and in vitro models for de- and remyelination in MS. The use of each of the models will depend on the research question. In vitro models provide the possibility to study direct effects on CNS cell types, without interference of other processes. Furthermore, access to CNS cell types is not hampered by the blood brain barrier. Furthermore, use of in *in vitro* models leads to a reduction of animal suffering. Nevertheless, we do not expect in *vitro* results to be directly translatable to the human situation and thus an intermediate step *in vivo* will be needed, but this can be on a limited scale when the range of conditions are narrowed by *in vitro* experiments.

In MS lesions, macrophages with the CA phenotype could inhibit repair or propagate lesion formation, since CA macrophages have been shown to be neurotoxic while AA activation abolished the neurotoxic effects. In MS lesions it could therefore be beneficial to reduce the CA phenotype and promote the AA phenotype. Possible mechanisms to skew the macrophage phenotype in the CNS are interesting to investigate, in order to design anti-inflammatory therapies. Here, we discuss these options.

6.1 Skewing of macrophage phenotype

Glucocorticoids are an accepted therapy during MS. Treatment with glucocorticoids might be a means of skewing the activational phenotype, since exposure to glucocorticoids induce a wound healing phenotype in macrophages *in vitro* [Mosser and Edwards, 2008; Gordon, 2003]. A glucocorticoid receptor ligand was found to attenuate experimental autoimmune neuritis, decrease the expression of inflammatory cytokines and iNOS and induce a M2 phenotype *in vitro* [Zhang et al., 2009].

Evidence for the possibility that substances in the periphery can influence CNS cells has been observed previously. In the CNS microglia have been shown to switch cytokine profile, from relatively anti-inflammatory to pro-inflammatory CA phenotype, after induction of Wallerian degeneration followed by systemic injection of LPS [Palin et al., 2008]. The peripheral LPS injection also led to a decrease in neurofilament staining, indicating that neurodegeneration is increased. Similar results were found with a mouse model for prion disease, more inflammation and neuronal apoptosis after systemic LPS injection [Cunningham et al., 2005]. Likewise, glucocorticoids and glatiramer acetate, when applied peripherally, could influence the phenotype of microglia and macrophages inside the CNS.

It would therefore be interesting to determine the effect of glucocorticoid treatment on the macrophage phenotype in the CNS. Furthermore, since in MS lesions the macrophages predominantly express markers of the CA phenotype, it would be useful to study whether AA macrophages that enter a pro-inflammatory environment would be able to keep their phenotype. Could AA macrophages be able to exert positive effects in a pro-inflammatory environment? These questions can be investigated using *in vitro* models, such as the spheroid model, representing the CNS environment.

6.2 Injection of skewed macrophages

Some investigation into direct treatment with AA macrophages has been performed and therapeutic effects have been observed. In a model for murine diabetes a reduction in renal and pancreatic injury was seen after treatment with *in vitro* generated AA macrophages [Zheng et al., 2011]. The injection of AA macrophages reduced disease in a model for colitis [Hunter et al., 2010]. Furthermore, axonal dieback induced by macrophages was reduced after the addition of multipotent adult progenitor cells, which induced the AA phenotype in macrophages *in vitro* [Busch et al., 2011]. During EAE, treatment with substances skewing the macrophage phenotype toward an AA phenotype, such as anti-CCL22 [Dogan et al., 2011] and 2-arachidonoylglycerol [Lourbopoulos et al., 2011], was found to ameliorate the disease course and increase the presence of macrophages with an AA phenotype in the lesions. In a model for relapsing EAE, the injection of AA macrophages, generated in vitro, reduced the development of relapses [Mikita et al., 2011]. Clinical EAE was reversed by the adoptive transfer of AA macrophages, which were induced in vitro with glatiramer acetate [Weber et al., 2007]. Our studies have shown that macrophage migration towards CNS cell types differs upon skewing [Vereyken et al., 2011] and that migration of macrophages in spheroids is limited and varies with skewing of the macrophages (Figure 4E). Microinjection of skewed macrophages into spheroids or co-culture of differently activated macrophages would allow more in depth analysis into the cellular mechanisms behind the effects reported in these studies.

7. Conclusion

Spheroid cultures are a suitable model to test the effects of novel therapeutics on remyelination, e.g. magnitude and speed. Furthermore, this model is very useful to study the mechanism of remyelination and the effects of demyelination, for example on axons. Using spheroid cultures, cells not endogenous to the CNS, like macrophages, can be introduced into the spheroids with relative ease [Loughlin et al., 1994; Loughlin et al., 1997; Pardo and Honegger, 2000] as we demonstrated. Both CA and AA macrophages can have beneficial effects in an MS lesion. The CA macrophages are very efficient in clearing debris, however, they are toxic to neurons. The AA macrophages secrete higher amounts of neurotrophins and are not neurotoxic, however they are less efficient in clearing debris. It would be of great value if an activational status in macrophages could be reached with an increased phagocytic capacity, without the production of neurotoxic substances such as ROS, NO and TNF-α, and with the secretion of growth factors. Future research should therefore focus on the functional activation status of macrophages stimulated with for example glucocorticoids, to enhance the secretion of growth factors and phagocytosis and limit secretion of neurotoxic substances.

8. Acknowledgements

We would like to extend our gratitude towards all who have contributed to the spheroid studies: Marije Bolijn, Priscilla Heijnen, Wia Baron, Sjef Copray, Elga de Vries, Amos Attali and Ilja Boor. Support grant: Dutch MS Research Foundation, grant number: 05-358c. Dutch Research Council (NWO (016.056.024))

9. References

Akira S, Uematsu S, Takeuchi O (2006) Pathogen recognition and innate immunity. *Cell* 124: 783-801

Albina JE, Mills CD, Henry WL, Jr., Caldwell MD (1990) Temporal expression of different pathways of 1-arginine metabolism in healing wounds. *J Immunol* 144: 3877-3880

Babior BM (1999) NADPH oxidase: an update. *Blood* 93: 1464-1476

Baer AS, Syed YA, Kang SU, Mitteregger D, Vig R, Ffrench-Constant C, Franklin RJ, Altmann F, Lubec G, Kotter MR (2009) Myelin-mediated inhibition of oligodendrocyte precursor differentiation can be overcome by pharmacological modulation of Fyn-RhoA and protein kinase C signalling. *Brain* 132: 465-481

Barkhof F, Filippi M, Miller DH, Scheltens P, Campi A, Polman CH, Comi G, Ader HJ, Losseff N, Valk J (1997) Comparison of MRI criteria at first presentation to predict conversion to clinically definite multiple sclerosis. *Brain* 120 (Pt 11): 2059-2069

Barnett MH, Prineas JW (2004) Relapsing and remitting multiple sclerosis: pathology of the newly forming lesion. *Ann Neurol* 55: 458-468

Barrette B, Hebert MA, Filali M, Lafortune K, Vallieres N, Gowing G, Julien JP, Lacroix S (2008) Requirement of myeloid cells for axon regeneration 1. *J Neurosci* 28: 9363-9376

Batchelor PE, Porritt MJ, Martinello P, Parish CL, Liberatore GT, Donnan GA, Howells DW (2002) Macrophages and Microglia Produce Local Trophic Gradients That Stimulate Axonal Sprouting Toward but Not beyond the Wound Edge 1. *Mol Cell Neurosci* 21: 436-453

Berglund CM, Aarum J, Haeberlein SL, Nyengaard JR, Hokfelt T, Sandberg K, Naslund J, Persson MA (2004) Characterization of long-term mouse brain aggregating cultures: evidence for maintenance of neural precursor cells. *J Comp Neurol* 474: 246-260

Birgbauer E, Rao TS, Webb M (2004) Lysolecithin induces demyelination in vitro in a cerebellar slice culture system. *J Neurosci Res* 78: 157-166

Bitsch A, Schuchardt J, Bunkowski S, Kuhlmann T, Bruck W (2000) Acute axonal injury in multiple sclerosis. Correlation with demyelination and inflammation. *Brain* 123 (Pt 6): 1174-1183

Bouhy D, Malgrange B, Multon S, Poirrier AL, Scholtes F, Schoenen J, Franzen R (2006) Delayed GM-CSF treatment stimulates axonal regeneration and functional recovery in paraplegic rats via an increased BDNF expression by endogenous macrophages. *FASEB J* 20: 1239-1241

Bourahoui A, De SJ, Guttierez R, Onraed B, Hennache B, Ferriby D, Stojkovic T, Vermersch P (2004) CSF isoelectrofocusing in a large cohort of MS and other neurological diseases. *Eur J Neurol* 11: 525-529

Bruck W, Bitsch A, Kolenda H, Bruck Y, Stiefel M, Lassmann H (1997) Inflammatory central nervous system demyelination: correlation of magnetic resonance imaging findings with lesion pathology. *Ann Neurol* 42: 783-793

Bruck W, Kuhlmann T, Stadelmann C (2003) Remyelination in multiple sclerosis. *J Neurol Sci* 206: 181-185

Bruck W, Porada P, Poser S, Rieckmann P, Hanefeld F, Kretzschmar HA, Lassmann H (1995) Monocyte/macrophage differentiation in early multiple sclerosis lesions. *Ann Neurol* 38: 788-796

Busch SA, Hamilton JA, Horn KP, Cuascut FX, Cutrone R, Lehman N, Deans RJ, Ting AE, Mays RW, Silver J (2011) Multipotent adult progenitor cells prevent macrophage-mediated axonal dieback and promote regrowth after spinal cord injury. *J Neurosci* 31: 944-953

Charcot M (1868) Histolgie de le sclerose en plaques. *Gaz Hop* 141: 554-558

Charles P, Reynolds R, Seilhean D, Rougon G, Aigrot MS, Niezgoda A, Zalc B, Lubetzki C (2002) Re-expression of PSA-NCAM by demyelinated axons: an inhibitor of remyelination in multiple sclerosis? *Brain* 125: 1972-1979

Compston A, Coles A (2008) Multiple sclerosis. *Lancet* 372: 1502-1517

Cordeiro-da-Silva A, Tavares J, Araujo N, Cerqueira F, Tomas A, Kong Thoo LP, Ouaissi A (2004) Immunological alterations induced by polyamine derivatives on murine splenocytes and human mononuclear cells. *Int Immunopharmacol* 4: 547-556

Correale J, de los Milagros Bassani Molinas (2002) Oligoclonal bands and antibody responses in multiple sclerosis. *J Neurol* 249: 375-389

Cunningham C, Wilcockson DC, Campion S, Lunnon K, Perry VH (2005) Central and systemic endotoxin challenges exacerbate the local inflammatory response and increase neuronal death during chronic neurodegeneration. *J Neurosci* 25: 9275-9284

de Groot CJ, Bergers E, Kamphorst W, Ravid R, Polman CH, Barkhof F, Van der Valk P. (2001) Post-mortem MRI-guided sampling of multiple sclerosis brain lesions: increased yield of active demyelinating and (p)reactive lesions. *Brain* 124: 1635-1645

DeLeo FR, Allen LA, Apicella M, Nauseef WM (1999) NADPH oxidase activation and assembly during phagocytosis. *J Immunol* 163: 6732-6740

Diemel LT, Wolswijk G, Jackson SJ, Cuzner ML (2004) Remyelination of cytokine- or antibody-demyelinated CNS aggregate cultures is inhibited by macrophage supplementation. *Glia* 45: 278-286

Dogan RN, Long N, Forde E, Dennis K, Kohm AP; Miller SD, Karpus WJ (2011) CCL22 regulates experimental autoimmune encephalomyelitis by controlling inflammatory macrophage accumulation and effector function. *J Leukoc Biol* 89: 93-104

Doring A, Yong VW (2011) The good, the bad and the ugly. Macrophages/microglia with a focus on myelin repair. *Front Biosci (Schol Ed)* 3: 846-856

Edwards JP, Zhang X, Frauwirth KA, Mosser DM (2006b) Biochemical and functional characterization of three activated macrophage populations. *J Leukoc Biol* 80: 1298-1307

Edwards JP, Zhang X, Frauwirth KA, Mosser DM (2006a) Biochemical and functional characterization of three activated macrophage populations. *J Leukoc Biol* 80: 1298-1307

Ercolini AM, Miller SD (2006) Mechanisms of immunopathology in murine models of central nervous system demyelinating disease. *J Immunol* 176: 3293-3298

Franklin RJ (2002) Why does remyelination fail in multiple sclerosis? *Nat Rev Neurosci* 3: 705-714

Franklin RJ, Ffrench-Constant C (2008) Remyelination in the CNS: from biology to therapy. *Nat Rev Neurosci* 9: 839-855

Gordon S (1986) Biology of the macrophage. *J Cell Sci Suppl* 4: 267-286

Gordon S (1998) The role of the macrophage in immune regulation. *Res Immunol* 149: 685-688

Gordon S (2003) Alternative activation of macrophages. *Nat Rev Immunol* 3: 23-35

Gordon S, Taylor PR (2005) Monocyte and macrophage heterogeneity. *Nat Rev Immunol* 5: 953-964

Gratchev A, Guillot P, Hakiy N, Politz O, Orfanos CE, Schledzewski K, Goerdt S (2001) Alternatively activated macrophages differentially express fibronectin and its splice variants and the extracellular matrix protein betaIG-H3. *Scand J Immunol* 53: 386-392

Henderson AP, Barnett MH, Parratt JD, Prineas JW (2009) Multiple sclerosis: distribution of inflammatory cells in newly forming lesions. *Ann Neurol* 66: 739-753

Hendriks JJ, Teunissen CE, de Vries HE, Dijkstra CD (2005) Macrophages and neurodegeneration. *Brain Res Brain Res Rev* 48: 185-195

Heppner FL, Greter M, Marino D, Falsig J, Raivich G, Hovelmeyer N, Waisman A, Rulicke T, Prinz M, Priller J, Becher B, Aguzzi A (2005) Experimental autoimmune encephalomyelitis repressed by microglial paralysis. *Nat Med* 11: 146-152

Hesse M, Modolell M, La Flamme AC, Schito M, Fuentes JM, Cheever AW, Pearce EJ, Wynn TA (2001) Differential regulation of nitric oxide synthase-2 and arginase-1 by type 1/type 2 cytokines in vivo: granulomatous pathology is shaped by the pattern of L-arginine metabolism. *J Immunol* 167: 6533-6544

Hibbs JB, Jr. (2002) Infection and nitric oxide. *J Infect Dis* 185 Suppl 1: S9-17

Honegger P, Richelson E (1976) Biochemical differentiation of mechanically dissociated mammalian brain in aggregating cell culture. *Brain Res* 109: 335-354

Huitinga I, Van Rooijen N, De Groot CJ, Uitdehaag BM, Dijkstra CD (1990) Suppression of experimental allergic encephalomyelitis in Lewis rats after elimination of macrophages. *J Exp Med* 172: 1025-1033

Hunter MM, Wang A, Parhar KS, Johnston MJ, van RN, Beck PL, McKay DM (2010) In vitro-derived alternatively activated macrophages reduce colonic inflammation in mice. *Gastroenterology* 138: 1395-1405

Janeway CA, Jr., Medzhitov R (2002) Innate immune recognition. *Annu Rev Immunol* 20: 197-216

John GR, Shankar SL, Shafit-Zagardo B, Massimi A, Lee SC, Raine CS, Brosnan CF (2002) Multiple sclerosis: re-expression of a developmental pathway that restricts oligodendrocyte maturation. *Nat Med* 8: 1115-1121

Junker A, Hohlfeld R, Meinl E (2011) The emerging role of microRNAs in multiple sclerosis. *Nat Rev Neurol* 7: 56-59

Katz D, Taubenberger JK, Cannella B, McFarlin DE, Raine CS, McFarland HF (1993) Correlation between magnetic resonance imaging findings and lesion development in chronic, active multiple sclerosis. *Ann Neurol* 34: 661-669

Kigerl KA, Gensel JC, Ankeny DP, Alexander JK, Donnelly DJ, Popovich PG (2009) Identification of two distinct macrophage subsets with divergent effects causing either neurotoxicity or regeneration in the injured mouse spinal cord. *J Neurosci* 29: 13435-13444

Kodelja V, Muller C, Tenorio S, Schebesch C, Orfanos CE, Goerdt S (1997) Differences in angiogenic potential of classically vs alternatively activated macrophages. *Immunobiology* 197: 478-493

Koning N, Bo L, Hoek RM, Huitinga I (2007) Downregulation of macrophage inhibitory molecules in multiple sclerosis lesions. *Ann Neurol* 62: 504-514

Kono H, Rock KL (2008) How dying cells alert the immune system to danger. *Nat Rev Immunol* 8: 279-289

Kotter MR, Li WW, Zhao C, Franklin RJ (2006) Myelin impairs CNS remyelination by inhibiting oligodendrocyte precursor cell differentiation. *J Neurosci* 26: 328-332

Kreider T, Anthony RM, Urban JF, Jr., Gause WC (2007) Alternatively activated macrophages in helminth infections. *Curr Opin Immunol* 19: 448-453

Kuhlmann T, Lingfeld G, Bitsch A, Schuchardt J, Bruck W (2002) Acute axonal damage in multiple sclerosis is most extensive in early disease stages and decreases over time. *Brain* 125: 2202-2212

Lassmann H, Bruck W, Lucchinetti C, Rodriguez M (1997) Remyelination in multiple sclerosis. *Mult Scler* 3: 133-136

Loughlin AJ, Copelman CA, Hall A, Armer T, Young BC, Landon DN, Cuzner ML (1997) Myelination and remyelination of aggregate rat brain cell cultures enriched with macrophages. *J Neurosci Res* 47: 384-392

Loughlin AJ, Honegger P, Woodroofe MN, Comte V, Matthieu JM, Cuzner ML (1994) Myelin basic protein content of aggregating rat brain cell cultures treated with cytokines and/or demyelinating antibody: effects of macrophage enrichment. *J Neurosci Res* 37: 647-653

Lourbopoulos A, Grigoriadis N, Lagoudaki R, Touloumi O, Polyzoidou E, Mavromatis I, Tascos N, Breuer A, Ovadia H, Karussis D, Shohami E, Mechoulam R, Simeonidou C (2011) Administration of 2-arachidonoylglycerol ameliorates both acute and chronic experimental autoimmune encephalomyelitis. *Brain Res* 1390: 126-141

Lublin FD, Reingold SC (1996) Defining the clinical course of multiple sclerosis: results of an international survey. National Multiple Sclerosis Society (USA) Advisory Committee on Clinical Trials of New Agents in Multiple Sclerosis. *Neurology* 46: 907-911

MacMicking J, Xie QW, Nathan C (1997) Nitric oxide and macrophage function. *Annu Rev Immunol* 15: 323-350

Mantovani A, Sica A, Sozzani S, Allavena P, Vecchi A, Locati M (2004b) The chemokine system in diverse forms of macrophage activation and polarization. *Trends Immunol* 25: 677-686

Mantovani A, Sica A, Sozzani S, Allavena P, Vecchi A, Locati M (2004a) The chemokine system in diverse forms of macrophage activation and polarization. *Trends Immunol* 25: 677-686

Martinez FO, Gordon S, Locati M, Mantovani A (2006) Transcriptional profiling of the human monocyte-to-macrophage differentiation and polarization: new molecules and patterns of gene expression. *J Immunol* 177: 7303-7311

Martinez FO, Sica A, Mantovani A, Locati M (2008) Macrophage activation and polarization. *Front Biosci* 13: 453-461

Matsushima GK, Morell P (2001) The neurotoxicant, cuprizone, as a model to study demyelination and remyelination in the central nervous system. *Brain Pathol* 11: 107-116

McDonald WI, Compston A, Edan G, Goodkin D, Hartung HP, Lublin FD, McFarland HF, Paty DW, Polman CH, Reingold SC, Sandberg-Wollheim M, Sibley W, Thompson A, van den NS, Weinshenker BY, Wolinsky JS (2001) Recommended diagnostic criteria for multiple sclerosis: guidelines from the International Panel on the diagnosis of multiple sclerosis. *Ann Neurol* 50: 121-127

Medzhitov R, Janeway CA, Jr. (2002) Decoding the patterns of self and nonself by the innate immune system. *Science* 296: 298-300

Mikita J, Dubourdieu-Cassagno N, Deloire MS, Vekris A, Biran M, Raffard G, Brochet B, Canron MH, Franconi JM, Boiziau C, Petry KG (2011) Altered M1/M2 activation patterns of monocytes in severe relapsing experimental rat model of multiple sclerosis. Amelioration of clinical status by M2 activated monocyte administration. *Mult Scler* 17: 2-15

Miller DH, Grossman RI, Reingold SC, McFarland HF (1998) The role of magnetic resonance techniques in understanding and managing multiple sclerosis. *Brain* 121 (Pt 1): 3-24

Miron VE, Ludwin SK, Darlington PJ, Jarjour AA, Soliven B, Kennedy TE, Antel JP (2010) Fingolimod (FTY720) enhances remyelination following demyelination of organotypic cerebellar slices. *Am J Pathol* 176: 2682-2694

Modolell M, Corraliza IM, Link F, Soler G, Eichmann K (1995) Reciprocal regulation of the nitric oxide synthase/arginase balance in mouse bone marrow-derived macrophages by TH1 and TH2 cytokines. *Eur J Immunol* 25: 1101-1104

Mosser DM (2003) The many faces of macrophage activation. *J Leukoc Biol* 73: 209-212

Mosser DM, Edwards JP (2008) Exploring the full spectrum of macrophage activation. *Nat Rev Immunol* 8: 958-969

Nathan C (2008) Metchnikoff's Legacy in 2008. *Nat Immunol* 9: 695-698

Nathan C, Shiloh MU (2000) Reactive oxygen and nitrogen intermediates in the relationship between mammalian hosts and microbial pathogens. *Proc Natl Acad Sci U S A* 97: 8841-8848

Nave KA (1994) Neurological mouse mutants and the genes of myelin. *J Neurosci Res* 38: 607-612

Nesbit GM, Forbes GS, Scheithauer BW, Okazaki H, Rodriguez M (1991) Multiple sclerosis: histopathologic and MR and/or CT correlation in 37 cases at biopsy and three cases at autopsy. *Radiology* 180: 467-474

Newman TA, Woolley ST, Hughes PM, Sibson NR, Anthony DC, Perry VH (2001) T-cell- and macrophage-mediated axon damage in the absence of a CNS-specific immune response: involvement of metalloproteinases. *Brain* 124: 2203-2214

Nielsen JM, Korteweg T, Barkhof F, Uitdehaag BM, Polman CH (2005) Overdiagnosis of multiple sclerosis and magnetic resonance imaging criteria. *Ann Neurol* 58: 781-783

O'Shea JJ, Murray PJ (2008) Cytokine signaling modules in inflammatory responses. *Immunity* 28: 477-487

Palin K, Cunningham C, Forse P, Perry VH, Platt N (2008) Systemic inflammation switches the inflammatory cytokine profile in CNS Wallerian degeneration. *Neurobiol Dis* 30: 19-29

Paolino E, Fainardi E, Ruppi P, Tola MR, Govoni V, Casetta I, Monetti VC, Granieri E, Carreras M (1996) A prospective study on the predictive value of CSF oligoclonal bands and MRI in acute isolated neurological syndromes for subsequent progression to multiple sclerosis. *J Neurol Neurosurg Psychiatry* 60: 572-575

Pardo B, Honegger P (2000) Differentiation of rat striatal embryonic stem cells in vitro: monolayer culture vs. three-dimensional coculture with differentiated brain cells. *J Neurosci Res* 59: 504-512

Polman CH, Reingold SC, Banwell B, Clanet M, Cohen JA, Filippi M, Fujihara K, Havrdova E, Hutchinson M, Kappos L, Lublin FD, Montalban X, O'Connor P, Sandberg-Wollheim M, Thompson AJ, Waubant E, Weinshenker B, Wolinsky JS (2011) Diagnostic criteria for multiple sclerosis: 2010 revisions to the McDonald criteria. *Ann Neurol* 69: 292-302

Polman CH, Reingold SC, Edan G, Filippi M, Hartung HP, Kappos L, Lublin FD, Metz LM, McFarland HF, O'Connor PW, Sandberg-Wollheim M, Thompson AJ, Weinshenker BG, Wolinsky JS (2005) Diagnostic criteria for multiple sclerosis: 2005 revisions to the "McDonald Criteria". *Ann Neurol* 58: 840-846

Popovich PG, Guan Z, Wei P, Huitinga I, van RN, Stokes BT (1999) Depletion of hematogenous macrophages promotes partial hindlimb recovery and neuroanatomical repair after experimental spinal cord injury. *Exp Neurol* 158: 351-365

Prineas JW, Barnard RO, Kwon EE, Sharer LR, Cho ES (1993) Multiple sclerosis: remyelination of nascent lesions. *Ann Neurol* 33: 137-151

Prineas JW, Connell F (1979) Remyelination in multiple sclerosis. *Ann Neurol* 5: 22-31

Pugliatti M, Sotgiu S, Rosati G (2002) The worldwide prevalence of multiple sclerosis. *Clin Neurol Neurosurg* 104: 182-191

Raine CS, Wu E (1993) Multiple sclerosis: remyelination in acute lesions. *J Neuropathol Exp Neurol* 52: 199-204

Rapalino O, Lazarov-Spiegler O, Agranov E, Velan GJ, Yoles E, Fraidakis M, Solomon A, Gepstein R, Katz A, Belkin M, Hadani M, Schwartz M (1998) Implantation of stimulated homologous macrophages results in partial recovery of paraplegic rats. *Nat Med* 4: 814-821

Rodriguez M, Lucchinetti CF (1999) Is apoptotic death of the oligodendrocyte a critical event in the pathogenesis of multiple sclerosis?. *Neurology* 53: 1615-1616

Romieu-Mourez R, Solis M, Nardin A, Goubau D, Baron-Bodo V, Lin R, Massie B, Salcedo M, Hiscott J (2006) Distinct roles for IFN regulatory factor (IRF)-3 and IRF-7 in the activation of antitumor properties of human macrophages. *Cancer Res* 66: 10576-10585

Shechter R, London A, Varol C, Raposo C, Cusimano M, Yovel G, Rolls A, Mack M, Pluchino S, Martino G, Jung S, Schwartz M (2009) Infiltrating blood-derived macrophages are vital cells playing an anti-inflammatory role in recovery from spinal cord injury in mice. *PLoS Med* 6: e1000113

Smith KJ, Kapoor R, Hall SM, Davies M (2001) Electrically active axons degenerate when exposed to nitric oxide. *Ann Neurol* 49: 470-476

Song E, Ouyang N, Horbelt M, Antus B, Wang M, Exton MS (2000) Influence of alternatively and classically activated macrophages on fibrogenic activities of human fibroblasts. *Cell Immunol* 204: 19-28

Stein M, Keshav S, Harris N, Gordon S (1992) Interleukin 4 potently enhances murine macrophage mannose receptor activity: a marker of alternative immunologic macrophage activation. *J Exp Med* 176: 287-292

Stirling DP, Khodarahmi K, Liu J, McPhail LT, McBride CB, Steeves JD, Ramer MS, Tetzlaff W (2004) Minocycline treatment reduces delayed oligodendrocyte death, attenuates axonal dieback, and improves functional outcome after spinal cord injury. *J Neurosci* 24: 2182-2190

Takeda K, Akira S (2005) Toll-like receptors in innate immunity. *Int Immunol* 17: 1-14

Teunissen CE, Dijkstra CD, Jasperse B, Barkhof F, Vanderstichele H, Vanmechelen E, Polman CH, Bo L (2006) Growth-associated protein 43 in lesions and cerebrospinal fluid in multiple sclerosis. *Neuropathol Appl Neurobiol* 32: 318-331

Teunissen CE, Iacobaeus E, Khademi M, Brundin L, Norgren N, Koel-Simmelink MJ, Schepens M, Bouwman F, Twaalfhoven HA, Blom HJ, Jakobs C, Dijkstra CD (2009) Combination of CSF N-acetylaspartate and neurofilaments in multiple sclerosis. *Neurology* 72: 1322-1329

Teunissen CE, Koel-Simmelink MJ, Pham TV, Knol JC, Khalil M, Trentini A, Killestein J, Nielsen J, Vrenken H, Popescu V, Dijkstra CD, Jimenez CR (2011) Identification of biomarkers for diagnosis and progression of MS by MALDI-TOF mass spectrometry. *Mult Scler* 17: 838-850

Teunissen CE, Steinbusch HW, Markerink-van Ittersum M., de Bruijn C., Axer H, de Vente J. (2000) Whole brain spheroid cultures as a model to study the development of nitric oxide synthase-guanylate cyclase signal transduction. *Brain Res Dev Brain Res* 125: 99-115

Trapp BD, Peterson J, Ransohoff RM, Rudick R, Mork S, Bo L (1998) Axonal transection in the lesions of multiple sclerosis. *N Engl J Med* 338: 278-285

Van den Bossche J., Bogaert P, Van Hengel J, Guerin CJ, Berx G, Movahedi K, Van den Bergh R., Pereira-Fernandes A, Geuns JM, Pircher H, Dorny P, Grooten J, De Baetselier P., Van Ginderachter JA (2009) Alternatively activated macrophages engage in homotypic and heterotypic interactions through IL-4 and polyamine-induced E-cadherin/catenin complexes. *Blood* 114: 4664-4674

van der Goes A., Boorsma W, Hoekstra K, Montagne L, De Groot CJ, Dijkstra CD (2005) Determination of the sequential degradation of myelin proteins by macrophages. *J Neuroimmunol* 161: 12-20

van der Valk, De Groot CJ (2000) Staging of multiple sclerosis (MS) lesions: pathology of the time frame of MS. *Neuropathol Appl Neurobiol* 26: 2-10

Vereyken EJ, Fluitsma DM, Bolijn MJ, Dijkstra CD, Teunissen CE (2009) An in vitro model for de- and remyelination using lysophosphatidyl choline in rodent whole brain spheroid cultures. *Glia* 57: 1326-1340

Vereyken EJ, Heijnen PD, Baron W, de Vries EH, Dijkstra CD, Teunissen CE (2011) Classically and alternatively activated bone marrow derived macrophages differ in cytoskeletal functions and migration towards specific CNS cell types. *J Neuroinflammation* 8: 58

Weber MS, Prod'homme T, Youssef S, Dunn SE, Rundle CD, Lee L, Patarroyo JC, Stuve O, Sobel RA, Steinman L, Zamvil SS (2007) Type II monocytes modulate T cell-mediated central nervous system autoimmune disease. *Nat Med* 13: 935-943

Wolswijk G (2000) Oligodendrocyte survival, loss and birth in lesions of chronic-stage multiple sclerosis. *Brain* 123 (Pt 1): 105-115

Wolswijk G (2002) Oligodendrocyte precursor cells in the demyelinated multiple sclerosis spinal cord. *Brain* 125: 338-349

Woodruff RH, Franklin RJ (1999) Demyelination and remyelination of the caudal cerebellar peduncle of adult rats following stereotaxic injections of lysolecithin, ethidium bromide, and complement/anti-galactocerebroside: a comparative study. *Glia* 25: 216-228

Zeyda M, Farmer D, Todoric J, Aszmann O, Speiser M, Gyori G, Zlabinger GJ, Stulnig TM (2007) Human adipose tissue macrophages are of an anti-inflammatory phenotype but capable of excessive pro-inflammatory mediator production. *Int J Obes (Lond)* 31: 1420-1428

Zhang X, Mosser DM (2008) Macrophage activation by endogenous danger signals. *J Pathol* 214: 161-178

Zhang Z, Zhang ZY, Schluesener HJ (2009) Compound A, a plant origin ligand of glucocorticoid receptors, increases regulatory T cells and M2 macrophages to attenuate experimental autoimmune neuritis with reduced side effects. *J Immunol* 183: 3081-3091

Zheng D, Wang Y, Cao Q, Lee VW, Zheng G, Sun Y, Tan TK, Wang Y, Alexander SI, Harris DC (2011) Transfused macrophages ameliorate pancreatic and renal injury in murine diabetes mellitus. *Nephron Exp Nephrol* 118: e87-e99

Ziemann U, Wahl M, Hattingen E, Tumani H (2011) Development of biomarkers for multiple sclerosis as a neurodegenerative disorder. *Prog Neurobiol*

9

Amyotrophic Lateral Sclerosis

David S. Shin[1], Ashley J. Pratt[2],
Elizabeth D. Getzoff[2] and J. Jefferson P. Perry[2,3]
[1]*Lawrence Berkeley National Laboratory,*
[2]*The Scripps Research Institute,*
[3]*Amrita University,*
[1,2]*USA*
[3]*India*

1. Introduction

Amyotrophic lateral sclerosis (ALS) is a fatal neurodegenerative motor neuron disease for which no successful treatment presently exists. ALS is also termed Charcot's disease (maladie de Charcot), after the French clinician Jean Martin Charcot who first described its features in 1869 (Charcot 1869) or Lou Gehrig's disease in the United States, after the New York Yankees baseball player afflicted with the condition. Within Europe ALS is often referred to as Motor Neuron Disease, describing the cells chiefly affected, although this term may also more generally refer to a wider group of motor neuron diseases.

ALS is characterized by the degeneration of motor cortex, brainstem and/or motor neurons associated with the spinal cord, resulting in muscle weakness and loss of voluntary muscle control. Progressive paralysis ensues, and respiratory failure is the usual cause of death. *Amyotrophic* refers to the lack (*a-*) of muscle (*-myo-*) nourishment (*-trophic*), resulting in wasting of the fibers; *Lateral* refers to the lateral corticospinal tract of affected neurons between the brain and spinal cord; *Sclerosis* is the resultant hardening of the tissue. The incidence of ALS globally ranges from 0.3 to 2.4 cases per 100,000 (Sathasivam 2010). Approximately 95% of ALS cases are random or sporadic (SALS), whereas 5 or more percent are inherited (familial ALS, FALS), with a subset of these arising from known genetic determinants.

Despite the initial description of the disorder about 150 years ago, and significant progress in the understanding of its pathology, ALS remains an ill-defined terminal disease with few medicinal options and an average duration of only a few years. Nonetheless, new developments in ALS research are slowly emerging in diagnostics, in elucidating molecular mechanisms behind the disease, and in generating treatments. Improved technologies and recent research insights, when coupled with meaningful collaborations between scientists and clinicians hold promise for exciting progress. Thus, we discuss here the current understanding of ALS in terms of its clinical presentation, and its molecular and cellular basis. In particular, we highlight new insights into the genetics of the inherited disease, with a focus on the mutant gene products Cu,Zn-superoxide dismutase (Cu,ZnSOD), Fused in Sarcoma/Translated in Lipsarcoma (FUS/TLS) and the Tar-DNA binding protein 43 (TDP-43). The standard care regimen will also be described, along with a focus on novel therapeutic strategies and developments for improving the outlook for patients with this terminal disease.

2. Clinical phenotype

The initial onset of ALS (both FALS and SALS) typically begins with one of several patterns. Seventy five percent of patients have "spinal onset," affecting the limbs (Kiernan et al. 2011). Within this group a "cervical" subset will have muscle weakness in the upper limbs, while symptoms of the "lumbar" subset will arise in the lower limbs. In ALS, affected cells include the upper motor neurons (UMN) in the motor cortex and/or lower motor neurons (LMN) in the brainstem and spinal cord. Presentation of pure UMN symptoms, sometimes referred to as primary lateral sclerosis (PLS), includes decelerated speech, weakness and spasticity, hyperreflexia, pseudobulbar affect (inappropriate emotionality including bursts of crying or laughing). Presentation of pure LMN symptoms, known as progressive muscular atrophy (PMA), includes severe weakness and hyperreflexia, in addition to loss of muscle tone, muscle atrophy, cramps and twitching (termed fasciculations) (Sathasivam 2010; Lomen-Hoerth 2008). A combination of UMN and LMN symptoms may also occur. Onset is usually asymmetrical, although progressive wasting and spreading will most likely ensue (Swash 1998).

Fewer patients have "bulbar onset" ALS, which targets muscles of the face and neck; this form is more common in women and the elderly (Forbes, Colville, and Swingler 2004; McCombe and Henderson 2010) and has a worse prognosis. Symptoms of the UMN-based bulbar variant (pseudobulbar palsy) include emotional responses (as mentioned above), slurred speech (dysarthria), excessive yawning and jerking of the jaw (Wicks 2007; Kuhnlein et al. 2008). The LMN-based affliction (bulbar palsy) manifests as tongue fasciculation resulting in dysarthria, drooling, difficulties in swallowing (dysphagia) and wasting of the tongue (Kuhnlein et al. 2008). Several rare, additional phenotypes exist, including a respiratory onset form, which shares the poorest prognosis with the bulbar onset form (Chio et al. 2011).

The characteristic clinical course of ALS is a progressive loss of voluntary movement, with symptoms spreading to more distant locations (Haverkamp, Appel, and Appel 1995), and the end result being paralysis and death from respiratory failure. Treatment with a ventilator may assist breathing and improve the quality of life (Radunovic et al. 2009). However, eventually the patient may enter a "locked-in" state, where communication is only possibly with the help of an electronic device, and ultimately, even oculomotor function may be impaired (Sharma et al. 2011). In addition to facial, limb and behavioral impairments, frontotemporal dementia (FTD) occurs in a subset of ALS patients (Murphy, Henry, and Lomen-Hoerth 2007), with negative implications for treatment and survival (Olney et al. 2005). Frontotemporal dementia (FTD) patients can also display ALS-like symptoms, suggesting that some aspects of these two diseases may overlap (Ferrari et al. 2011). Unfortunately, treatment of ALS is mostly palliative; the sole approved drug, riluzole (as discussed in section 4), extends life for only a few months (Miller et al. 2007). Typically, half of diagnosed ALS patients will succumb to the disease within about 3 years, 20-25% within 5 years and a small minority can survive 10 years and beyond (Talbot 2009; Testa et al. 2004; Forsgren et al. 1983). Post-mortem staining of the degenerating tissues in motor neurons of the motor cortex, brainstem and spinal cord with eosin and hematoxylin may reveal Bunina bodies and/or ubiquitin-positive-inclusions of the skein-like or hyaline form (most commonly the Lewy body-like variety), among others (Leigh et al. 1991). Thus, the underlying multi-pathway cellular dyshomeostasis leading to the complicated, heterogeneous clinical phenotypes associated with ALS and its variants so far remains mysterious and is under intense investigation.

The distinction between familial and sporadic cases of ALS is not always clear-cut, due to incomplete genetic penetrance, complicating environmental factors and diagnostic difficulties. FALS has been attributed to approximately 5% of ALS cases (Byrne and Hardiman 2010; Talbot 2010), although higher levels in certain geographical regions have been reported (Haberlandt 1959; Murros and Fogelholm 1983). It has been suggested that even rates for the familial disease as high as 13.5% might be underestimates (Andersen 2006), due to the complicating variable of reduced penetrance in some families, causing miscategorization of some FALS cases as SALS (Williams, Floate, and Leicester 1988). FALS is usually inherited in a Mendelian, autosomal dominant manner (Veltema, Roos, and Bruyn 1990), with autosomal recessive and X-linked modes of inheritance occurring rarely (Donkervoort and Siddique 1993; Andersen et al. 1996). The clinical symptoms of FALS and SALS are generally similar, but may be more homogeneous within individual FALS-afflicted families than between them (Horton, Eldridge, and Brody 1976). The mean age of onset at about 48-52 years for FALS (Mulder et al. 1986; Li, Alberman, and Swash 1988) is earlier than the mean at approximately 56 years for SALS (Li, Alberman, and Swash 1988; Haverkamp, Appel, and Appel 1995) and the survival period is also shorter for FALS than for SALS (Mulder et al. 1986). A small minority of ALS patients exhibit juvenile onset (usually before age 25), which is generally characterized by longer survival (Aggarwal and Shashiraj 2006; Ben Hamida, Hentati, and Ben Hamida 1990). Juvenile-onset ALS can occur in an autosomal dominant form, linked to several known genes (Blair et al. 2000) or in a form that may be recessive or sporadic (Hadano et al. 2001).

The lifetime risk of ALS is about 1 in 400, [in the United Kingdom (Alonso et al. 2009)], yet due to the very short survival rate of about 3 years (Donkervoort and Siddique 1993), the disease prevalence is low, ranging from only 0.8 per 100,000 people (in Mexico) to 8.4 per 100,000 (in Sweden) (Olivares, Esteban, and Alter 1972; Gunnarsson and Palm 1984). The yearly incidence of ALS globally varies only slightly worldwide, from as few as 0.3 diagnoses per 100,000 persons in Hong Kong-China (Fong et al. 1996) to 2.4 cases per 100,000 in Finland (Fong et al. 1996), excepting a few, documented, high-occurrence clusters [e.g. an ALS-Parkinsonism-like disease frequency in Guam of up to 100 times greater than average in the middle of the 20th century (Steele and McGeer 2008)]. More studies of non-Caucasian populations are needed to evaluate ALS rates across all ethnic groups (Cronin, Hardiman, and Traynor 2007). The gender ratio for ALS varies somewhat between studies, and with factors such as age and ethnicity (McCombe and Henderson 2010; Abhinav et al. 2007) but consistently shows an increased risk for males. This variability may be due to regional, environmental or genetic differences among patients or, to a decrease in the skewing of ALS cases toward men over time (Worms 2001). Interestingly, the ratio also tends more toward gender equality in FALS than in SALS (Mulder et al. 1986; Li, Alberman, and Swash 1988).

No diagnostic test for ALS is currently available. The Revised El Escorial criteria (Brooks et al. 2000), developed by the World Federation of Neurology, are a set of findings used in the diagnosis of ALS. They categorize the case as "definite," "probable" or "possible," based on clinical UMN and LMN observations and electrophysiological data. These criteria are commonly used for participation in clinical trials, although they have been suggested to be inappropriate for general clinical practice (Andersen et al. 2005) and not sensitive enough as an early diagnostic tool (Kiernan et al. 2011). Earlier diagnosis is in fact highly associated with a longer survival (Testa et al. 2004; Haverkamp, Appel, and Appel 1995), although the median duration between first symptoms and diagnosis was found to be about a year for many cases (Chio 1999; Spuler et al. 2011). Another measure sometimes used in research or private practice is the revised ALS Functional Rating Scale (ALSFRS-R), a scoring tool to monitor the disease progression of patients (Cedarbaum et al. 1999). These measures and others [e.g. the Awaji criteria, (de Carvalho et al. 2008)] are undoubtedly useful. However, objective laboratory tests (e.g. for ALS-specific blood or cerebrospinal fluid biomarkers) would represent a major stride in diagnosis, and some progress is underway in this area (Turner et al. 2009), though validation is still needed.

Current diagnosis of ALS is typically by process of elimination. The trained clinician will assess the presence of UMN and/or LMN symptoms and any evidence of disease progression, then test to eliminate potentially overlapping syndromes. For FALS, the presence of an affected family member can aid diagnosis, and trigger genetic testing, if appropriate (Andersen 2000). Due to the heterogeneity of presentation (Chio et al. 2011), the exclusion of ALS mimics is a very important part of diagnosis. Conditions with overlapping symptoms may include spinal disease or injury (e.g. compression), enzyme or vitamin deficiency (B-12 etc.), cancers, myopathy, neuropathy, infections such as Lyme or HIV, thyroid problems, myasthenia gravis, Kennedy's disease, Tay-Sachs diseases, lead poisoning and multiple sclerosis, among others (Sathasivam 2010; Lomen-Hoerth 2008; Traynor et al. 2000; Silani et al. 2011). Elimination of these ALS mimics is non-trivial, especially since misdiagnosis is very common (Chio 1999; Traynor et al. 2000). Conversely, false positive diagnosis of ALS (estimated at around 10%) can also have marked impacts on patient prognosis and treatment (Davenport et al. 1996; Ludolph and Knirsch 1999). Magnetic resonance imaging (MRI) is one of the most commonly performed diagnostic tests to image the condition of the brain and neck, to eliminate injury as a cause of symptoms. Electromyography (EMG) and nerve conduction studies are useful for evaluating muscle and nerve status. Blood tests (to determine blood count, erythrocyte sedimentation, specific enzyme abnormalities such as creatine kinase) are also useful (Talbot 2009). Less commonly, CSF tests, psychological tests and muscle biopsies are performed to rule out other conditions. Therefore, diagnosis is made by careful examination of the clinical presentation coupled to evaluation by laboratory tests.

3. Pathophysiology

Despite a multitude of genetic, biochemical, cellular and clinical investigations, current ALS research suggests that there is no definitive single cause for the disease and/or that the cellular pathways involved employ much complexity. Thus, further research is required on all fronts to elucidate the underlying pathophysiological mechanisms. We focus on several key disease-implicated proteins, and discuss advances and controversies in our understanding of how mutations may give rise to the disease. We include our own studies on ALS-linked mutations in Cu,Zn superoxide dismutase (SOD), which account for a very significant proportion of genetically defined FALS cases. We also address other genetic factors and environmental influences that have been implicated in ALS.

3.1 Genetic factors
Many recent significant advances in ALS research result from investigations of genetic lesions and their consequent biological defects leading to the disease. Most of these genetic

abnormalities in ALS alter expressed proteins through missense and nonsense mutations, but some genetic linkages are presently not yet connected to a specific underlying protein defect. ALS cases arising from genetic defects have been further divided into subtypes dependent on gene mapping, linkage analysis and phenotype (Table 1). The more characterized subtypes are referred to as ALS1 through ALS14. We have also included in Table 1 several other genes implicated in ALS susceptibility (Al-Chalabi et al. 1999; He and Hays 2004; Munch et al. 2005; Munch et al. 2004). Below, we describe the distribution of >130 distinct mutations in ALS1 (Cu,ZnSOD) within the protein structure, and provide current hypotheses for how this multitude of distinct substitutions affect Cu,ZnSOD structure and function, leading to an ALS phenotype. We also focus on proteins involved in predominately sporadic ALS cases. In particular, we highlight recent results that point to mutation-induced dysfunctions of ALS6 (FUS/TLS) and ALS10 TDP-43 (also involved in certain familial ALS cases), two proteins that are involved in DNA/RNA synthesis and gene regulation, implicating a role for RNA metabolic defects in the disease.

ALS Sub-type	Gene	MIM Gene Number	Locus	Protein	MIM Pheno-type	Age of Onset	Notes
ALS1	SOD1	147450	21q22.1 | 21q22.11	Cu,Zn superoxide dismutase	105400	Adult	AD, AR, Sp
ALS2	ALS2	606352	2q33.1	Alsin	205100	Juvenile	AR
ALS3	-	-	18q21	-	606640	Adult	AD
ALS4	SETX	608465	9q34.13	Senataxin	602433	Juvenile	AD
ALS5	SPG11	-	15q15-q21.1	Spatacsin	602099	Any age	AR
ALS6	FUS	137070	16p11.2	Fused in sarcoma	608030	Adult	AD, AR, Sp
ALS7	-	-	20p13	-	608031	Adult	AD
ALS8	VAPB	605704	20q13.33	VAMP-associated protein B	608627	Adult	AD
ALS9	ANG	105850	14q11.1-q11.2	Angiogenin	611895	Adult	AD, Sp
ALS10	TARDBP	605078	1p36.22	TDP-43	612069	Adult	AD, Sp
ALS11	FIG4	609390	6q21	Phosphoinositide 5-phosphatase	612577	Adult	AD
ALS12	OPTN	602432	10p13	Optineurin	613435	Adult	AD, AR, Sp
ALS13	ATXN2	601517	12q24.1	Ataxin-2	183090	-	Suscept
ALS14	VCP	601023	9p13.3	Valosin-containing protein	613954	Adult	AD
-	DCTN	601143	2p13	Dynactin	105400	-	Suscept
-	NEFH	162230	22q12.2	Heavy neurofilament subunit	105400	-	Suscept
-	PRPH	105400	12q12-q13	Peripherin	105400	-	Suscept
-	UBQLN2	-	Xp11.2	Ubiquilin	-	Any age	X-linked

Table 1. ALS subtypes. ALS phenotypes map to many chromosomal loci, and often to specific proteins implicated in the disease. Data for this table were compiled from the Online Mendelian Inheritance in Man® (MIM) website (http://omim.org) and other sources (Pasinelli and Brown 2006; Ticozzi et al. 2011; Boillee, Vande Velde, and Cleveland 2006; Deng et al. 2011) MIM gene and phenotype numbers are included for reference. Abbreviations in Notes column: AD, autosomal dominant; AR, autosomal recessive; Sp, sporadic; Suscept, aids susceptibility to ALS; X-linked, Chromosome X linkage

3.1.1 Cu,Zn superoxide dismutase

Cu,ZnSOD was first isolated from bovine erythrocytes in the late 1930s (Mann and Keilin 1938). The protein was then termed hemocuprein for its copper content, apparent from the blue color of the crystalline protein. In the 1950s, Cu,ZnSOD was purified from brain (Porter and Folch 1957), where it accounts for approximately 1% of neuronal cytosolic protein (Siddique and Deng 1996). McCord and Fridovich biochemically characterized the protein in 1969, and discovered that it catalyzed the dismutation of superoxide radicals to hydrogen peroxide and oxygen (McCord and Fridovich 1969). Reactive oxygen species, such as superoxide, were subsequently linked to aging and to many diseases. This cytosolic protein was discovered to be unusually stable, surviving organic extraction in the original purifications (McCord and Fridovich 1969) and maintaining enzymatic activity under harsh conditions, such as denaturants and heat (Forman and Fridovich 1973; Malinowski and Fridovich 1979; Hallewell et al. 1991). Our labs routinely use heat denaturation of host proteins when purifying Cu,ZnSOD from heterologous expression systems (Shin et al. 2009). This unusual enzymatic stability could be involved ALS etiology.

Members of our groups have analyzed the biochemical, biophysical and structural properties of wild-type and ALS-linked mutant Cu,ZnSOD proteins. The first Cu,ZnSOD X-ray crystal structure (Tainer et al. 1982; Tainer et al. 1983), revealing the fold and structure-based mechanism of catalysis, was from the bovine enzyme and was later followed by our crystal structure of human Cu,ZnSOD (Figure 1) (Parge, Hallewell, and Tainer 1992).

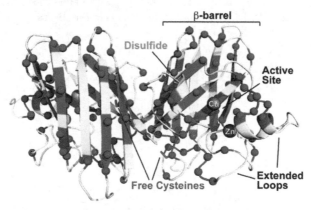

Fig. 1. Human Cu,ZnSOD crystal structure (PDB ID 1PU0) and known ALS mutation sites. Cu,ZnSOD exists as a homodimer and each subunit consists of a single Greek-key motif barrel-like domain, flanked by extended loops that form the active site cleft and house catalytic Cu and Zn ions (large labeled spheres). The smaller red spheres denote Cα ALS mutation site positions mapped onto this cartoon representation of the protein. The conserved disulfide bond (green) in each subunit conveys stability, while free cysteine residues (magenta) are implicated in irreversible unfolding

Our latest published structures of Cu,ZnSOD (Shin et al. 2009) were derived from the eukaryotic thermophile *Alvinella pompejana*, a deep-sea thermal vent worm that we and others discovered contains particularly stable proteins (Burjanadze 2000; Henscheid et al. 2005; Kashiwagi et al. 2010; Piccino et al. 2004). *Alvinella pompejana* Cu,ZnSOD allowed us to obtain both the first sub-angstrom resolution crystal structure of Cu,ZnSOD, and a co-crystal structure with the H_2O_2 product. These structures revealed that the copper ion likely moves within the active site during catalysis (Shin et al. 2009). Structural and computational analyses showed that electrostatic guidance (Getzoff et al. 1992; Getzoff et al. 1983; Perry et al. 2010) aids catalysis, allowing Cu,ZnSOD to be one of the fastest enzymes known.

Our initial structural studies on human Cu,ZnSOD were conducted prior to the discovery that ALS was correlated with mutations in Cu,ZnSOD (Deng et al. 1993; Rosen 1993). Greater than 130 Cu,ZnSOD mutations, occuring at ~70 of the 153 amino acids that comprise a single subunit of human Cu,ZnSOD (Figure 1), are now implicated in causing ALS; the vast majority of these are autosomal dominant in inheritance. These Cu,ZnSOD associated ALS mutations also constitute the majority of ALS cases that have been genetically defined, approximately 20% of FALS cases and ~1-3% of SALS cases. Mapping of the ALS mutations onto the human Cu,ZnSOD structure prompted our suggestion of a 'framework destabilization' hypothesis (Deng et al. 1993). This destabilization hypothesis suggests that ALS SOD mutations promote local unfolding events in Cu,ZnSOD that can drive self-aggregation and potentially aberrant interactions with other proteins, dysregulating the normal cellular functions of this highly abundant protein in neuronal cells.

Alternative hypotheses include a gain of function mechanism, for example a change of SOD chemistry so that the enzyme performs other reactions (such as peroxidation and increased tyrosine nitration), or exhibits an increase or decrease in catalytic activity (Beckman et al. 1993; Brown 1995; Crow et al. 1997; Rosen 1993; Wiedau-Pazos et al. 1996; Wong and Borchelt 1995; Zhang et al. 2002). However, support for these other hypotheses is unclear. Certain mutations are known to make a more active enzyme, while others produce a less active protein, and some have with relatively unchanged chemistry. Some mutations (such as H46R and H48Q) remove copper binding, rendering the protein non-catalytic, thus suggesting that gain of enzymatic function or increased activity is unlikely. Transgenic mice harboring SOD1 mutations present ALS-like symptoms (Gurney et al. 1994), but transgenic SOD1 knockout mice do not (Reaume et al. 1996). This indicates that a loss of normal catalytic activity or a gain of abnormal activity may not be important in propagating ALS. Also, activity-altering mutations would be expected to be focused in and around the active site, rather than occurring across the entire Cu,ZnSOD fold.

Protein aggregates are observed within neural cells from Alzheimer's, Huntington's and Parkinson's individuals (Dobson 2001; Soto 2001; Wanker 2000). Likewise, proteinaceous aggregates were discovered in neurons of ALS patients (Leigh et al. 1991). We observed *in vitro* that purified FALS A4V and H43R mutants form fibrous aggregates, and that two free cysteines within the protein are not required for this aggregation. These two ALS mutants bound Congo Red and Thioflavin T dyes that typically bind amyloid-like β-sheet structures (Figure 2) (DiDonato et al. 2003). Notably, the kinetics of forming aggregates and the binding affinity for dyes were more enhanced for the more clinically aggressive mutant A4V mutant. In cellular inclusions, aggregates were found to be immunoreactive for Cu,ZnSOD, and did not dissociate readily in the presence of detergents or reductants (Bruijn et al. 1998; Durham et al. 1997). Also, the detection of Cu,ZnSOD-containing inclusions often precedes ALS-like symptoms, and the aggregates are similar to Lewy bodies found in Parkinson's disease (Johnston et al. 2000; Kato et al. 2001).

ALS mutant SODs interact and/or co-precipitate with additional proteins to form the inclusions observed in cells from ALS patients; these inclusions resemble those characteristic of other neurodegenerative disease. These associated proteins include 1) proteins involved in stress response pathways, namely Derlin-1 (Nishitoh et al. 2008) and Rac1 (Harraz et al. 2008), 2) chromogramin proteins associated with neurosectretory vesicles (Urushitani et al. 2006), 3) the cytosolic chaperone Hsc70 (Wang et al. 2009), 4) the SOD copper chaperone (Kato et al. 2001), and 5) the dynein complex heavy chain, which is used in neural retrograde transport (Kieran et al. 2005; Zhang et al. 2007). Thus, local destabilizing SOD1 mutations, leading to interactions and/or co-precipitation of these proteins within aggregates, may impact normal cellular functions. It was also recently discovered that neural membrane fluidity was altered in transgenic ALS mice that harbor a FALS SOD mutation (Miana-Mena et al. 2011). The authors hypothesize that membranes may be altered through lipid peroxidation, yet misfolded SODs may also play a role by interacting with membranes. Other hypotheses for the involvement of mutant SOD in ALS include disruption of the ubiquitin and proteosome system, altering mitochondrial function, playing a role in glutamatergic neurotransmission leading to excitotoxicity, and interference with axonal transport systems (Bastos et al. 2011; Kiernan et al. 2011; Ticozzi et al. 2011). Thus, we suggest that the framework destabilization hypothesis, unlike other suggested hypotheses, provides a unified mechanism for ALS mutant phenotype: This hypothesis encompasses the widespread distribution of ALS mutation sites within the protein, and is further supported by the observed *in vitro* aggregation results and the cellular analyses that are also in keeping with other aggregation-prone neurodegenerative diseases.

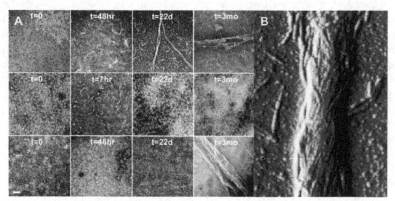

Fig. 2. FALS SOD mutants promote the formation of filamentous aggregates. (A) Electron micrographs of H43R and A4V fibers reveals diameters of 2-15 nm implying a loss of dimer assembly specificity. Samples of H43R (top row), A4V (middle row) and wild-type (bottom row), all in the C6A, C111S SOD background lacking free Cys, were subjected to conditions designed to perturb the SOD fold. The scale bar = 40 nm. (B) Atomic force micrograph (phase mode) of large H43R bundles. Adapted from (DiDonato et al. 2003)

3.1.2 FUS/TLS

The *FUS* gene, representing the ALS6 subtype of amyotrophic lateral sclerosis, encodes the "fused in sarcoma" protein, initially characterized as one of the fusion proteins generated by carcinogenic oncogenes (Crozat et al. 1993; Rabbitts et al. 1993). The alternative name TLS stands for "translocation in liposarcoma", and the gene product is often referred to as FUS/TLS, as we will do for the remainder of this chapter. FUS/TLS is a 526 amino acid protein of the TET family (which stands for Translocated in liposarcoma/Ewing's sarcoma/TATA-binding protein-associated factor 15). FUS/TLS binds both DNA and RNA, and like Cu,ZnSOD, is ubiquitously expressed. The protein is divided into distinct motifs and regions, which are responsible for different functions [see Figure 3 and the following reviews (Dormann and Haass 2011; Lagier-Tourenne and Cleveland 2009; Perry, Shin, and Tainer 2010)]. FUS/TLS plays a role in transcription activities within the cell via interactions with a variety of proteins, including transcription factors and hormone receptors (Cassiday and Maher 2002; Lagier-Tourenne and Cleveland 2009) (Cassiday and Maher 2002; Lagier-Tourenne and Cleveland 2009; Law, Cann, and Hicks 2006). FUS/TLS may also function in DNA damage responses by binding to non-coding RNA elements transcribed by the 5' regulatory region of the cell-cycle kinase cyclin D1 gene. This binding event recruits FUS/TLS to interact with and inhibit CREB-binding protein and p300 histone acetelytransferase, further repressing cyclin D1-mediated transcription (Perry, Shin, and Tainer 2010). FUS/TLS has also been implicated in RNA processing, such as splicing, transport and maturation (Lagier-Tourenne and Cleveland 2009). In neurons, FUS/TLS is transported to dendritic spines upon activation of glutamate receptor mGluR5 (Fujii et al. 2005).

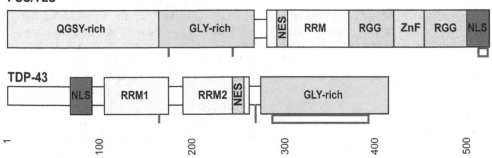

Fig. 3. Schematic diagrams of the FUS/TLS and TDP-43 proteins. Both proteins contain similar motifs, bind DNA and RNA, and are involved in both ALS and FTD. (Top) FUS/TLS contains QGSY- and Gly-rich regions, an RNA recognition motif (RRM) with a nuclear export signal (NES), a pair of RGG-motifs flanking a Zinc-finger (ZnF), and a nuclear localization signal (NLS). (Bottom) The TDP-43 protein has its NLS at the N-terminus, two RRM motifs with the latter containing an NES, and a C-terminal Gly-rich region. Red bars indicate ALS mutation sites, and red boxes indicate ALS hotspots that contain multiple ALS mutation sites. Numbers below indicate amino acid positions

The *FUS* gene was implicated in ALS after the discovery that a locus within chromosome 16 was linked to both autosomal dominant (Ticozzi et al. 2011; Vance et al. 2009) and recessive manifestations of the disease (Kwiatkowski et al. 2009). FUS mutations have since been identified in patients with sporadic ALS, and according to recent reviews [see (Kiernan et al. 2011; Ticozzi et al. 2011)], *FUS* mutants are estimated to account for approximately 4-5% of FALS and 1% of SALS cases. Interestingly, mutations in FUS/TLS are also involved in FTD [see (Mackenzie, Rademakers, and Neumann 2010)]. The disease-promoting mechanisms in mutant *FUS*-mediated ALS are not understood, but aggregate formation has been observed (Deng et al. 2010; Vance et al. 2009; Dormann and Haass 2011). The FUS/TLS mutations tend to cluster mainly at the C-terminal glycine-rich region and NLS (Dormann and Haass 2011; Lagier-Tourenne and Cleveland 2009; Perry, Shin, and Tainer 2010), instead of throughout the entire structure as observed in Cu,ZnSOD. Similar to Cu,ZnSOD mutant pathology is the observation that inclusions containing FUS/TLS are found within the cytosol within diseased neural cells (Dormann et al. 2010). Interestingly, NLS mutations that yield a greater concentration of FUS/TLS within the cytosol correlate with a more rapid onset and aggressiveness of the disease. Also, some of the most severe NLS mutations cause substitutions in amino acids required for an interaction with transportin, a nuclear import receptor (Dormann et al. 2010). Mutant cytosolic FUS/TLS may also be incorporated into stress granules that may serve as an inclusion precursor (Dormann and Haass 2011)).

Additionally, FUS/TLS has been predicted to contain prion-like regions within its amino-acid sequence, which may also contribute to the formation of aggregates (Udan and Baloh 2011).

3.1.3 TDP-43

TDP-43, named for binding to TAR DNA of the human immunodeficiency type 1 virus, is also a DNA and RNA binding protein like FUS/TLS. TDP-43 is encoded by the *TARDBP* gene, and is classified as the ALS10 subtype. TDP-43 is composed of 414 residues, and includes functional motifs shared with FUS/TLS (Figure 3). Functions for TDP-43 include transcriptional regulator (Abhyankar, Urekar, and Reddi 2007; Ayala, Misteli, and Baralle 2008), and TDP-43 was also implicated in binding UG-repeat sequences, resulting in pathogenic consequences that include cystic fibrosis (Mantovani et al. 2007). Like FUS/TLS, TDP-43 has been implicated in both ALS and FTD pathology (Arai et al. 2006; Mackenzie, Rademakers, and Neumann 2010; Dormann and Haass 2011; Perry, Shin, and Tainer 2010). Presently, over 35 mutations in TDP-43 have been implicated in these two diseases, including ~0.5-2% of sporadic ALS cases (Arai et al. 2006) and ~3-5% of autosomal dominant FALS cases (Lagier-Tourenne and Cleveland 2009; Ticozzi et al. 2011). TDP-43 aggregates are also found within diseased neural cells, where the protein is found to be highly ubiquinated and phosphorylated, as well as being truncated (Arai et al. 2006; Neumann et al. 2006). These aggregates are generally localized to the cytoplasm, while nuclear levels of TDP-43 are significantly diminished. Interestingly, analysis of the aggregates suggests that these deposits are not composed of amyloid-like structures (Kwong et al. 2008). Cu,ZnSOD is not found within the TDP-43 or the FUS/TLS aggregates; however, a recent report states that mutant Cu,ZnSOD interacts with TDP-43 (Higashi et al. 2010), and was shown to co-immunoprecipitate with FUS/TLS for a function in stabilizing histone deactylase 6 (HDAC6) mRNA (Kim et al. 2010). ALS mutations in TDP-43 appear to enhance this interaction with FUS/TLS (Ling et al. 2010). Therefore, additional research is required to clearly define these provisional links between TDP-43, FUS/TLS and/or Cu,ZnSOD in ALS pathology.

The majority of mutations found within TDP-43 ALS patients are missense mutations toward the C-terminal end of the protein, beginning at the glycine-rich segment. Recent research has identified the possibility that like FUS/TLS, TDP-43 also contains a prion-like element at its C-terminus. This region contains Gln and Asn residues similar to yeast Q/N prion domains. This represents yet another structural element that may initiate the formation of aggregates within ALS10 type cells. Currently, research on the function of TDP-43 and its roles in various pathologies including ALS and FTD is on the rise. Changes in TDP-43 structure and stability behind its ALS pathology may also influence the expression and activities of various cellular machinery within neural cells [see detailed reviews: (Dormann and Haass 2011; Lagier-Tourenne and Cleveland 2009; Lagier-Tourenne, Polymenidou, and Cleveland 2010; Perry, Shin, and Tainer 2010; Swarup et al. 2011)].

3.1.4 Other ALS subtypes

Research is being initiated on the defective genes for the other, more rare, ALS subtypes [see more detailed reviews (Boillee, Vande Velde, and Cleveland 2006; Kiernan et al. 2011; Pasinelli and Brown 2006; Strong et al. 2007; Ticozzi et al. 2011) for further information on these lesser-characterized ALS subtypes]. Many proteins encoded by these ALS subtype genes share the ability to modulate gene expression and/or RNA metabolism; this includes the *ANG* (ALS9) and *SETX* (ALS4) gene products, along with those of *FUS/TLS, TDP-43* and *SOD1* (Strong 2010). Also, the VAPB (ALS8) mutant shares the ability to form aggregates (Suzuki et al. 2009). Notably, the native alsin protein encoded by the *ALS2* gene has been observed to offer protection against Cu,ZnSOD mutational effects in certain cells (Hadano et al. 2007). Many mutations in *ALS2* are nonsense mutations that lead to truncations in the gene product, which can destabilize the protein, resulting in proteasomal degradation (Yamanaka et al. 2003). Another study suggests that alsin loss may cause neurons to be more vulnerable to excitotoxicity, via glutamate receptors (Lai et al. 2006). Co-localization has not yet been observed between Cu,ZnSOD and FUS/TLS or TDP-43. However, optineurin, which is encoded by *OPTN* and represents ALS12, does appear to colocalize with Cu,ZnSOD, FUS/TLS and TDP-43 [see (Ito et al. 2011)], and the interaction of optineruin with at least with the former two, appears to be mutually exclusive. A comprehensive study of a five generation family with ALS lead to the discovery that mutations in UBQLN2, which encodes the ubiquitin-like protein ubiquilin 2, cause dominant X-linked juvenile and adult-onset ALS and ALS/dementia (Deng et al. 2011). Also, excitingly, two very recent research findings have identified the largely uncharacterized locus 9p21 *C9ORF72* gene product to be linked to a significant proportion of dominant cases of ALS/FTD (Renton et al, 2011; DeJesus-Hernandez et al. 2011) Thus, it currently appears that genetic lesions may lead to ALS by different pathways, and continued research will be needed to establish whether there are one, several or many more general mechanistic themes that lead to the ALS phenotypes.

3.2 Other factors
Non-genetic risk factors for ALS, including environmental factors and physical injury, are being actively pursued. Although the effects of these risks of ALS are difficult to deconvolute (e.g. the prevalence of ALS in athletes), the involvement of these factors may enhance underlying, genetic predispositions to the disease, or may indeed have a direct link to ALS.

3.2.1 Diet/Lifestyle
The role of diet in ALS was assessed when considerably higher prevalence levels of ALS were noted in certain Western Pacific populations (50-100-fold). Non-genetic causes for these ALS cases have been suggested to be due to high levels of β-methyl-amino-L-alanine. This non-standard amino acid is highly concentrated in a certain seed that is consumed by animals that provide food for the inhabitants of Guam (Bastos et al. 2011; Ince and Codd 2005). A recent study has highlighted adverse effects from high levels of branched-chain amino acids (BCAAs) on the ion channels of mice. The researchers discovered an increased sodium current within motor neurons, resembling that observed in the transgenic Cu,ZnSOD G93A mouse model for ALS. The increased sodium current promotes hyperexcitability of the cells, which may lead to excitotoxicity, subsequent calcium influx and apoptosis (Carunchio et al. 2010; Manuel and Heckman 2011). BCAAs are commonly used as a supplement by athletes, and therefore might account for the increased incidence of ALS seen in Italian soccer (Chio et al. 2005) and American football (Abel 2007) players.

Smoking was proposed as another potential risk factor for ALS (Kamel et al. 1999), and continues to provoke interest (Armon 2009). Several studies reported no ill effects of smoking on ALS (Schmidt et al. 2010) (Okamoto et al. 2009), others implicated a gender-specific effect (Alonso et al. 2010), and a recent study of 832 ALS patients suggested smoking increased ALS incidence by ~1.4 fold (Wang et al. 2011).

3.2.2 Injury and trauma

Neuronal injury may result in excessive stimulation by α-amino-hydroxy-5-methylisoxasole-4 propionic acid (AMPA), glutamate or kainite, leading to excitotoxcity and downstream apoptosis (Perry, Shin, and Tainer 2010; Beal 1992). Thus, head trauma may be linked to the increased incidence of ALS observed in Italian soccer players, American football players, and military personnel, all of whom more commonly have head injuries (Horner et al. 2008; Miranda et al. 2008). Other forms of trauma, such as electrical shock, have also been correlated to ALS [for a broader list and additional details, see the review by (Bastos et al. 2011)].

3.2.3 Environmental toxins

Exposure to environmental toxins is actively investigated as a potential contributing factor to ALS. Several metals have been implicated in increased risk for ALS after occupational exposure to lead, residency in areas with high levels of selenium, and accidental contact with mercury (Bastos et al. 2011). Inhabitants of Guam who exhibit ALS-like symptoms have been exposed to potentially high levels of aluminum (Wicklund 2005). More complex molecules implicated in increased risk of ALS include formaldehyde, pesticides that are suspected to cause ALS in Italian soccer players, and chemical agents to which military personnel have been subjected. Yet, a causative effect between ALS and such factors is difficult to establish. One reason for this is the relatively small sample size in some of these studies. A second reason is the difficulty in deconvoluting which specific factor or combination of factors contributed to the disease, as in the case for the soccer players. Third, some of the ALS patients within the studies may have had an undetected genetic defect, and the additional environmental factor accelerated the course of the disease.

4. Therapeutic progress

The only approved treatment for ALS is riluzole, which functions to reduce glutamate-induced excitotoxicity in ALS individuals, and is licensed by Sanofi-Aventis with the brand name Rilutek. Riluzole only modestly slows the progression of ALS, with a 9% gain in the probability of surviving one year, and a small beneficial effect for limb function, but not muscle strength (Miller et al. 2007). Several other drugs that gave positive results in animal models failed in human trials. However, additional clinical trials now underway are aimed at producing new ALS therapies by using varied strategic approaches that go beyond the modulation of glutamate levels [reviewed in (Zoccolella, Santamato, and Lamberti 2009)(see http://clinicaltrials.gov)]. Exciting progress in this regard includes the commencement of a phase I clinical trial by Neuralstem that aims to establish the safety and feasibility of using stem cells to treat ALS, by injecting these cells directly into the spinal cord (see http://neurology.emory.edu/ALS/Stem%20Cell.html). This development is based on initial studies showing that human fetal neuronal stem cells could delay the onset and progression in a rat model of ALS (Xu et al. 2006).

The Northeast ALS consortium (NEALS), a non-profit consortium bringing together scientific and clinical investigators from now 97 institutions across in the United States, Puerto Rico, Canada and Ireland, forms a central component of many of the clinical trials (http://www.alsconsortium.org). For example, as part of NEALS, a stage III trial of ceftriaxone, which has been recently observed to modulate glutamate uptake, is being conducted by Massachusetts General Hospital with the National Institute of Neurological

Disorders and Stroke. Ceftriaxone is a semi-synthetic cephalosporin antibiotic, originally approved by the FDA for treating bacterial infections. Combination therapies are also being analyzed, including a phase II a trial by Phoenix Neurological Associates LTD of riluzole in conjunction with tretionin and pioglitazone. Tretinoin, used to treat acute promyelocytic leukemia (Sanz 2006), is a retinoic acid derivative, and as such may have neuroprotective properties (Choi et al. 2009; Lee et al. 2009). The oral anti-diabetic pioglitazone has anti-inflammatory properties that showed positive responses in an ALS mouse model (Schutz et al. 2005). Tamoxifen is currently in stage II clinical trials for treating ALS, based on an observation by clinicians that an ALS patient also receiving tamoxifen for breast cancer had an unusually mild form of the disease (see http://www.alsa.org/research/clinical-trials/trial-tamoxifen.html). Tamoxifen may also help protect cells from glutamate toxicity (Maenpaa et al. 2002) in addition to inhibiting protein kinase C mediated spinal inflammation and prolonging life expectancy in a mouse model of ALS (Traynor et al. 2006; Zoccolella, Santamato, and Lamberti 2009).

Several other compounds with neuroprotective activities are undergoing clinical trials. These include rasagiline, which was reported to have neuroprotective properties in an ALS mouse model (Waibel et al. 2004). Rasagiline is currently used as a therapy for Parkinson's disease, functioning as a selective inhibitor of monoamine oxidase B, and is now under phase II clinical trials for ALS treatment by the University of Kansas. Neuraltus Pharmaceuticals is targeting an anti-inflammatory response through transforming macrophage cells from a neurotoxic to a protective state, with the compound 'NP001' that is now in phase II clinical trials (see http://www.neuraltus.com). Biogen Idec and Knopp Biosciences have an interesting small molecule therapeutic, dexpramipexole, which also has a neuroprotective function, through increasing the efficiency of mitochondria in neurons (Gribkoff and Bozik 2008). Dexpramipexole is the R(+) enantiomer of an already licensed compound, pramipexole, which is used for the treatment of both Parkinson's disease and restless legs syndrome. Pramipexole functions as a non-ergot dopaminergic autoreceptor antagonist, but has dose-limiting side effects that include orthostatic hypotension and hallucination, due its dopaminergic receptor activity. Dempramipexole, on the other hand, has a much lower affinity for dopaminergic receptors, and in phase II trials was well tolerated at levels considerably higher than the maximum daily dose of pramipexole (Bozik et al. 2011). Dexpramipexole also showed positive trends in slowing functional decline and improving survivability in phase II, and is now undergoing a multi-national phase III study.

Approaches specifically targeting Cu,ZnSOD include arimoclomol, a compound developed by CytRx corporation, that activates chaperones to perturb protein aggregation. Arimoclomol was observed to extend life in an ALS mutant Cu,ZnSOD mouse model (indirectly supporting the framework destabilization model for Cu,ZnSOD mutations), and is currently at the Phase II/III stage (Kalmar et al. 2008). Cornell University and the Muscular Dystrophy Association are studying pyrimethamine, an anti-malarial drug shown in one study to substantially reduce Cu,ZnSOD levels in mice (Lange 2008), although a separate study at the University of Massachusetts Medical School did not observe this pyrimethamine effect in either cells or animal models of disease (Wright et al. 2010). Moving away from small molecule based therapies, Isis Pharmaceuticals is taking an siRNA approach to combat FALS mutant Cu,ZnSOD, with Isis-SOD1RX entering into phase I clinical trials. Isis-SOD1RX is antisense oligonucleotide to SOD1 that is infused directly into the cerebral spinal fluid, due to an inability to pass the blood brain barrier. This siRNA was shown to reduce both Cu,ZnSOD protein and mRNA levels throughout the brain and spinal cord in animal models (Smith et al. 2006).

Other recent therapeutic approaches target muscle deficiencies in ALS. Cytokinetics developed 'CK-2107357', an activator of the fast skeletal muscle troponin complex, increasing cellular sensitivity to calcium, which results in an increase in skeletal muscle force and a decrease in the time to muscle fatigue. In phase IIa trials, CK-2107357 showed evidence of clinical effect, as well as being suitably safe and tolerated. Acceleron Pharma is developing ACE-031, a protein therapeutic that builds muscle and increases strength by inhibiting signaling through the activin type IIb cell surface receptor (Cadena et al. 2010). ACE-031 increased skeletal muscle mass and strength in disease models of amyotrophic lateral sclerosis (ALS), muscular dystrophy, glucocorticoid-induced muscle loss and age-related muscle loss (sarcopenia). An extended phase II clinical trial in Canada for Duchenne Muscular Dystrophy was recently terminated, and is pending further analysis of safety data.

5. Future research

Evidently, much work remains on all fronts from uncovering disease mechanisms to developing new therapies for ALS. The very recent publication determining that mutations in ubiquilin 2 are a cause of dominantly inherited X-linked ALS and ALS/dementia has opened up a new area of ALS research (Deng et al. 2011). Ubiquilin 2 functions as part of the protein degradation pathway, revealing pathological roles for this pathway in ALS and suggesting new therapeutic opportunities for treating ALS, since ubiquilin 2 was found in skein-like inclusions of a wide variety of ALS cases (Deng et al. 2011). Another area of important focus is improvement of animal models for ALS, as the utility of these has come into question (Benatar 2007; Bedlack, Traynor, and Cudkowicz 2007). One problem is that treatment in these animal models typical begins before the onset of disease symptoms, whereas this is not possible for ALS individuals, due to a lack of understanding of causative factors and potential differences in pathogenic mechanisms between SALS and FALS. Notably, when guidelines on improving animal study criteria were implemented, therapeutic benefits from a host of compounds that included ceftiaxone and even riluzole were no longer observed (Scott et al. 2008), further highlighting issues with the use and understanding of current models. Improved experimental ALS models will also be of use to further our understanding of the causative factors of SALS, such as potentially toxic effects of smoking on motor neurons. Future therapeutic studies also need to take into consideration overcoming problems within clinical trials, such as the small sample sizes and short durations of study, making assessment of milder effects that are expected with many of the therapeutics more challenging.

Once key advance that is likely to influence the future direction of research is the generation of ALS stem cells from adult skin cells from an individual with ALS (Dimos et al. 2008). Now, stem cells from different patients can be isolated and used to grow different motor neuron cell lines for more detailed analyses, or potentially for high-throughput screening.

6. Conclusions

There has been some exciting progress in our understanding of ALS, including recent developments in the genetics and molecular mechanisms behind this most common form of motor neuron disease. New discoveries include the identification of two ALS-linked proteins, FUS/TLS and TDP-43, which are involved in DNA/RNA metabolism. However, we still have to clearly establish whether aggregation or loss of the wild-type functions of either of these two proteins is the underlying cause of the disease phenotype. Studies behind the pathogenicity of Cu,ZnSOD mutations in ALS are also continuing, with the recent data supporting an initial concept that mutation-induced structural instability of the protein drives aggregation events, which ultimately prove toxic to the neuronal cell. Encouragingly, several distinct therapeutic strategies are in play aiming to at least delay the progression of the disease. These strategies range from small molecule inhibitors, some of which are in later stages of clinical trials, to siRNA and stem cell based approaches. We hope that the rapid pace of research findings and the ongoing clinical trials will shortly produce novel therapies that can help fight against this terrible disease.

7. Acknowledgments

A.J.P. is grateful to the N.S.F. and the Skaggs Institute for Chemical Biology at The Scripps Research Institute for pre-doctoral funding, and E.D.G would like to acknowledge funding from NIH grant GM39345.

8. References

Abel, E. L. 2007. Football increases the risk for Lou Gehrig's disease, amyotrophic lateral sclerosis. *Percept Mot Skills* 104 (3 Pt 2):1251-4.

Abhinav, K., B. Stanton, C. Johnston, J. Hardstaff, R. W. Orrell, R. Howard, J. Clarke, M. Sakel, M. A. Ampong, C. E. Shaw, P. N. Leigh, and A. Al-Chalabi. 2007. Amyotrophic lateral sclerosis in South-East England: a population-based study. The South-East England register for amyotrophic lateral sclerosis (SEALS Registry). *Neuroepidemiology* 29 (1-2):44-8.

Abhyankar, M. M., C. Urekar, and P. P. Reddi. 2007. A novel CpG-free vertebrate insulator silences the testis-specific SP-10 gene in somatic tissues: role for TDP-43 in insulator function. *J Biol Chem* 282 (50):36143-54.

Aggarwal, A., and Shashiraj. 2006. Juvenile amyotrophic lateral sclerosis. *Indian J Pediatr* 73 (3):225-6.

Al-Chalabi, A., P. M. Andersen, P. Nilsson, B. Chioza, J. L. Andersson, C. Russ, C. E. Shaw, J. F. Powell, and P. N. Leigh. 1999. Deletions of the heavy neurofilament subunit tail in amyotrophic lateral sclerosis. *Hum Mol Genet* 8 (2):157-64.

Alonso, A., G. Logroscino, S. S. Jick, and M. A. Hernan. 2009. Incidence and lifetime risk of motor neuron disease in the United Kingdom: a population-based study. *Eur J Neurol* 16 (6):745-51.

Alonso, A., G. Logroscino, S. S. Jick, and M. A. Hernan. 2010. Association of smoking with amyotrophic lateral sclerosis risk and survival in men and women: a prospective study. *BMC Neurol* 10:6.

Andersen, P. M. 2000. Genetic factors in the early diagnosis of ALS. *Amyotroph Lateral Scler Other Motor Neuron Disord* 1 Suppl 1:S31-42.

Andersen, P. M. 2006. Amyotrophic lateral sclerosis associated with mutations in the CuZn superoxide dismutase gene. *Curr Neurol Neurosci Rep* 6 (1):37-46.

Andersen, P. M., G. D. Borasio, R. Dengler, O. Hardiman, K. Kollewe, P. N. Leigh, P. F. Pradat, V. Silani, B. Tomik, and EFNS Task Force Diag Management. 2005. EFNS task force on management of amyotrophic lateral sclerosis: guidelines for diagnosing and clinical care of patients and relatives - An evidence-based review with good practice points. *European Journal of Neurology* 12 (12):921-938.

Andersen, P. M., L. Forsgren, M. Binzer, P. Nilsson, V. Ala-Hurula, M. L. Keranen, L. Bergmark, A. Saarinen, T. Haltia, I. Tarvainen, E. Kinnunen, B. Udd, and S. L. Marklund. 1996. Autosomal recessive adult-onset amyotrophic lateral sclerosis associated with homozygosity for Asp90Ala CuZn-superoxide dismutase mutation. A clinical and genealogical study of 36 patients. *Brain* 119 (Pt 4):1153-72.

Arai, T., M. Hasegawa, H. Akiyama, K. Ikeda, T. Nonaka, H. Mori, D. Mann, K. Tsuchiya, M. Yoshida, Y. Hashizume, and T. Oda. 2006. TDP-43 is a component of ubiquitin-positive tau-negative inclusions in frontotemporal lobar degeneration and amyotrophic lateral sclerosis. *Biochem Biophys Res Commun* 351 (3):602-11.

Armon, C. 2009. Smoking may be considered an established risk factor for sporadic ALS. *Neurology* 73 (20):1693-1698.

Ayala, Y. M., T. Misteli, and F. E. Baralle. 2008. TDP-43 regulates retinoblastoma protein phosphorylation through the repression of cyclin-dependent kinase 6 expression. *Proc Natl Acad Sci U S A* 105 (10):3785-9.

Bastos, A. F., M. Orsini, D. Machado, M. P. Mello, S. Nader, J. G. Silva, A. M. da Silva Catharino, M. R. de Freitas, A. Pereira, L. L. Pessoa, F. R. Sztajnbok, M. A. Leite, O. J. Nascimento, and V. H. Bastos. 2011. Amyotrophic lateral sclerosis: one or multiple causes? *Neurol Int* 3 (1):e4.

Beal, M. F. 1992. Mechanisms of excitotoxicity in neurologic diseases. *FASEB J* 6 (15):3338-44.

Beckman, J. S., M. Carson, C. D. Smith, and W. H. Koppenol. 1993. ALS, SOD and peroxynitrite. *Nature* 364 (6438):584.

Bedlack, R. S., B. J. Traynor, and M. E. Cudkowicz. 2007. Emerging disease-modifying therapies for the treatment of motor neuron disease/amyotropic lateral sclerosis. *Expert Opin Emerg Drugs* 12 (2):229-52.

Ben Hamida, M., F. Hentati, and C. Ben Hamida. 1990. Hereditary motor system diseases (chronic juvenile amyotrophic lateral sclerosis). Conditions combining a bilateral pyramidal syndrome with limb and bulbar amyotrophy. *Brain* 113 (Pt 2):347-63.

Benatar, M. 2007. Lost in translation: treatment trials in the SOD1 mouse and in human ALS. *Neurobiol Dis* 26 (1):1-13.

Blair, I. P., C. L. Bennett, A. Abel, B. A. Rabin, J. W. Griffin, K. H. Fischbeck, D. R. Cornblath, and P. F. Chance. 2000. A gene for autosomal dominant juvenile amyotrophic lateral sclerosis (ALS4) localizes to a 500-kb interval on chromosome 9q34. *Neurogenetics* 3 (1):1-6.

Boillee, S., C. Vande Velde, and D. W. Cleveland. 2006. ALS: a disease of motor neurons and their nonneuronal neighbors. *Neuron* 52 (1):39-59.

Bozik, M. E., J. L. Mather, W. G. Kramer, V. K. Gribkoff, and E. W. Ingersoll. 2011. Safety, Tolerability, and Pharmacokinetics of KNS-760704 (Dexpramipexole) in Healthy Adult Subjects. *J Clin Pharmacol* 51 (8):1177-85.

Brooks, B. R., R. G. Miller, M. Swash, and T. L. Munsat. 2000. El Escorial revisited: revised criteria for the diagnosis of amyotrophic lateral sclerosis. *Amyotroph Lateral Scler Other Motor Neuron Disord* 1 (5):293-9.

Brown, R. H., Jr. 1995. Amyotrophic lateral sclerosis: recent insights from genetics and transgenic mice. *Cell* 80 (5):687-92.

Bruijn, L. I., M. K. Houseweart, S. Kato, K. L. Anderson, S. D. Anderson, E. Ohama, A. G. Reaume, R. W. Scott, and D. W. Cleveland. 1998. Aggregation and motor neuron toxicity of an ALS-linked SOD1 mutant independent from wild-type SOD1. *Science* 281 (5384):1851-4.

Burjanadze, T. V. 2000. New analysis of the phylogenetic change of collagen thermostability. *Biopolymers* 53 (6):523-8.

Byrne, S. C., and O. Hardiman. 2010. Rate of Familial Amyotrophic Lateral Sclerosis - A Systematic Review and Meta-Analysis. *Neurology* 74 (9):A56-A56.

Cadena, S. M., K. N. Tomkinson, T. E. Monnell, M. S. Spaits, R. Kumar, K. W. Underwood, R. S. Pearsall, and J. L. Lachey. 2010. Administration of a soluble activin type IIB receptor promotes skeletal muscle growth independent of fiber type. *J Appl Physiol* 109 (3):635-42.

Carunchio, I., L. Curcio, M. Pieri, F. Pica, S. Caioli, M. T. Viscomi, M. Molinari, N. Canu, G. Bernardi, and C. Zona. 2010. Increased levels of p70S6 phosphorylation in the G93A mouse model of Amyotrophic Lateral Sclerosis and in valine-exposed cortical neurons in culture. *Exp Neurol* 226 (1):218-30.

Cassiday, L. A., and L. J. Maher, 3rd. 2002. Having it both ways: transcription factors that bind DNA and RNA. *Nucleic Acids Res* 30 (19):4118-26.

Cedarbaum, J. M., N. Stambler, E. Malta, C. Fuller, D. Hilt, B. Thurmond, A. Nakanishi, and Bdnf Als Study Grp. 1999. The ALSFRS-R: a revised ALS functional rating scale that incorporates assessments of respiratory function. *Journal of the Neurological Sciences* 169 (1-2):13-21.

Charcot, J.M. 1869. Deux cas d'atrophie musculaire progressive avec lesions de la substance grise et des faisceaux antero-lateraux de la moelle epiniere. *Arch Physiol Neurol Pathol* 2:744-754.

Chio, A. 1999. ISIS Survey: an international study on the diagnostic process and its implications in amyotrophic lateral sclerosis. *J Neurol* 246 Suppl 3:III1-5.

Chio, A., G. Benzi, M. Dossena, R. Mutani, and G. Mora. 2005. Severely increased risk of amyotrophic lateral sclerosis among Italian professional football players. *Brain* 128 (Pt 3):472-6.

Chio, A., A. Calvo, C. Moglia, L. Mazzini, and G. Mora. 2011. Phenotypic heterogeneity of amyotrophic lateral sclerosis: a population based study. *J Neurol Neurosurg Psychiatry* 82 (7):740-6.

Choi, B. K., J. H. Kim, J. S. Jung, Y. S. Lee, M. E. Han, S. Y. Baek, B. S. Kim, J. B. Kim, and S. O. Oh. 2009. Reduction of ischemia-induced cerebral injury by all-trans-retinoic acid. *Exp Brain Res* 193 (4):581-9.

Cronin, S., O. Hardiman, and B. J. Traynor. 2007. Ethnic variation in the incidence of ALS: a systematic review. *Neurology* 68 (13):1002-7.

Crow, J. P., Y. Z. Ye, M. Strong, M. Kirk, S. Barnes, and J. S. Beckman. 1997. Superoxide dismutase catalyzes nitration of tyrosines by peroxynitrite in the rod and head domains of neurofilament-L. *J Neurochem* 69 (5):1945-53.

Crozat, A., P. Aman, N. Mandahl, and D. Ron. 1993. Fusion of CHOP to a novel RNA-binding protein in human myxoid liposarcoma. *Nature* 363 (6430):640-4.

Davenport, R. J., R. J. Swingler, A. M. Chancellor, and C. P. Warlow. 1996. Avoiding false positive diagnoses of motor neuron disease: lessons from the Scottish Motor Neuron Disease Register. *J Neurol Neurosurg Psychiatry* 60 (2):147-51.

de Carvalho, M., R. Dengler, A. Eisen, J. D. England, R. Kaji, J. Kimura, K. Mills, H. Mitsumoto, H. Nodera, J. Shefner, and M. Swash. 2008. Electrodiagnostic criteria for diagnosis of ALS. *Clin Neurophysiol* 119 (3):497-503.

Dejesus-Hernandez M., I.R. Mackenzie, B.F. Boeve, A.L. Boxer, M. Baker, N.J. Rutherford, A.M. Nicholson, N.A. Finch, H. Flynn, J. Adamson, N. Kouri, A. Wojtas, P. Sengdy,

G.Y. Hsuing, A. Karydas A., W.W. Seeley, K.A. Josephs, G. Coppola, D.H. Geshwind, Z.K. Wszolek, H. Feldman, D.S. Knopman, R.C. Petersen, B.L. Miller, D.W. Dickson, K.B. Boylan, N.R. Graff-Radford and R. Rademakers. 2011. Expanded GGGGCC Hexanucleotide Repeat in Noncoding Region of C9ORF72 Causes Chromosome 9p-Linked FTD and ALS. *Neuron* Epub Sept 21.

Deng, H. X., W. Chen, S. T. Hong, K. M. Boycott, G. H. Gorrie, N. Siddique, Y. Yang, F. Fecto, Y. Shi, H. Zhai, H. Jiang, M. Hirano, E. Rampersaud, G. H. Jansen, S. Donkervoort, E. H. Bigio, B. R. Brooks, K. Ajroud, R. L. Sufit, J. L. Haines, E. Mugnaini, M. A. Pericak-Vance, and T. Siddique. 2011. Mutations in UBQLN2 cause dominant X-linked juvenile and adult-onset ALS and ALS/dementia. *Nature*.

Deng, H. X., A. Hentati, J. A. Tainer, Z. Iqbal, A. Cayabyab, W. Y. Hung, E. D. Getzoff, P. Hu, B. Herzfeldt, R. P. Roos, and et al. 1993. Amyotrophic lateral sclerosis and structural defects in Cu,Zn superoxide dismutase. *Science* 261 (5124):1047-51.

Deng, H. X., H. Zhai, E. H. Bigio, J. Yan, F. Fecto, K. Ajroud, M. Mishra, S. Ajroud-Driss, S. Heller, R. Sufit, N. Siddique, E. Mugnaini, and T. Siddique. 2010. FUS-immunoreactive inclusions are a common feature in sporadic and non-SOD1 familial amyotrophic lateral sclerosis. *Ann Neurol* 67 (6):739-48.

DiDonato, M., L. Craig, M. E. Huff, M. M. Thayer, R. M. Cardoso, C. J. Kassmann, T. P. Lo, C. K. Bruns, E. T. Powers, J. W. Kelly, E. D. Getzoff, and J. A. Tainer. 2003. ALS mutants of human superoxide dismutase form fibrous aggregates via framework destabilization. *J Mol Biol* 332 (3):601-15.

Dimos, J. T., K. T. Rodolfa, K. K. Niakan, L. M. Weisenthal, H. Mitsumoto, W. Chung, G. F. Croft, G. Saphier, R. Leibel, R. Goland, H. Wichterle, C. E. Henderson, and K. Eggan. 2008. Induced pluripotent stem cells generated from patients with ALS can be differentiated into motor neurons. *Science* 321 (5893):1218-21.

Dobson, C. M. 2001. Protein folding and its links with human disease. *Biochem Soc Symp* (68):1-26.

Donkervoort, S., and T. Siddique. 1993. Amyotrophic Lateral Sclerosis Overview. *In: Pagon RA, Bird TD, Dolan CR, Stephens K, editors. GeneReviews [Internet]. Seattle (WA): University of Washington, Seattle; 1993-. [updated 2009 Jul 28]*.

Dormann, D., and C. Haass. 2011. TDP-43 and FUS: a nuclear affair. *Trends Neurosci*.

Dormann, D., R. Rodde, D. Edbauer, E. Bentmann, I. Fischer, A. Hruscha, M. E. Than, I. R. Mackenzie, A. Capell, B. Schmid, M. Neumann, and C. Haass. 2010. ALS-associated fused in sarcoma (FUS) mutations disrupt Transportin-mediated nuclear import. *EMBO J* 29 (16):2841-57.

Durham, H. D., J. Roy, L. Dong, and D. A. Figlewicz. 1997. Aggregation of mutant Cu/Zn superoxide dismutase proteins in a culture model of ALS. *J Neuropathol Exp Neurol* 56 (5):523-30.

Ferrari, R., D. Kapogiannis, E. D. Huey, and P. Momeni. 2011. FTD and ALS: A Tale of Two Diseases. *Curr Alzheimer Res*.

Fong, K. Y., Y. L. Yu, Y. W. Chan, R. Kay, J. Chan, Z. Yang, M. C. Kwan, K. P. Leung, P. C. Li, T. H. Lam, and R. T. Cheung. 1996. Motor neuron disease in Hong Kong Chinese: epidemiology and clinical picture. *Neuroepidemiology* 15 (5):239-45.

Forbes, R. B., S. Colville, and R. J. Swingler. 2004. The epidemiology of amyotrophic lateral sclerosis (ALS/MND) in people aged 80 or over. *Age Ageing* 33 (2):131-4.

Forman, H. J., and I. Fridovich. 1973. On the stability of bovine superoxide dismutase. The effects of metals. *J Biol Chem* 248 (8):2645-9.

Forsgren, L., B. G. Almay, G. Holmgren, and S. Wall. 1983. Epidemiology of motor neuron disease in northern Sweden. *Acta Neurol Scand* 68 (1):20-9.

Fujii, R., S. Okabe, T. Urushido, K. Inoue, A. Yoshimura, T. Tachibana, T. Nishikawa, G. G. Hicks, and T. Takumi. 2005. The RNA binding protein TLS is translocated to dendritic spines by mGluR5 activation and regulates spine morphology. *Curr Biol* 15 (6):587-93.

Getzoff, E. D., D. E. Cabelli, C. L. Fisher, H. E. Parge, M. S. Viezzoli, L. Banci, and R. A. Hallewell. 1992. Faster superoxide dismutase mutants designed by enhancing electrostatic guidance. *Nature* 358 (6384):347-51.

Getzoff, E. D., J. A. Tainer, P. K. Weiner, P. A. Kollman, J. S. Richardson, and D. C. Richardson. 1983. Electrostatic recognition between superoxide and copper, zinc superoxide dismutase. *Nature* 306 (5940):287-90.

Gribkoff, V. K., and M. E. Bozik. 2008. KNS-760704 [(6R)-4,5,6,7-tetrahydro-N6-propyl-2, 6-benzothiazole-diamine dihydrochloride monohydrate] for the treatment of amyotrophic lateral sclerosis. *CNS Neurosci Ther* 14 (3):215-26.

Gunnarsson, L.-G., and Palm. 1984. Motor Neuron Disease and Heavy Manual Labor: An Epidemiologic Survey of Värmland County, Sweden. *Neuroepidemiology* 3 (4):195-206.

Gurney, M. E., H. F. Pu, A. Y. Chiu, M. C. Dalcanto, C. Y. Polchow, D. D. Alexander, J. Caliendo, A. Hentati, Y. W. Kwon, H. X. Deng, W. J. Chen, P. Zhai, R. L. Sufit, and T. Siddique. 1994. Motor-Neuron Degeneration in Mice That Express a Human Cu,Zn Superoxide-Dismutase Mutation. *Science* 264 (5166):1772-1775.

Haberlandt, W. F. 1959. Genetic aspects of amyotrophic lateral sclerosis and progressive bulbar paralysis. *Acta Genet Med Gemellol (Roma)* 8:369-74.

Hadano, S., C. K. Hand, H. Osuga, Y. Yanagisawa, A. Otomo, R. S. Devon, N. Miyamoto, J. Showguchi-Miyata, Y. Okada, R. Singaraja, D. A. Figlewicz, T. Kwiatkowski, B. A. Hosler, T. Sagie, J. Skaug, J. Nasir, R. H. Brown, S. W. Scherer, G. A. Rouleau, M. R. Hayden, and J. E. Ikeda. 2001. A gene encoding a putative GTPase regulator is mutated in familial amyotrophic lateral sclerosis 2 (vol 29, pg 166, 2001). *Nature Genetics* 29 (3):352-352.

Hadano, S., R. Kunita, A. Otomo, K. Suzuki-Utsunomiya, and J. E. Ikeda. 2007. Molecular and cellular function of ALS2/alsin: implication of membrane dynamics in neuronal development and degeneration. *Neurochem Int* 51 (2-4):74-84.

Hallewell, R. A., K. C. Imlay, P. Lee, N. M. Fong, C. Gallegos, E. D. Getzoff, J. A. Tainer, D. E. Cabelli, P. Tekamp-Olson, G. T. Mullenbach, and et al. 1991. Thermostabilization of recombinant human and bovine CuZn superoxide dismutases by replacement of free cysteines. *Biochem Biophys Res Commun* 181 (1):474-80.

Harraz, M. M., J. J. Marden, W. Zhou, Y. Zhang, A. Williams, V. S. Sharov, K. Nelson, M. Luo, H. Paulson, C. Schoneich, and J. F. Engelhardt. 2008. SOD1 mutations disrupt redox-sensitive Rac regulation of NADPH oxidase in a familial ALS model. *J Clin Invest* 118 (2):659-70.

Haverkamp, L. J., V. Appel, and S. H. Appel. 1995. Natural history of amyotrophic lateral sclerosis in a database population. Validation of a scoring system and a model for survival prediction. *Brain* 118 (Pt 3):707-19.

He, C. Z., and A. P. Hays. 2004. Expression of peripherin in ubiquinated inclusions of amyotrophic lateral sclerosis. *J Neurol Sci* 217 (1):47-54.

Henscheid, K. L., D. S. Shin, S. C. Cary, and J. A. Berglund. 2005. The splicing factor U2AF65 is functionally conserved in the thermotolerant deep-sea worm Alvinella pompejana. *Biochim Biophys Acta* 1727 (3):197-207.

Higashi, S., Y. Tsuchiya, T. Araki, K. Wada, and T. Kabuta. 2010. TDP-43 physically interacts with amyotrophic lateral sclerosis-linked mutant CuZn superoxide dismutase. *Neurochem Int* 57 (8):906-13.

Horner, R. D., S. C. Grambow, C. J. Coffman, J. H. Lindquist, E. Z. Oddone, K. D. Allen, and E. J. Kasarskis. 2008. Amyotrophic lateral sclerosis among 1991 Gulf War veterans: evidence for a time-limited outbreak. *Neuroepidemiology* 31 (1):28-32.

Horton, W. A., R. Eldridge, and J. A. Brody. 1976. Familial motor neuron disease. Evidence for at least three different types. *Neurology* 26 (5):460-5.

Ince, P. G., and G. A. Codd. 2005. Return of the cycad hypothesis - does the amyotrophic lateral sclerosis/parkinsonism dementia complex (ALS/PDC) of Guam have new implications for global health? *Neuropathol Appl Neurobiol* 31 (4):345-53.

Ito, H., K. Fujita, M. Nakamura, R. Wate, S. Kaneko, S. Sasaki, K. Yamane, N. Suzuki, M. Aoki, N. Shibata, S. Togashi, A. Kawata, Y. Mochizuki, T. Mizutani, H. Maruyama, A. Hirano, R. Takahashi, H. Kawakami, and H. Kusaka. 2011. Optineurin is co-localized with FUS in basophilic inclusions of ALS with FUS mutation and in basophilic inclusion body disease. *Acta Neuropathol* 121 (4):555-7.

Johnston, J. A., M. J. Dalton, M. E. Gurney, and R. R. Kopito. 2000. Formation of high molecular weight complexes of mutant Cu, Zn-superoxide dismutase in a mouse model for familial amyotrophic lateral sclerosis. *Proc Natl Acad Sci U S A* 97 (23):12571-6.

Kalmar, B., S. Novoselov, A. Gray, M. E. Cheetham, B. Margulis, and L. Greensmith. 2008. Late stage treatment with arimoclomol delays disease progression and prevents protein aggregation in the SOD1 mouse model of ALS. *J Neurochem* 107 (2):339-50.

Kamel, F., D. M. Umbach, T. L. Munsat, J. M. Shefner, and D. P. Sandler. 1999. Association of cigarette smoking with amyotrophic lateral sclerosis. *Neuroepidemiology* 18 (4):194-202.

Kashiwagi, S., I. Kuraoka, Y. Fujiwara, K. Hitomi, Q. J. Cheng, J. O. Fuss, D. S. Shin, C. Masutani, J. A. Tainer, F. Hanaoka, and S. Iwai. 2010. Characterization of a Y-Family DNA Polymerase eta from the Eukaryotic Thermophile Alvinella pompejana. *J Nucleic Acids* 2010.

Kato, S., H. Sumi-Akamaru, H. Fujimura, S. Sakoda, M. Kato, A. Hirano, M. Takikawa, and E. Ohama. 2001. Copper chaperone for superoxide dismutase co-aggregates with superoxide dismutase 1 (SOD1) in neuronal Lewy body-like hyaline inclusions: an immunohistochemical study on familial amyotrophic lateral sclerosis with SOD1 gene mutation. *Acta Neuropathol* 102 (3):233-8.

Kieran, D., M. Hafezparast, S. Bohnert, J. R. Dick, J. Martin, G. Schiavo, E. M. Fisher, and L. Greensmith. 2005. A mutation in dynein rescues axonal transport defects and extends the life span of ALS mice. *J Cell Biol* 169 (4):561-7.

Kiernan, M. C., S. Vucic, B. C. Cheah, M. R. Turner, A. Eisen, O. Hardiman, J. R. Burrell, and M. C. Zoing. 2011. Amyotrophic lateral sclerosis. *Lancet* 377 (9769):942-55.

Kim, S. H., N. P. Shanware, M. J. Bowler, and R. S. Tibbetts. 2010. Amyotrophic lateral sclerosis-associated proteins TDP-43 and FUS/TLS function in a common biochemical complex to co-regulate HDAC6 mRNA. *J Biol Chem* 285 (44):34097-105.

Kuhnlein, P., H. J. Gdynia, A. D. Sperfeld, B. Lindner-Pfleghar, A. C. Ludolph, M. Prosiegel, and A. Riecker. 2008. Diagnosis and treatment of bulbar symptoms in amyotrophic lateral sclerosis. *Nature Clinical Practice Neurology* 4 (7):366-374.

Kwiatkowski, T. J., Jr., D. A. Bosco, A. L. Leclerc, E. Tamrazian, C. R. Vanderburg, C. Russ, A. Davis, J. Gilchrist, E. J. Kasarskis, T. Munsat, P. Valdmanis, G. A. Rouleau, B. A.

Hosler, P. Cortelli, P. J. de Jong, Y. Yoshinaga, J. L. Haines, M. A. Pericak-Vance, J. Yan, N. Ticozzi, T. Siddique, D. McKenna-Yasek, P. C. Sapp, H. R. Horvitz, J. E. Landers, and R. H. Brown, Jr. 2009. Mutations in the FUS/TLS gene on chromosome 16 cause familial amyotrophic lateral sclerosis. *Science* 323 (5918):1205-8.

Kwong, L. K., K. Uryu, J. Q. Trojanowski, and V. M. Lee. 2008. TDP-43 proteinopathies: neurodegenerative protein misfolding diseases without amyloidosis. *Neurosignals* 16 (1):41-51.

Lagier-Tourenne, C., and D. W. Cleveland. 2009. Rethinking ALS: the FUS about TDP-43. *Cell* 136 (6):1001-4.

Lagier-Tourenne, C., M. Polymenidou, and D. W. Cleveland. 2010. TDP-43 and FUS/TLS: emerging roles in RNA processing and neurodegeneration. *Hum Mol Genet* 19 (R1):R46-64.

Lai, C., C. Xie, S. G. McCormack, H. C. Chiang, M. K. Michalak, X. Lin, J. Chandran, H. Shim, M. Shimoji, M. R. Cookson, R. L. Huganir, J. D. Rothstein, D. L. Price, P. C. Wong, L. J. Martin, J. J. Zhu, and H. Cai. 2006. Amyotrophic lateral sclerosis 2-deficiency leads to neuronal degeneration in amyotrophic lateral sclerosis through altered AMPA receptor trafficking. *J Neurosci* 26 (45):11798-806.

Lange, D. 2008. Abstract C46: pyrimethamine as a therapy for SOD1 associated FALS: Early findings. *Amyotroph. Lateral Scler.* 9 ((Suppl. 1)):45-47.

Law, W. J., K. L. Cann, and G. G. Hicks. 2006. TLS, EWS and TAF15: a model for transcriptional integration of gene expression. *Brief Funct Genomic Proteomic* 5 (1):8-14.

Lee, H. P., G. Casadesus, X. Zhu, H. G. Lee, G. Perry, M. A. Smith, K. Gustaw-Rothenberg, and A. Lerner. 2009. All-trans retinoic acid as a novel therapeutic strategy for Alzheimer's disease. *Expert Rev Neurother* 9 (11):1615-21.

Leigh, P. N., H. Whitwell, O. Garofalo, J. Buller, M. Swash, J. E. Martin, J. M. Gallo, R. O. Weller, and B. H. Anderton. 1991. Ubiquitin-immunoreactive intraneuronal inclusions in amyotrophic lateral sclerosis. Morphology, distribution, and specificity. *Brain* 114 (Pt 2):775-88.

Li, T. M., E. Alberman, and M. Swash. 1988. Comparison of sporadic and familial disease amongst 580 cases of motor neuron disease. *J Neurol Neurosurg Psychiatry* 51 (6):778-84.

Ling, S. C., C. P. Albuquerque, J. S. Han, C. Lagier-Tourenne, S. Tokunaga, H. Zhou, and D. W. Cleveland. 2010. ALS-associated mutations in TDP-43 increase its stability and promote TDP-43 complexes with FUS/TLS. *Proc Natl Acad Sci U S A* 107 (30):13318-23.

Lomen-Hoerth, C. 2008. Amyotrophic lateral sclerosis from bench to bedside. *Semin Neurol* 28 (2):205-11.

Ludolph, A. C., and U. Knirsch. 1999. Problems and pitfalls in the diagnosis of ALS. *Journal of the Neurological Sciences* 165 Suppl 1:S14-20.

Mackenzie, I. R., R. Rademakers, and M. Neumann. 2010. TDP-43 and FUS in amyotrophic lateral sclerosis and frontotemporal dementia. *Lancet Neurol* 9 (10):995-1007.

Maenpaa, H., M. Mannerstrom, T. Toimela, L. Salminen, P. Saransaari, and H. Tahti. 2002. Glutamate uptake is inhibited by tamoxifen and toremifene in cultured retinal pigment epithelial cells. *Pharmacol Toxicol* 91 (3):116-22.

Malinowski, D. P., and I. Fridovich. 1979. Subunit association and side-chain reactivities of bovine erythrocyte superoxide dismutase in denaturing solvents. *Biochemistry* 18 (23):5055-60.

Mann, T., and D. Keilin. 1938. Haemocuprein and hepatocuprein, copper-protein compounds of blood and liver in mammals. *Proceedings of the Royal Society of London Series B-Biological Sciences* 126 (844):303-315.

Mantovani, V., P. Garagnani, P. Selva, C. Rossi, S. Ferrari, M. Cenci, N. Calza, V. Cerreta, D. Luiselli, and G. Romeo. 2007. Simple method for haplotyping the poly(TG) repeat in individuals carrying the IVS8 5T allele in the CFTR gene. *Clin Chem* 53 (3):531-3.

Manuel, M., and C. J. Heckman. 2011. Stronger is not always better: could a bodybuilding dietary supplement lead to ALS? *Exp Neurol* 228 (1):5-8.

McCombe, P. A., and R. D. Henderson. 2010. Effects of gender in amyotrophic lateral sclerosis. *Gend Med* 7 (6):557-70.

McCord, J. M., and I. Fridovich. 1969. Superoxide dismutase. An enzymic function for erythrocuprein (hemocuprein). *J Biol Chem* 244 (22):6049-55.

Miana-Mena, F. J., E. Piedrafita, C. Gonzalez-Mingot, P. Larrode, M. J. Munoz, E. Martinez-Ballarin, R. J. Reiter, R. Osta, and J. J. Garcia. 2011. Levels of membrane fluidity in the spinal cord and the brain in an animal model of amyotrophic lateral sclerosis. *J Bioenerg Biomembr* 43 (2):181-6.

Miller, R. G., J. D. Mitchell, M. Lyon, and D. H. Moore. 2007. Riluzole for amyotrophic lateral sclerosis (ALS)/motor neuron disease (MND). *Cochrane Database Syst Rev* (1):CD001447.

Miranda, M. L., M. Alicia Overstreet Galeano, E. Tassone, K. D. Allen, and R. D. Horner. 2008. Spatial analysis of the etiology of amyotrophic lateral sclerosis among 1991 Gulf War veterans. *Neurotoxicology* 29 (6):964-70.

Mulder, D. W., L. T. Kurland, K. P. Offord, and C. M. Beard. 1986. Familial adult motor neuron disease: amyotrophic lateral sclerosis. *Neurology* 36 (4):511-7.

Mulder, D. W., L. T. Kurland, K. P. Offord, and C. M. Beard. 1986. Familial Adult Motor-Neuron Disease - Amyotrophic-Lateral-Scelerosis. *Neurology* 36 (4):511-517.

Munch, C., A. Rosenbohm, A. D. Sperfeld, I. Uttner, S. Reske, B. J. Krause, R. Sedlmeier, T. Meyer, C. O. Hanemann, G. Stumm, and A. C. Ludolph. 2005. Heterozygous R1101K mutation of the DCTN1 gene in a family with ALS and FTD. *Ann Neurol* 58 (5):777-80.

Munch, C., R. Sedlmeier, T. Meyer, V. Homberg, A. D. Sperfeld, A. Kurt, J. Prudlo, G. Peraus, C. O. Hanemann, G. Stumm, and A. C. Ludolph. 2004. Point mutations of the p150 subunit of dynactin (DCTN1) gene in ALS. *Neurology* 63 (4):724-6.

Murphy, J., R. Henry, and C. Lomen-Hoerth. 2007. Establishing subtypes of the continuum of frontal lobe impairment in amyotrophic lateral sclerosis. *Arch Neurol* 64 (3):330-4.

Murros, K., and R. Fogelholm. 1983. Amyotrophic lateral sclerosis in Middle-Finland: an epidemiological study. *Acta Neurol Scand* 67 (1):41-7.

Neumann, M., D. M. Sampathu, L. K. Kwong, A. C. Truax, M. C. Micsenyi, T. T. Chou, J. Bruce, T. Schuck, M. Grossman, C. M. Clark, L. F. McCluskey, B. L. Miller, E. Masliah, I. R. Mackenzie, H. Feldman, W. Feiden, H. A. Kretzschmar, J. Q. Trojanowski, and V. M. Lee. 2006. Ubiquitinated TDP-43 in frontotemporal lobar degeneration and amyotrophic lateral sclerosis. *Science* 314 (5796):130-3.

Nishitoh, H., H. Kadowaki, A. Nagai, T. Maruyama, T. Yokota, H. Fukutomi, T. Noguchi, A. Matsuzawa, K. Takeda, and H. Ichijo. 2008. ALS-linked mutant SOD1 induces ER stress- and ASK1-dependent motor neuron death by targeting Derlin-1. *Genes Dev* 22 (11):1451-64.

Okamoto, K., T. Kihira, T. Kondo, G. Kobashi, M. Washio, S. Sasaki, T. Yokoyama, Y. Miyake, N. Sakamoto, Y. Inaba, and M. Nagai. 2009. Lifestyle factors and risk of amyotrophic lateral sclerosis: a case-control study in Japan. *Ann Epidemiol* 19 (6):359-64.

Olivares, L., E. S. Esteban, and M. Alter. 1972. Mexican "resistance" to amyotrophic lateral sclerosis. *Arch Neurol* 27 (5):397-402.

Olney, R. K., J. Murphy, D. Forshew, E. Garwood, B. L. Miller, S. Langmore, M. A. Kohn, and C. Lomen-Hoerth. 2005. The effects of executive and behavioral dysfunction on the course of ALS. *Neurology* 65 (11):1774-7.

Parge, H. E., R. A. Hallewell, and J. A. Tainer. 1992. Atomic structures of wild-type and thermostable mutant recombinant human Cu,Zn superoxide dismutase. *Proc Natl Acad Sci U S A* 89 (13):6109-13.

Pasinelli, P., and R. H. Brown. 2006. Molecular biology of amyotrophic lateral sclerosis: insights from genetics. *Nature Reviews Neuroscience* 7 (9):710-723.

Perry, J. J. P., D. S. Shin, and J. A. Tainer. 2010. Amyotrophic Lateral Sclerosis. *Diseases of DNA Repair* 685:9-20.

Perry, J. J., D. S. Shin, E. D. Getzoff, and J. A. Tainer. 2010. The structural biochemistry of the superoxide dismutases. *Biochim Biophys Acta* 1804 (2):245-62.

Piccino, P., F. Viard, P. M. Sarradin, N. Le Bris, D. Le Guen, and D. Jollivet. 2004. Thermal selection of PGM allozymes in newly founded populations of the thermotolerant vent polychaete Alvinella pompejana. *Proceedings of the Royal Society of London Series B-Biological Sciences* 271 (1555):2351-2359.

Porter, H., and J. Folch. 1957. Cerebrocuprein I. A copper-containing protein isolated from brain. *J Neurochem* 1 (3):260-71.

Rabbitts, T. H., A. Forster, R. Larson, and P. Nathan. 1993. Fusion of the dominant negative transcription regulator CHOP with a novel gene FUS by translocation t(12;16) in malignant liposarcoma. *Nat Genet* 4 (2):175-80.

Radunovic, A., D. Annane, K. Jewitt, and N. Mustfa. 2009. Mechanical ventilation for amyotrophic lateral sclerosis/motor neuron disease. *Cochrane Database Syst Rev* (4):CD004427.

Reaume, A. G., J. L. Elliott, E. K. Hoffman, N. W. Kowall, R. J. Ferrante, D. F. Siwek, H. M. Wilcox, D. G. Flood, M. F. Beal, R. H. Brown, Jr., R. W. Scott, and W. D. Snider. 1996. Motor neurons in Cu/Zn superoxide dismutase-deficient mice develop normally but exhibit enhanced cell death after axonal injury. *Nat Genet* 13 (1):43-7.

Renton A.E., E. Majounie, A. Waite, J. Simón-Sánchez, S. Rollinson, J.R. Gibbs, J.C. Schymick, H. Laaksovirta, J.C. van Swieten, L. Myllykangas, H. Kalimo, A. Paetau, Y. Abramzon, A.M. Remes, A. Kagnovich, S.W. Scholz, J. Duckworth, J. Ding, D.W. Harmer, D.G. Hernandez, J.O. Johnson, K. Mok, M. Ryten, D. Trabzuni, R.J. Guerreiro, R.W. Orrell, J. Neal, A. Murray, J. Pearson, I.E. Jansen, D. Sondervan, H. Seelaar, D. Blake, K. Young, N. Halliwell, J.B. Callister, G. Toulson, A. Richardson, A. Gerhard, J. Snowden, D. Mann, D. Neary, M.A. Nalls, T. Peuralinna, L. Jansson, V.M. Isoviita, A.L. Kaivorinne, M.Hölttä-Vuori, E. Ikonen, R. Sulkava, M. Benatar, J. Wuu, A. Chiò, G. Restagno, G. Borghero, M. Sabatelli; The ITALSGEN Consortium, D. Heckerman, E. Rogaeva, L. Zinman, J.D. Rothstein, M. Sendtner, C. Drepper, E.E. Eichler, C. Alkan, Z. Abdullaev, S.D. Pack, A. Dutra, E. Pak , J. Hardy, A. Singleton, N.M. Williams , P. Heutink, S. Pickering-Brown, H.R. Morris, P.J. Tienari and B.J. Traynor. 2011. A Hexanucleotide Repeat Expansion in C9ORF72 Is the Cause of Chromosome 9p21-Linked ALS-FTD. *Neuron.* Epub Sept 21.

Rosen, D. R. 1993. Mutations in Cu/Zn superoxide dismutase gene are associated with familial amyotrophic lateral sclerosis. *Nature* 364 (6435):362.

Sanz, M. A. 2006. Treatment of acute promyelocytic leukemia. *Hematology Am Soc Hematol Educ Program*:147-55.

Sathasivam, S. 2010. Motor neurone disease: clinical features, diagnosis, diagnostic pitfalls and prognostic markers. *Singapore Medical Journal* 51 (5):367-373.

Schmidt, S., L. C. Kwee, K. D. Allen, and E. Z. Oddone. 2010. Association of ALS with head injury, cigarette smoking and APOE genotypes. *Journal of the Neurological Sciences* 291 (1-2):22-9.

Schutz, B., J. Reimann, L. Dumitrescu-Ozimek, K. Kappes-Horn, G. E. Landreth, B. Schurmann, A. Zimmer, and M. T. Heneka. 2005. The oral antidiabetic pioglitazone protects from neurodegeneration and amyotrophic lateral sclerosis-like symptoms in superoxide dismutase-G93A transgenic mice. *J Neurosci* 25 (34):7805-12.

Scott, S., J. E. Kranz, J. Cole, J. M. Lincecum, K. Thompson, N. Kelly, A. Bostrom, J. Theodoss, B. M. Al-Nakhala, F. G. Vieira, J. Ramasubbu, and J. A. Heywood. 2008. Design, power, and interpretation of studies in the standard murine model of ALS. *Amyotroph Lateral Scler* 9 (1):4-15.

Sharma, R., S. Hicks, C. M. Berna, C. Kennard, K. Talbot, and M. R. Turner. 2011. Oculomotor dysfunction in amyotrophic lateral sclerosis: a comprehensive review. *Arch Neurol* 68 (7):857-61.

Shin, D. S., M. Didonato, D. P. Barondeau, G. L. Hura, C. Hitomi, J. A. Berglund, E. D. Getzoff, S. C. Cary, and J. A. Tainer. 2009. Superoxide dismutase from the eukaryotic thermophile Alvinella pompejana: structures, stability, mechanism, and insights into amyotrophic lateral sclerosis. *J Mol Biol* 385 (5):1534-55.

Siddique, T., and H. X. Deng. 1996. Genetics of amyotrophic lateral sclerosis. *Human Molecular Genetics* 5:1465-1470.

Silani, V., S. Messina, B. Poletti, C. Morelli, A. Doretti, N. Ticozzi, and L. Maderna. 2011. The diagnosis of Amyotrophic lateral sclerosis in 2010. *Arch Ital Biol* 149 (1):5-27.

Smith, R. A., T. M. Miller, K. Yamanaka, B. P. Monia, T. P. Condon, G. Hung, C. S. Lobsiger, C. M. Ward, M. McAlonis-Downes, H. Wei, E. V. Wancewicz, C. F. Bennett, and D. W. Cleveland. 2006. Antisense oligonucleotide therapy for neurodegenerative disease. *J Clin Invest* 116 (8):2290-6.

Soto, C. 2001. Protein misfolding and disease; protein refolding and therapy. *FEBS Lett* 498 (2-3):204-7.

Spuler, S., A. Stroux, F. Kuschel, A. Kuhlmey, and F. Kendel. 2011. Delay in diagnosis of muscle disorders depends on the subspecialty of the initially consulted physician. *BMC Health Serv Res* 11:91.

Steele, J. C., and P. L. McGeer. 2008. The ALS/PDC syndrome of Guam and the cycad hypothesis. *Neurology* 70 (21):1984-90.

Strong, M. J. 2010. The evidence for altered RNA metabolism in amyotrophic lateral sclerosis (ALS). *J Neurol Sci* 288 (1-2):1-12.

Strong, M. J., K. Volkening, R. Hammond, W. Yang, W. Strong, C. Leystra-Lantz, and C. Shoesmith. 2007. TDP43 is a human low molecular weight neurofilament (hNFL) mRNA-binding protein. *Mol Cell Neurosci* 35 (2):320-7.

Suzuki, H., K. Kanekura, T. P. Levine, K. Kohno, V. M. Olkkonen, S. Aiso, and M. Matsuoka. 2009. ALS-linked P56S-VAPB, an aggregated loss-of-function mutant of VAPB, predisposes motor neurons to ER stress-related death by inducing aggregation of co-expressed wild-type VAPB. *J Neurochem* 108 (4):973-985.

Swarup, V., D. Phaneuf, C. Bareil, J. Robertson, G. A. Rouleau, J. Kriz, and J. P. Julien. 2011. Pathological hallmarks of amyotrophic lateral sclerosis/frontotemporal lobar degeneration in transgenic mice produced with TDP-43 genomic fragments. *Brain*.

Swash, M. 1998. Early diagnosis of ALS/MND. *Journal of the Neurological Sciences* 160 Suppl 1:S33-6.

Tainer, J. A., E. D. Getzoff, K. M. Beem, J. S. Richardson, and D. C. Richardson. 1982. Determination and analysis of the 2 A-structure of copper, zinc superoxide dismutase. *J Mol Biol* 160 (2):181-217.

Tainer, J. A., E. D. Getzoff, J. S. Richardson, and D. C. Richardson. 1983. Structure and mechanism of copper, zinc superoxide dismutase. *Nature* 306 (5940):284-7.

Talbot, K. 2009. Motor neuron disease: the bare essentials. *Pract Neurol* 9 (5):303-9.

Talbot, K. 2010. Do twin studies still have anything to teach us about the genetics of amyotrophic lateral sclerosis? *J Neurol Neurosurg Psychiatry* 81 (12):1299-300.

Testa, D., R. Lovati, M. Ferrarini, F. Salmoiraghi, and G. Filippini. 2004. Survival of 793 patients with amyotrophic lateral sclerosis diagnosed over a 28-year period. *Amyotroph Lateral Scler Other Motor Neuron Disord* 5 (4):208-12.

Ticozzi, N., C. Tiloca, C. Morelli, C. Colombrita, B. Poletti, A. Doretti, L. Maderna, S. Messina, A. Ratti, and V. Silani. 2011. Genetics of familial Amyotrophic lateral sclerosis. *Arch Ital Biol* 149 (1):65-82.

Traynor, B. J., L. Bruijn, R. Conwit, F. Beal, G. O'Neill, S. C. Fagan, and M. E. Cudkowicz. 2006. Neuroprotective agents for clinical trials in ALS: a systematic assessment. *Neurology* 67 (1):20-7.

Traynor, B. J., M. B. Codd, B. Corr, C. Forde, E. Frost, and O. Hardiman. 2000. Amyotrophic lateral sclerosis mimic syndromes - A population-based study. *Archives of Neurology* 57 (1):109-113.

Turner, M. R., M. C. Kiernan, P. N. Leigh, and K. Talbot. 2009. Biomarkers in amyotrophic lateral sclerosis. *Lancet Neurol* 8 (1):94-109.

Udan, M., and R. H. Baloh. 2011. Implications of the prion-related Q/N domains in TDP-43 and FUS. *Prion* 5 (1):1-5.

Urushitani, M., A. Sik, T. Sakurai, N. Nukina, R. Takahashi, and J. P. Julien. 2006. Chromogranin-mediated secretion of mutant superoxide dismutase proteins linked to amyotrophic lateral sclerosis. *Nat Neurosci* 9 (1):108-18.

Vance, C., B. Rogelj, T. Hortobagyi, K. J. De Vos, A. L. Nishimura, J. Sreedharan, X. Hu, B. Smith, D. Ruddy, P. Wright, J. Ganesalingam, K. L. Williams, V. Tripathi, S. Al-Saraj, A. Al-Chalabi, P. N. Leigh, I. P. Blair, G. Nicholson, J. de Belleroche, J. M. Gallo, C. C. Miller, and C. E. Shaw. 2009. Mutations in FUS, an RNA processing protein, cause familial amyotrophic lateral sclerosis type 6. *Science* 323 (5918):1208-11.

Veltema, A. N., R. A. Roos, and G. W. Bruyn. 1990. Autosomal dominant adult amyotrophic lateral sclerosis. A six generation Dutch family. *J Neurol Sci* 97 (1):93-115.

Waibel, S., A. Reuter, S. Malessa, E. Blaugrund, and A. C. Ludolph. 2004. Rasagiline alone and in combination with riluzole prolongs survival in an ALS mouse model. *J Neurol* 251 (9):1080-4.

Wang, H., E. J. O'Reilly, M. G. Weisskopf, G. Logroscino, M. L. McCullough, M. J. Thun, A. Schatzkin, L. N. Kolonel, and A. Ascherio. 2011. Smoking and risk of amyotrophic lateral sclerosis: a pooled analysis of 5 prospective cohorts. *Arch Neurol* 68 (2):207-13.

Wang, J., G. W. Farr, C. J. Zeiss, D. J. Rodriguez-Gil, J. H. Wilson, K. Furtak, D. T. Rutkowski, R. J. Kaufman, C. I. Ruse, J. R. Yates, 3rd, S. Perrin, M. B. Feany, and A. L. Horwich. 2009. Progressive aggregation despite chaperone associations of a mutant SOD1-YFP in transgenic mice that develop ALS. *Proc Natl Acad Sci U S A* 106 (5):1392-7.

Wanker, E. E. 2000. Protein aggregation in Huntington's and Parkinson's disease: implications for therapy. *Mol Med Today* 6 (10):387-91.

Wicklund, M. P. 2005. Amyotrophic lateral sclerosis: possible role of environmental influences. *Neurol Clin* 23 (2):461-84.

Wicks, P. 2007. Excessive yawning is common in the bulbar-onset form of ALS. *Acta Psychiatr Scand* 116 (1):76; author reply 76-7.

Wiedau-Pazos, M., J. J. Goto, S. Rabizadeh, E. B. Gralla, J. A. Roe, M. K. Lee, J. S. Valentine, and D. E. Bredesen. 1996. Altered reactivity of superoxide dismutase in familial amyotrophic lateral sclerosis. *Science* 271 (5248):515-8.

Williams, D. B., D. A. Floate, and J. Leicester. 1988. Familial motor neuron disease: differing penetrance in large pedigrees. *Journal of the Neurological Sciences* 86 (2-3):215-30.

Wong, P. C., and D. R. Borchelt. 1995. Motor neuron disease caused by mutations in superoxide dismutase 1. *Curr Opin Neurol* 8 (4):294-301.

Worms, P. M. 2001. The epidemiology of motor neuron diseases: a review of recent studies. *J Neurol Sci* 191 (1-2):3-9.

Wright, P. D., M. Huang, A. Weiss, J. Matthews, N. Wightman, M. Glicksman, and R. H. Brown, Jr. 2010. Screening for inhibitors of the SOD1 gene promoter: pyrimethamine does not reduce SOD1 levels in cell and animal models. *Neurosci Lett* 482 (3):188-92.

Xu, L., J. Yan, D. Chen, A. M. Welsh, T. Hazel, K. Johe, G. Hatfield, and V. E. Koliatsos. 2006. Human neural stem cell grafts ameliorate motor neuron disease in SOD-1 transgenic rats. *Transplantation* 82 (7):865-75.

Yamanaka, K., C. Vande Velde, E. Eymard-Pierre, E. Bertini, O. Boespflug-Tanguy, and D. W. Cleveland. 2003. Unstable mutants in the peripheral endosomal membrane component ALS2 cause early-onset motor neuron disease. *Proc Natl Acad Sci U S A* 100 (26):16041-6.

Zhang, F., A. L. Strom, K. Fukada, S. Lee, L. J. Hayward, and H. Zhu. 2007. Interaction between familial amyotrophic lateral sclerosis (ALS)-linked SOD1 mutants and the dynein complex. *J Biol Chem* 282 (22):16691-9.

Zhang, H., J. Joseph, M. Gurney, D. Becker, and B. Kalyanaraman. 2002. Bicarbonate enhances peroxidase activity of Cu,Zn-superoxide dismutase. Role of carbonate anion radical and scavenging of carbonate anion radical by metalloporphyrin antioxidant enzyme mimetics. *J Biol Chem* 277 (2):1013-20.

Zoccolella, S., A. Santamato, and P. Lamberti. 2009. Current and emerging treatments for amyotrophic lateral sclerosis. *Neuropsychiatr Dis Treat* 5:577-95.

Permissions

The contributors of this book come from diverse backgrounds, making this book a truly international effort. This book will bring forth new frontiers with its revolutionizing research information and detailed analysis of the nascent developments around the world.

We would like to thank Raymond Chuen-Chung CHANG, PhD, for lending his expertise to make the book truly unique. He has played a crucial role in the development of this book. Without his invaluable contribution this book wouldn't have been possible. He has made vital efforts to compile up to date information on the varied aspects of this subject to make this book a valuable addition to the collection of many professionals and students.

This book was conceptualized with the vision of imparting up-to-date information and advanced data in this field. To ensure the same, a matchless editorial board was set up. Every individual on the board went through rigorous rounds of assessment to prove their worth. After which they invested a large part of their time researching and compiling the most relevant data for our readers. Conferences and sessions were held from time to time between the editorial board and the contributing authors to present the data in the most comprehensible form. The editorial team has worked tirelessly to provide valuable and valid information to help people across the globe.

Every chapter published in this book has been scrutinized by our experts. Their significance has been extensively debated. The topics covered herein carry significant findings which will fuel the growth of the discipline. They may even be implemented as practical applications or may be referred to as a beginning point for another development. Chapters in this book were first published by InTech; hereby published with permission under the Creative Commons Attribution License or equivalent.

The editorial board has been involved in producing this book since its inception. They have spent rigorous hours researching and exploring the diverse topics which have resulted in the successful publishing of this book. They have passed on their knowledge of decades through this book. To expedite this challenging task, the publisher supported the team at every step. A small team of assistant editors was also appointed to further simplify the editing procedure and attain best results for the readers.

Our editorial team has been hand-picked from every corner of the world. Their multi-ethnicity adds dynamic inputs to the discussions which result in innovative outcomes. These outcomes are then further discussed with the researchers and contributors who give their valuable feedback and opinion regarding the same. The feedback is then collaborated with the researches and they are edited in a comprehensive manner to aid the understanding of the subject.

Apart from the editorial board, the designing team has also invested a significant amount of their time in understanding the subject and creating the most relevant covers. They scrutinized every image to scout for the most suitable representation of the subject and create an appropriate cover for the book.

The publishing team has been involved in this book since its early stages. They were actively engaged in every process, be it collecting the data, connecting with the contributors or procuring relevant information. The team has been an ardent support to the editorial, designing and production team. Their endless efforts to recruit the best for this project, has resulted in the accomplishment of this book. They are a veteran in the field of academics and their pool of knowledge is as vast as their experience in printing. Their expertise and guidance has proved useful at every step. Their uncompromising quality standards have made this book an exceptional effort. Their encouragement from time to time has been an inspiration for everyone.

The publisher and the editorial board hope that this book will prove to be a valuable piece of knowledge for researchers, students, practitioners and scholars across the globe.

List of Contributors

Teodora Dzhambazova, Violeta Kondakova, Ivan Tsvetkov and Rossitza Batchvarova
AgroBioInstitute, Bulgaria

Jacqueline Bayliss, Romana Stark, Alex Reichenbach and Zane B. Andrews
Department of Physiology, Monash University, Australia

Barbara Yang, Kuen-Hua You, Shing-Chuen Wang, Hau-Ren Chen and Cheng-I Lee
Department of Life Science, National Chung Cheng University, Taiwan, ROC

Jiapu Zhang
Centre in Informatics and Applied Optimization & Graduate School of Sciences, Informatics
Technology and Engineering, University of Ballarat, Mount Helen, VIC 3353, Australia

Thomas W. Bebee and Dawn S. Chandler
The Center for Childhood Cancer at the Research Institute at Nationwide Children's
Hospital, Columbus, Ohio, USA
The Department of Pediatrics, The Ohio State University, Columbus, Ohio, USA

Venkata Ramesh Dasari and Krishna Kumar Veeravalli
Departments of Cancer Biology and Pharmacology, University of Illinois College of Medicine
at Peoria, Peoria, Illinois, USA

Jasti S. Rao
Departments of Cancer Biology and Pharmacology, University of Illinois College of Medicine
at Peoria, Peoria, Illinois, USA
Neurosurgery, University of Illinois College of Medicine at Peoria, Peoria, Illinois, USA

Dan Fassett and Dzung H. Dinh
Neurosurgery, University of Illinois College of Medicine at Peoria, Peoria, Illinois, USA
Illinois Neurological Institute, University of Illinois College of Medicine at Peoria, Peoria,
Illinois, USA

Bruno S. Mietto, Rodrigo M. Costa and Silmara V. de Lima
Program of Basic and Clinical Neuroscience, Brazil

Ana M. B. Martinez
Institute of Medical Biochemistry, Federal University of Rio de Janeiro, Brazil

Sérgio T. Ferreira
Program of Basic and Clinical Neuroscience, Brazil
Institute of Medical Biochemistry, Federal University of Rio de Janeiro, Brazil

E.J.F. Vereyken, C.D. Dijkstra and C.E. Teunissen
VU University Medical Center, Amsterdam, The Netherlands

David S. Shin
Lawrence Berkeley National Laboratory, USA

Ashley J. Pratt and Elizabeth D. Getzoff
The Scripps Research Institute, USA

J. Jefferson P. Perry
The Scripps Research Institute, USA
Amrita University, India

Printed in the USA
CPSIA information can be obtained
at www.ICGtesting.com
JSHW011353221024
72173JS00003B/270